D1064689

Head and Neck Injuries in Football

MECHANISMS, TREATMENT, AND PREVENTION

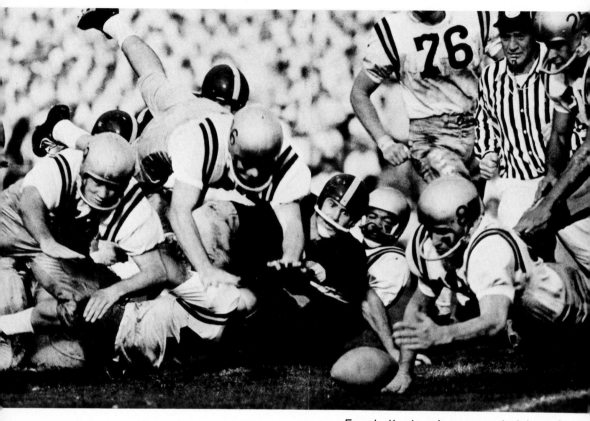

Football, already at great heights of popularity, grew tremendously during the decade, partly because of the new emphasis on power, speed, and all-out pursuit: a fumbled ball seemed like the focus of lines of intense magnetic force.

(*SPORTS ILLUSTRATED* photo by John G. Zimmerman © Time Inc.)

Head and Neck Injuries in Football

MECHANISMS, TREATMENT, AND PREVENTION

Richard C. Schneider, M.D.

Professor and Head,
Section of Neurosurgery, Department of Surgery
University of Michigan Medical Center
Ann Arbor, Michigan

The Williams & Wilkins Company / Baltimore

Copyright ©, 1973
The Williams & Wilkins Company
428 E. Preston Street
Baltimore, Md. 21202, U.S.A.

All rights reserved. This book is protected by copyright. No part of this book may be reproduced in any form or by any means, including photocopying, or utilized by any information storage and retrieval system without written permission from the copyright owner.

Made in the United States of America

Library of Congress Catalog Card Number 73-4197
SBN 683-07573-X

Composed and printed at the
Waverly Press, Inc.
Mt. Royal and Guilford Aves.
Baltimore, Md. 21202, U.S.A.

617.14
S 359 h

To my wife

MADELEINE T. SCHNEIDER

the devoted coach and
the quietly effective quarterback
for this neurosurgeon

Preface

The football fields of our nation have been a vast proving ground or laboratory for the study of the tragic neurologic sequelae of head and neck trauma in man. There has been an opportunity to study the films of the games and determine the actual mechanisms of injury. The evaluation of such football plays and players has been responsible for the initial observations made concerning the "tear-drop" cervical fracture with its anterior cervical cord compression and its chronic instability and spinal deformity. Two syndromes were defined from these observations and studies. The first was the "acute anterior spinal cord injury syndrome," a set of symptoms which suggested that urgent surgery should be performed, and "the acute central cervical cord injury," a pattern indicating that early operation was unnecessary and recovery might occur using conservative immobilization treatment.

This work has stimulated our Clinic to enter the investigative field of trauma with the development of a sophisticated impact track by Mr. Elwyn Gooding. Experimentally Dr. Hank Gosch has been able to create in the anesthetized animal the same central lesions at the second cervical spinal cord level as occur in man on direct vertex and occipital impacts. Dr. Glenn Kindt and Mr. Elwyn Gooding have been able to use this track to develop an excellent method of comparing the impact absorption characteristics of various types of headgear. Although these studies are not completed, they are far superior to other current methods of grossly dropping a weight on a helmet from a height or swinging weight against the headgear and recording a single oscillographic pattern.

The result of these experiences has enabled the development of the new double crown pneumatic helmet with a more flexible outer shell, which should prove more effective in preventing head injury than less resilient ones with poor inner suspensions.

Most significant, however, must be the realization that many minor to moderate cerebral concussions and contusions, intracranial blood clots, and fractured cervical spines with tetraplegia could be avoided by enforcing the rule that "spearing" and "stick-blocking" must be outlawed. The data published above support this statement and some athletic directors, coaches, and officials must realize the decision is theirs to avert some of such tragedies.

The author has presented much of this material portraying these tragic situations in football in more than one-half of the United States. One of the most frequent questions asked after such a lecture is: "If you had a son (this author does not have one) would you encourage or permit him to play football?" The carefully considered answer has been: "*If* the boy was of high school age, or older, with the proper physique, conditioning, and balanced mental capacity; *if* the boy was supplied with the proper protective equipment; *if* he were to be taught the proper coaching techniques with the avoidance of stick-blocking or spearing; *if* his coach was a perceptive thoughtful man, who regarded each lad as his own son; *if* the boy had the desire—I would then encourage him to play football."

Veiled in anonymity within the following pages are the case histories of the two opposing professional quarterbacks of the 1972 Super Bowl, Roger Staubach and Bob Griese, when they were playing as stars on collegiate teams. Fortunately their injuries were minor and because of their intelligence and training they have continued successfully in their professional careers learning how to absorb the severe physical contact. Fine athletes, such as these, exemplify the best in the game of football. Their dedication to physical conditioning, their ability to tolerate frustration and accept adversity with a courage to return, compete, and excel, and their sense of fair play, discipline, and self-respect are their hallmarks. Any young man who can live up to these ideals, which currently are too often lacking, should compete well in the game of life. The calculated risks are worth it.

Richard C. Schneider

Acknowledgements

This work must be regarded as a composite effort of a multitude of people over a 12 year period. Therefore perhaps I may be pardoned for the extensive list of acknowledgements.

This book has been supported to a major degree through the generosity of the late Hon. Alvin M. Bentley and his wife, Mrs. Arvella Bentley. Their contributions have enabled the construction of that part of the Neurosurgical Research Laboratory which has been responsible for the important experimental and the clinically applied investigative work to be reported in the following pages.

In recent years two grants have been kindly made by the Committee on Injuries and Fatalities of the National Collegiate Athletic Association. These have supported this Laboratory for the continuing performance of the experimental studies in the hope of eventually providing additional safety to all football players.

I am greatly indebted to a distinguished and dedicated group of several former University of Michigan football alumni, Messrs. Robert J. Brown, Paul G. Goebel, Sr. and Douglas Roby, who recently participated in their half-century alumni team celebration. Together they joined two other kind benefactors, Mr. Edward E. Rothman and Dr. Edgar A. Kahn, in aiding in the development of the prototype of the pneumatic inner crown support helmet. This project was initiated by Dr. Kahn, the Emeritus Head of the Section of Neurological Surgery to whom I personally am grateful for a most enjoyable and rewarding 25 year association. I acknowledge with deep gratitude the many hours spent by Mr. Joseph J. Keeley, Associate Director, and Mr. David M. Plawchan, Project Representative, of the Office of Research Administration in aiding in the details of the helmet research project.

To two contributors and associates, Dr. Elizabeth C. Crosby, the Head of the Neurosurgical Laboratory for years, and Miss Hazel D. Calhoun, I am deeply indebted for their aid in the difficult and time consuming task of compilation of the index. Throughout the years Dr. Crosby has served as a constant source of stimulation and inspiration to those members of the Neurosurgical Service who have been privileged to have learned from her teachings and to have participated with her in the research program. It is a pleasure to have this opportunity to personally thank her for kindness, understanding, and many fine contributions to the Section. To Miss Calhoun I am most grateful for her aid in EEG recordings on every case of convulsive seizures treated surgically by the Section of Neurosurgery as well as for her extensive work on this book.

I am especially indebted to my secretary, Mrs. Kay Neff, who effortlessly managed to stave off so many of the nonessentials of the everyday routine. Somehow she managed to check the photography, the references, consult on the manuscript, and in a final surge draw together the loose ends to complete the book. To Mrs. Doris Reuter I am deeply grateful for the typing and retyping of the manuscript and her review of the references. She has no peer in her constant goal of seeking nothing less than perfection. Mrs. Ruth Trimm, my former secretary of 18 years, was indispensable in the task of gathering statistics and helping to compile data at the onset of this project.

Mr. Edgar L. Sherman, the Supervisor, and Mr. Robert Bensinger of the Medical Photography Department have been most cooperative in somehow providing remarkably good photographs from less than acceptable negatives. The difficult problem of removing significant excerpts from third and fourth generation movies was remarkably achieved by Mr. Aubert Lavistida and Mr. Douglas W. Rideout of the Audiovisual Education Department. Their graciousness in the face of constant revisions I shall never forget. The Medical Illustration Department under the Directorship of Mr. Gerald P. Hodge and his associates, Mr. Albert Teoli, Mrs. Evelyn Sullivan, Mr. Dennis Lee, and Mr. Nikki Tan, have given generously of their many talents in illustrating the book.

The author is deeply indebted to Mrs. Laura B. Hawke and Miss Helen F. Meranda, medical librarians at the University of Michigan Medical Center, for their immeasurable aid in providing references and reviewing the bibliography.

Finally, I wish to particularly express my gratitude to Mrs. Ruby Richardson and Mr. Dick M. Hoover for their counsel in preparation of the book and The Williams & Wilkins Company for its publication.

Special acknowledgement is made of the fine cooperation rendered by the Executive Committees of the Harvey Cushing Society (currently the American Association of Neurological Surgeons) and the Congress of Neurological Surgeons and their respective memberships for supplying data in the football survey. Without their aid much of this study would not have been possible.

The following group of people have been directly responsible for making available the material in the questionnaire used in this study and have contributed in the follow-up of cases or aided in many other ways in the preparation of this monograph. This list is composed of neurosurgical colleagues, pathologists, team physicians, athletic directors, coaches, trainers, attorneys, newsmen, photographers, high school principals, hospital record room librarians, police, manufacturers, and other people from many walks of life to whom this author is deeply indebted. More than a few of the people on the list may have forgotten a long distance telephone call or a brief note which has provided so much information and help to this author. It is hoped that their combined efforts will specifically afford a better understanding of the mechanisms of injury to football players, create new efforts to prevent damage to the brain and spinal cord, and provide an improvement in the treatment of these injured athletes. Any failure to list the name of a contributor has not been by design but is merely a sin of omission due to the long interval of study and preparation of this book.

Dr. Walter D. Abbott
Dr. George Ablin
Dr. Akio Aburano
Dr. John H. Adametz
Dr. John E. Adams
Dr. Eben Alexander, Jr.
Dr. Clifford Allen
Dr. LeRoy Allen
Dr. Fred L. Allman, Jr.
Dr. Carter Anderson, Jr.
Dr. Robert Andre
Dr. Bartley Antine
Sister Agnes Arn
Mr. David C. Arnold
Dr. Neal I. Aronson
Dr. George M. Austin
Dr. Milton Avol

Dr. Arthur H. Bacon
Dr. Robert W. Bailey
Dr. John T. Bakody
Mr. Paul T. Baldwin
Dr. Karl G. Balthasar
Dr. Charles Baran
Mr. Frank Bargstrom
Dr. Thomas G. Barnes
Mr. J. G. Barry
Dr. Robert C. Bassett
Dr. Stanley Batkin
Dr. Arthur Battista
Dr. Francis Bayer
Dr. J. F. Beachler, Jr.
Dr. J. B. Beaird, Jr.
Dr. Martin J. Bellinger
Mr. William Bender, Jr.
Mr. Milbry E. Benedict
Mr. Don Bilsborough
Dr. Edward J. Bishop
Dr. Samuel P. W. Black
Dr. Carl S. Blyth
Mr. C. D. Boehme
Dr. John W. Bossard
Dr. Miles Bouton
Dr. Francis C. Boyer
Dr. Charles E. Brackett
Dr. A. D. Brickler
Dr. Carl Brinkman
Mr. Paul Brown
Mr. Thorne Brown
Mr. Edmund B. Brownell
Mr. and Mrs. Roy Brownell
Dr. A. W. Burek
Dr. Dennis Burke
Dr. Cecil R. Burket
Dr. Joseph Burnet

Dr. James Butcher
Mr. Walter Byers

Dr. W. P. Callahan
Dr. Mario J. Campagna
Mr. Donald B. Canham
Dr. Joe Melville Capps
Dr. Pedro C. Caram
Dr. Francis A. Carmichael, Jr.
Dr. Kenneth L. Casey
Dr. Ernest L. Cashion
Mr. John Castignola
Mr. Roberto Chavira
Dr. Harvey Chenault
Mr. Arthur Chetwynd
Dr. Edwin F. Chobot, Jr.
Dr. Shelley N. Chou
Mr. Richard Clark
Dr. Kenneth S. Clarke
Dr. Cully A. Cobb, Jr.
Dr. James Collins
Dr. William F. Collins, Jr.
Dr. William Combs
Dr. Donald Cooper
Dr. Thomas Y. Cooper
Dr. Asbury Coward (Capt., USN)
Dr. Fred Crescente
Mr. Herbert O. Crisler
Mr. Kenneth L. Crocker
Dr. George C. Culbreth
Dr. Charles W. Cure

Dr. Gustave J. Dammin
Dr. Courtland S. Davis, Jr.
Dr. Joseph H. Davis
Dr. Don DeBlanc
Mr. James Decker
Dr. Richard C. Deming
Dr. Robert H. Denham, Jr.
Mr. Donald Derby
Mr. Norman Des Jardins
Dr. Richard L. DeSaussure
Dr. Robert E. Dicks
Dr. Henry W. Dodge, Jr.
Dr. Ronald A. Dolan
Dr. William D. Dolan
Dr. Joseph F. Dorsey
Dr. Charles E. Dowman
Dr. John B. Doyle, Jr.
Mr. Donald Dufek
Dr. Hobart H. Dumke
Dr. Howard S. Dunbar
Dr. Jack Dunn, Jr.

Mr. Floyd R. Eastwood
Dr. Arthur Ecker

Mr. William T. Eddington
Dr. Albert J. Ehlert
Dr. George Ehni
Mr. Chalmers W. Elliott
Mr. William Elson
Mr. Les F. Etter
Dr. Marco T. Eugenio
Mr. Forest Evashevski

Mr. Clifford Fagan
Dr. Saeed M. Farhat
Dr. Robert Farris*
Dr. John A. Faulkner
Dr. Martin C. Feferman
Dr. Avner I. Feldman
Dr. Robert Fennell
Dr. James S. Feurig
Dr. William C. Fisher
Mr. J. D. Fitzgerald
Dr. Stevenson Flanigan
Mr. Henry Fonde
Dr. James C. Fox
Dr. Lyle A. French

Mr. A. S. Gaither
Dr. J. Garber Galbraith
Dr. W. James Gardner
Dr. John T. Garner
Dr. Richard W. Garrity
Dr. H. Harvey Gass
Dr. Francis Gaydosh
Dr. William J. German
Dr. A. Yale Gerol
Dr. Robert Gerow
Dr. F. Gary Gieseke
Mr. Frank Gindey
Dr. Harold J. Goald
Dr. James B. Golden
Dr. Purdue L. Gould
Dr. William A. Gracie, Jr.
Dr. George H. Gray, Jr.
Dr. Robert C. Greenwood
Dr. John G. Griffin
Dr. Robert A. Groff
Dr. E. S. Gurdjian

Dr. Benjamin Haddad
Dr. John W. Hanbery
Mr. Raymond I. Harris
Mr. Henry Hatch
Dr. Douglas C. Hawkes
Dr. Robert A. Hayne
Mr. Thomas E. Healion
Mr. J. Griffin Heard
Dr. Fred V. Hein

Dr. William Helme
Dr. Marshall G. Henry
Mr. George E. Hess
Dr. Wallace I. Hess
Dr. William J. Hester
Dr. Henry Hodd
Dr. Lucien R. Hodges
Dr. Theodore F. Hoff
Mr. Will Hofheinz
Dr. George Hoke
Dr. Hal C. Holland
Mr. Robert C. Hollway
Dr. Donald J. Holmes
Dr. Henry L. Hood
Dr. J. Patrick Hooker
Dr. Storer P. Humphreys
Mr. James E. Hunt
Dr. William E. Hunt
Dr. Samuel E. Hunter
Mr. Pete Hurst
Dr. William Hurteau

Dr. Joseph A. Jachimczyk
Dr. Anthony Jefferson
Dr. Howard Jennings
Dr. Michael Jerva
Mrs. Dorothy Johnson
Dr. H. P. Jubelt

Lt. Col. Ludwig G. Kempe, M.C., U.S. Army
Dr. Jack S. Kennedy
Dr. Merle F. Killian
Dr. Robert B. King
Mr. Delaney Kiphuth
Dr. Homer D. Kirgis
Dr. William C. Kite, Jr.
Dr. David G. Kline
Dr. George H. Koepke
Mr. William Koponen
Dr. Marvin A. Korbin
Dr. Theodore Kurze

Mr. James LaBlonde
Dr. Peter Ladewig
Dr. Aldo Lainin
Dr. Austin Lamberts
Dr. James M. Lansche
Mr. Grant S. Lashbrook
Father Leary
Dr. Warren H. Leimbach
Dr. Lloyd Lemmen
Dr. Paul M. Lin
Dr. George Lipesya
Dr. William R. Lipscomb
Dr. A. C. Lisle, Jr.

* Deceased.

Dr. Carl F. List*
Dr. Raeburn C. Llewellyn
Dr. George S. Loquvam
Dr. Edgar S. Lotspeich
Dr. Herbert Lourie
Mr. William Lowder
Dr. James C. Luce

Dr. Homer G. McClintock
Mr. Thomas B. McDonald
Dr. James Eugene McIntosh
Mr. J. Lindsy McLean, Jr.
Mr. Guy J. Mackey
Dr. Marion Mann
Dr. Simon E. Markowich
Dr. Thomas M. Marshall
Dr. Luther C. Martin
Mr. T. J. Mason
Dr. Donald D. Matson
Dr. Norman Matthews
Dr. William F. Meacham
Dr. John Mealey, Jr.
Dr. Walter A. Meier
Dr. W. J. S. Melvin
Mr. Albert J. Meyer
Dr. Walter B. Meyer
Dr. Franklin C. Miles
Dr. Leroy J. Miller
Dr. W. T. Mitchell, Jr.
Mr. Robert P. Molitor
Mr. Jack Mollenkopf
Dr. Henry J. Monotoye
Dr. William H. Mosberg, Jr.
Dr. Peter D. Moyes
Dr. Robert H. Mudd
Dr. Charles E. Mueller, Jr.
Dr. John J. Mueller
Gen. Paul W. Myers, M.C., USAF

Dr. Robert L. Nafzgar
Dr. Tom M. Nash
Dr. James W. Nellen
Mr. David Nelson
Mr. J. A. Nelson
Dr. Richard E. Newquist
Dr. James B. Nichols, Jr.
Dr. Richard G. Nilges
Dr. Hal Norgaard
Dr. Horace Norrell
Dr. George R. Nugent
Dr. Frank E. Nulsen

Dr. Francis H. O'Brien
Dr. Frank B. O'Connell
Dr. William S. Ogle

Dr. C. Kent Olson
Mr. Bennie G. Oosterbaan
Dr. Frank J. Otenasek

Mr. Lenwood Paddock
Dr. Harley P. Palmer
Mrs. Wilma B. Park
Dr. Dwight Parkinson
Mr. Ara Parseghian
Dr. Fremont Peck
Dr. Irwin Perlmutter
Dr. Pedro P. Polakoff, II
Dr. Claude Pollard, Jr.
Dr. Marvin J. Powell
Dr. Robert H. Pudenz
Mr. Ronald L. Pulliam

Dr. Thomas R. Quigley

Dr. Stephen E. Reid
Dr. Edward Reifel
Dr. Frank Reilly
Mr. Allan M. Renfrew
Mr. Robert Riger
Dr. Elliot Rinzler
Dr. Morris H. Rivers
Dr. Ernst Rodin
Dr. J. Speed Rogers
Dr. Stacy Rollins, Jr.
Lt. Cmdr. Norman Ronis, M.C., USN
Dr. Kenneth D. Rose
Dr. Charles W. Rossel
Dr. Stuart N. Rowe
Dr. Allan J. Ryan

Mr. Harold S. Sawyer
Dr. Robert H. Saxton
Mr. Glenn E. Schembechler
Dr. George Schemm
Dr. Edwin R. Schmidt
Mr. Joe Schmidt
Dr. Paul F. Schrode
Dr. John E. Schwab
Dr. James P. Schweinfurth
Dr. Jess T. Schwidde
Mr. Steve Sebo
Dr. Roy J. Secrest
Mr. Clark Shaughnessy
Dr. Norman C. Shealy
Dr. C. Hunter Shelden
Mr. William Shepherd
Dr. John Shillito, Jr.
Dr. H. Jack Siefert
Dr. F. Miles Skultety
Dr. Harry W. Slade

* Deceased.

Dr. Alexander Slepian
Dr. Donald B. Slocum
Dr. George Smith
Dr. Richard A. Smith
Dr. I. Joshua Speigel
Dr. Donald E. Stafford
Dr. Donald L. Stainsby
Dr. Elvin H. Stanton
Dr. Ralph Stephens
Mr. James E. Stephenson
Dr. John D. Stewart
Dr. Bernard B. Stone
Dr. Jim Lewis Story
Dr. Averill Stowell
Dr. Winslow P. Stratemeyer
Dr. Ralph L. Seuchting
Dr. Oscar Sugar
Mr. Robert Sullivan
Dr. Garrett M. Swain
Dr. Homer S. Swanson
Dr. Henry H. Sweets, Jr.

Dr. Z. E. Taheri
Dr. James A. Taren
Dr. Joseph A. Tarkington
Dr. Ronald R. Tasker
Mr. Theodore Tedora
Dr. Robert Tennant
Mr. George H. Thompson
Dr. John M. Thompson
Dr. David A. Tilly
Dr. Robert S. Tolmach

Dr. Bruce Trembly
Dr. R. Paul Tucker

Dr. Gordon van den Noort
Dr. Hubert Velten
Dr. Philip Vogel

Dr. Francis S. Walker
Dr. Jacques B. Wallach
Dr. Gordon T. Wannamaker
Mr. Murray Warmath
Dr. Robert A. Waters
Mr. Francis H. Watt
Dr. Preston S. Weadon
Dr. Edgar N. Weaver
Dr. Walter Wegner
Dr. Edward C. Weiford
Dr. Lawrence Weinberger
Mr. Donald A. Weir
Dr. Carl H. Wells
Dr. Nicholas Wetzel
Dr. Robert Weyand
Dr. Benjamin B. Whitcomb
Dr. E. T. White
Dr. James C. White
Dr. John D. White
Capt. Roy D. Wilkerson, M.C., U.S. Army
Dr. Edward N. Willey
Dr. Chester Williams
Dr. Robert P. Woods

Dr. Julian R. Youmans

Richard C. Schneider, M.D.
Ann Arbor, Michigan

Contributors

Hazel D. Calhoun, B.A., M.A.
> Assistant Professor in Electroencephalographic Technology, Section of Electroencephalography, Department of Psychiatry and Section of Neurological Surgery, University of Michigan Medical Center *(Chapter 10)*

Elizabeth C. Crosby, Ph.D., Sc.D.
> Professor Emeritus of Anatomy, Department of Anatomy, University of Michigan; Head of the Laboratory of Neurosurgery Research, University of Michigan Medical Center; Professor Emeritus of Anatomy, Department of Anatomy, University of Alabama *(Chapter 9)*

Elwyn R. Gooding
> Research Associate, Laboratory of Neurosurgical Research, Section of Neurosurgery, University of Michigan Medical Center *(Chapters 14 and 15)*

Hank H. Gosch, M.D.
> Assistant Professor, Section of Neurosurgery, Department of Surgery, University of Michigan Medical Center *(Chapter 14)*

Glenn W. Kindt, M.D.
> Associate Professor, Section of Neurosurgery, Department of Surgery, University of Michigan Medical Center *(Chapter 15)*

Kenneth A. Kooi, M.S., M.D.
> Professor of Electroencephalography in the Departments of Neurology and Psychiatry, University of Michigan Medical Center *(Chapter 10)*

Frederick C. Kriss, M.D.
> Neurosurgical Consultant, St. Mary's Hospital Medical Center, Madison General Hospital, University Hospital, Madison, Wisconsin; Clinical Associate Professor,

Department of Neurosurgery, University of Wisconsin. Formerly, Instructor of Neurosurgery, Section of Neurosurgery, Department of Surgery, University of Michigan Medical Center *(Chapter 11)*

Robert A. Moore, M.D.

Medical Director, Mesa Vista Hospital, San Diego, and Associate Clinical Professor of Psychiatry, University of California at San Diego School of Medicine. Formerly, Assistant Professor of Psychiatry, Department of Psychiatry, University of Michigan Medical Center *(Chapter 8)*

Gerald A. O'Connor, M.D.

Clinical Assistant Professor of Orthopedic Surgery, University of Michigan and Team Physician for the University of Michigan *(Chapter 13)*

Richard C. Schneider, M.D.

Professor and Head, Section of Neurosurgery, Department of Surgery, University of Michigan Medical Center; formerly a member of the Committee on the Medical Aspects of Sports, American Medical Association 1962-1971; formerly a member of the Board of Control of Intercollegiate Athletics, University of Michigan, 1964-1968 *(chapters 1 through 16)*

Contents

Introduction

To undertake the writing of a monograph on head and neck injuries spanning the spectrum of potential readers from the trainer, coach, team physician group, then the medical student or physician interested in trauma, and finally the specialists in neurosurgery and orthopedic surgery is extremely difficult. There is the obvious danger that the material presented may be, on the one hand, too complex for the layman or, on the other, too simplistic for the more sophisticatedly trained specialist. Nevertheless the attempt has been made to provide sufficient information at both ends of this span to make this book valuable to all who are concerned in the great game of football. The general discussion has been for the most part presented in the largest type. The case histories are published in a finer print. The very specialized portions of the material, such as the neuroanatomical details, have been recorded, for the most part, in the finest type. Hopefully this apportionment will enable the reader to do the selective reading as required for his specific needs.

With the exception of four figures, which have been so identified, all of the photographs of x-rays, pathologic specimens, etc. have been taken from football players actually injured in football. Lastly, there is but one of the 55 cases presented which could not be followed to absolute actual documentation from the records, for part of the information was culled from reports by the news media.

An interesting and informative book *You Have to Pay the Price* by former Army and Dartmouth Coach Earl Blaik and sports writer Tim Cohane was published in 1960. It is recommended reading for information and historical data concerning our national sport, football. These authors emphasize the blood, the sweat, the tears, the anxieties, and the frustrations associated with the game. This is "the price." Within its covers the classic statement may be found: "Football games are not won by the faint aroma of good fellowship," a fact which is evident in many sports, but this is particularly true regarding contact sports such as football. The main thesis of the present publication is to review the neurosurgical aspects of the problem with the great question of "Does one have to pay the price?" namely, that of severe permanent injury or death. Football is a rough sport, which in some instances may prove to be disastrous. The player who elects to participate in the sport must do so with the complete understanding that he does so at his own risk. The parent who lends his support and gives permission for a son to play the game must realize these dangers and accept this responsibility. If serious injury to his son does occur, he should not cast about seeking to place the blame on someone else. A certain number of serious injuries are bound to occur, but it should be the goal of every physician, coach, trainer, and sports equipment manufacturer to do everything possible to avoid such catastrophies.

Football, like the automobile, has emerged in the last decade with a tremendous increase in power and speed (Frontispiece). Just as there have been changes in car models during these years, a variety of alterations of football rules and equipment have been made to enable football to be a more exciting spectator sport. Unfortunately man's intellectual capacity seems to be unable to keep pace with some of these innovations whether they are related to the use of automobiles or to playing the game of football. For example, coaches and trainers must use the new safeguards, such as the helmet and face guard, intelligently to provide proper protection for the player. The current coaching and training techniques, which have evolved, have employed the equipment as an offensive weapon and therefore its usefulness not only has been negated to a major degree but even has been the source of serious injury and death.

In recent years the ever increasing interest in athletic injuries has resulted in a compilation of data relative to the incidence and types of severe or fatal injuries in football. Efforts have been made to apply these studies to the proper treatment and the prevention of such injuries. Much of the credit for this achievement must be attributed to the efforts of the Committee on Injuries and Fatalities of the American Football Coaches Association which has for the past 40 years led the way. The tedious and painstaking annual accumulation and the analysis of the data acquired by the members of this organization are presented annually at its meeting. Dr. Carl Blyth, Chairman of the above Committee, reported that 96% of the fatal injuries in the 1966 season were due to head and spinal lesions. The current Chairman, Dr. Donald Cooper, reported 29 fatal head and spinal injuries in 1970. In any given year this is not significant, but there has been a slowly progressive upward trend. Because of the number of head, spine, and spinal cord injuries, it seemed important that the fatal injury statistics should be evaluated from a neurosurgical standpoint. Thus this report reviews in detail the serious and fatal injuries occurring during the five year interval from the 1959 to the 1964 season. It is apparent that there must have been many other football players who sustained serious but non-fatal injuries and were treated successfully by neurosurgeons during this time. Through the kindness and cooperation of the Executive Committees of the Harvey Cushing Society and the Congress of Neurological Surgeons, it was possible to forward football injury questionnaires to 1013 neurosurgeons covering their experience for this same five year period with not only the fatal but also the non-fatal injuries being listed. It required three years to follow up the patients and to complete the study. There is every reason to believe that these statistics are still valid today; consequently, in the interval the author has been involved in collecting further information about players, who fit into specific categories, and has promoted further experimental and clinical research.

Six hundred and nineteen replies were received making a 61.1% return of questionnaires which obviously is far short of providing a complete picture. Many neurosurgeons in practice do not have complete cross reference diagnostic files in their offices. For example, this author himself forgot to include the names of several football player patients with serious injuries and realizes that any number of busy neurosurgical colleagues may have done likewise. In another instance one group of seven neurologic surgeons, who have a very well organized office, were kind enough to extract their records of such injuries from the files covering a period from January 1960 through March 1963. If one omits their 26 cases of cerebral concussion, since this is a minor type of injury, there were 20 other cases which exhibited some major neurosurgical disability, such as subdural hematomas, transverse myelitis cases, etc., in this group. It obviously would be a great imposition to request complete details concerning each of these cases so they could be included in this report, for this group of patients would be a study in itself. Inasmuch as this author did not have complete data, these neurosurgical cases have not been included in this report. All of the material presented here has been checked as carefully as possible against hospital and medical records and, where indicated, medical examiners' and coroners' reports. Since the compilation of this study, it has become progressively difficult to procure such data. Almost all the player identification symbols in the following pages, such as the numerals, have been obliterated or altered as completely as possible to preserve anonymity. In a few cases where the individual is identifiable, signed permissions have been freely granted in the hope of aiding other football players.

chapter one

Statistical Data

A graph depicting the number of direct fatalities occurring in football from the 1931 through the 1970 seasons (Fig. 1) shows that since 1956 almost a plateau had been reached for the number of fatalities incurred until the 1964 season when there was a sudden upsurge of deaths. In surveying the group of direct fatalities sustained during the 1947 to 1969 interval, there has been a slowly progressive shift with a proportional diminution of the incidence of abdominal and internal injuries and a corresponding elevation of the mortality rate due to head and spinal cord injuries. (However, it must be remembered that the number of participants in football has increased annually.)

It was not pertinent to record separately in our survey the reports collected from each of 39 of the United States and from five of the Canadian Provinces. However, six of the seven states with the greatest number of serious or fatal injuries, totaling 101, with 32 deaths, were in the Midwest and the West (Fig. 2). The first four of these states were among the most populous in our country. However, below the line on the chart two more of our most heavily populated states are listed which are in the East, and their record of serious and fatal injuries, 12, with 8 deaths, seemed in comparison to be considerably less in number. (The term "serious" neurosurgical injury refers to such lesions as: lacerations of the brain, blood clots within the brain or on its surface or its membranous coverings, ruptured discs, partially or totally transected spinal cords with paralysis for life or death itself, etc.) An investigation of the differences of football coaching techniques between these two regions of our country might be of some interest and value. It is alleged that *"spearing"* and *"stick-blocking,"* i.e., using the head as a weapon by thrusting it into a player on the ground or planting it in the oncoming ball carrier's midsection, respectively, is more frequently taught the farther southward and westward one travels. This is hearsay, requires confirmation, and will no doubt elicit a vigorous denial.

The sources of these football injuries and deaths may be of some interest (Fig. 3). Since at the time of this survey it was estimated there were 780,000 high school football players annually, 141 very serious or fatal football injuries seemed a

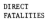

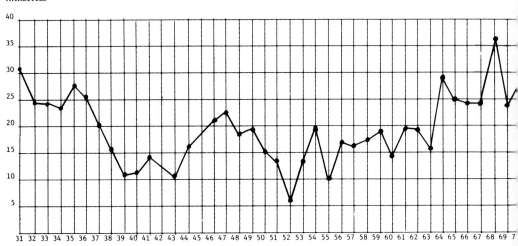

*No study was made in 1942.   Source: Table I – Fatalities Directly Due To Football

Fig. 1. Reprinted from C. S. Blyth and D. C. Arnold: The Thirty-ninth Annual Survey of Football Fatalities 1931–1970.

"The incidence of direct fatalities for 1970 was 2.00 per 100,000 participants for high schools and colleges combined. There were 26 fatalities among 1,275,000 players (1,200,000 high school players plus 75,000 college players)."

According to the above report the second week in October was the peak time of occurrence for such deaths directly attributable to football. During this particular season 77% were due to head and spinal injuries. Fifty-five percent of the fatalities were recorded in the 16 to 18 year level with 36% occurring in defensive play. Thirty-two percent of the players who died sustained their injury while tackling the opponent.

The number of fatalities is not great. However, there is no way of calculating the incidence of and types of morbidity such as neurologic deficit from the many non-fatal craniocerebral or spine and spinal cord injuries.

	Injury	Deaths
CALIFORNIA	22	(3)
TEXAS	21	(9)
MICHIGAN	14	(5)
OHIO	13	(7)
FLORIDA	11	(3)
INDIANA	10	(4)
KANSAS	10	(1)
NEW YORK	6	(4)
PENNSYLVANIA	6	(4)
TOTAL	113	(40)

Fig. 2. Above the line on the chart are the most populous states in the Midwest, Far West, and one state in the South which had a total of 101 serious injuries with 32 fatalities. Two of the most populous states in the East are shown below the line with a total of 12 severe injuries with 8 deaths. [Reprinted from Schneider (1) by permission of The Congress of Neurological Surgeons.]

HIGH SCHOOL	141
COLLEGE	34
SAND LOT	26
PROFESSIONAL	14
SEMI-PRO	3
ELEMENTARY	1
(UNKNOWN)	6
TOTAL	225

Fig. 3. The source and numbers of various football injuries are shown. Note the relatively small number of sandlot players, who wear no equipment, compared to the high school, college, and professional athletes who are well protected by proper equipment. [Reprinted from Schneider (1) by permission of The Congress of Neurological Surgeons.]

rather small proportion. Similarly 34 serious and fatal injuries in a group in which there were more than 70,000 college football participants seemed relatively slight. The proportion of injuries was greater in professional football where an estimated 4500 men play annually with 14 severely injured or killed. The 26 injuries or fatalities sustained in sandlot football were in individuals who had not been wearing any football equipment. If one deducts the sum of these first three categories from the estimated total of 2.5 million people who played football in the United States annually at that time, this sandlot group comprised approximately 1,645,000 players, by far the greatest number of participants. Since it required three years to compile all of the data, these numbers of football players in each category and the grand total have markedly increased. *It is this sandlot group which is commonly believed by many people to have the greatest number of fatalities because of the lack of proper protection. In all of the other classifications noted, the players were fully equipped with presumed adequate protection for the game.* It may be said the sandlot player does not play nearly as hard, i.e., not striking with as great force, as the high school, college, or professional athlete wearing adequate equipment and protection. The question may well be raised: Do the other groups of players, who are well outfitted, play harder with a false sense of security because of their equipment or may the present rules possibly increase the perils of the sport?

Reference

1. Schneider, R. C.: Serious and Fatal Neurosurgical Football Injuries. *Clin. Neurosurg.*, *12:* 226, 1966.

chapter two

Anatomy of the Head*

It seems pertinent to present a rather simplified review of the anatomy of the head in order that the following material may be more meaningful. (To the medical student and qualified physician the author apologizes for the rather simplistic coverage of the topic.)

Scalp

The scalp (4) consists of five layers: hair and skin, the subcutaneous connective tissue, the aponeurosis or galea, a loose layer of connective tissue, and the pericranium. These five layers serve as a protective coating for the bony structure and the scalp tends to slide over the skull when it is struck a tangential blow.

Skull

The skull (3) has been described as a "rigid bony box" having three principal contents: the cerebrospinal fluid, the blood, and the brain. There is one main exit from the skull or cranium and that is through the foramen magnum or "large window" at its base (Fig. 4A). Through this aperture, the medulla and spinal cord pass, entering the bony spinal canal in the neck. The bones of the adult skull are constructed of firm outer and inner layers or tables. Interspersed between them is a layer of softer bone, or "marrow," containing blood channels. Some of these larger vascular pathways are visible on skull x-rays. In the forepart of the skull are situated the frontal sinuses which are air cavities which communicate with the nose and the upper respiratory passages. In the floor of the frontal area are located the roofs of the orbits. Between them in the midline of the skull is a very thin, bony plate, the cribriform plate, through which pass the filaments or projections of the olfactory nerves which carry the sense of smell from the upper part of the nose and nasopharynx to the brain. Immediately under and posterior to the cribriform plate, the ethmoid sinuses and sphenoid sinus

---

* Reprinted by permission from M. Houts, Editor: *Courtroom Medicine*, Chap. 14, p. 511, © 1958, Matthew Bender & Company, Inc.

5

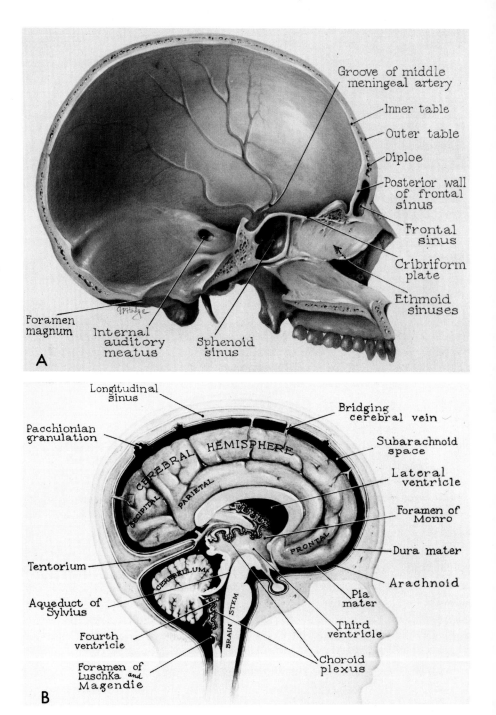

Fig. 4A. The skull is seen in sagittal section illustrating some important anatomical landmarks. (Reprinted by permission from M. Houts, Editor: *Courtroom Medicine*, Chap. 14, p. 516, © 1958, Matthew Bender & Company, Inc.)

Fig. 4B. A sagittal section of the brain shows some of the normal anatomical relationships between the skull, meninges (dura mater, arachnoid and pia mater), and brain. (Reprinted by permission from M. Houts, Editor: *Courtroom Medicine*, Chap. 14, p. 511, © 1958, Matthew Bender & Company, Inc.)

are found; these are mucous membrane-lined cavities or structures communicating with the nasal cavity.

Another very important region in the skull is that of the internal auditory meatus, the bony canal serving as a portal for the seventh nerve (the facial) which supplies muscles for the movement of the same side of the face and the eighth nerve (the acoustic) which is concerned with the functions of hearing and balance on the same side of the body.

In the skull there are suture lines, which are wavy, irregular lines formed where the bones of the skull eventually unite or fuse together. There are other channels in the skull which are fairly constant. Most prominent in importance is the middle meningeal artery groove which extends through the region of the temple or temporal area; and, as it extends upward through the thin inner table of bone, it threads forward and backward as two main branches. This is the major extra-dural arterial vessel which is imbedded within the bony tables of the skull. Two other grooves may be present. These are found on either side of the middle of the back of the head, extending from the center of the skull toward either ear. They contain the transverse or lateral venous sinuses, two major channels carrying venous blood from the brain posteriorly and downward toward the heart.

Brain Coverings or Meninges

Directly inside the skull, three layers of membranes are encountered, collectively called the meninges (Fig. 4B) (1). The outermost, the dura mater, is tough and fibrous and hugs the inner table of the skull to which it is intimately adherent at certain points. The dura serves as a strong protective covering for the brain. Within it are situated several large blood vessels, the venous sinuses, whose function is described above. The largest of these is the longitudinal or superior sagittal sinus, which begins in the center of the forward part of the skull and extends directly backward in the midline to the posterior portion of the skull where it joins with the transverse or lateral venous sinuses (Fig. 4B). The confluens of the sinuses is that point in midline in the posterior end of the skull where all the venous channels or sinuses meet. Suspended vertically from the midline under the superior longitudinal sinus is a flap of tough, fibrous tissue—a prolongation of the dura—designated the falx (5), which partially divides the cranium into two equal lateral chambers. At the base of the brain is another fibrous layer lying in a horizontal plane, the tentorium, which is a partial partition between the middle and posterior compartments, or fossae, of the skull. Through its foremost point runs a curved opening through which the lowermost portion of the brain, the brain stem, descends into the posterior compartment or fossa. The posterior part of the tentorium fuses with the dura to incorporate the confluens of the sinuses and hence supports and contains the transverse or lateral sinuses (3).

The second of the three meninges, or membranes, is the arachnoid. This is a much finer, tissue paper-thin, transparent structure which lies immediately under the dura. The arachnoid, in general, lies around the inner margins of the dura;

and between the two layers there is a potential space which is ordinarily of little significance, for it is traversed only by the bridging blood vessels and small vascular structures known as Pacchionian granulations. Beneath the arachnoid is found a very important space, the subarachnoid space, which surrounds the brain and contains the cerebrospinal fluid, a clear, watery fluid which acts as a water cushion, protecting the brain. It is traversed by the bridging blood vessels and Pacchionian granulations described above.

The third and last important membrane is the pia mater, which is a very fine, transparent, and fairly tough structure, intimately associated with the surface of the brain, dipping into the various gullies, or sulci, and rising up over the crests, or convolutions.

Brain

The brain itself is composed for the most part of two massive, paired structures, the cerebral hemispheres, which are mirror images of each other. These lie above the tentorium in the anterior and middle compartments or the fossae of the skull. Beneath the tentorium, in the posterior compartment, or fossa, lie two paired structures, cerebellar hemispheres, with a smaller midline component, the vermis of the cerebellum. At the base lies the brain stem which extends from the middle compartment downward and through an aperture in the tentorium, into the posterior fossa to the foramen magnum, the opening at the base of the skull. The uppermost end of the spinal cord begins here and extends into the spinal canal.

The paired cerebral hemispheres are described as having four main components: the frontal, parietal, occipital, and temporal portions or lobes (Fig. 4B). The back part or most posterior portion of the frontal lobe contains an area designated as the "motor strip" which extends laterally along one of the larger fissures. This motor strip contains a major portion of the brain cells responsible for discrete movements of the face, trunk, and extremities of the opposite side of the body. Just behind this fissure, in the forward part of the parietal lobe, is another important area, the "sensory strip" which contains brain cells responsible for sensation in the face, trunk, and extremities of the opposite side of the body. Although there are second motor areas in other parts of the brain, which, when stimulated, contribute more gross movements, a further discussion of them is inappropriate here (1).

If a cut is made directly through the center of the brain in a vertical plane, the chambers or ventricles of the brain will thereby be exposed (Fig. 4B). On either side of the midline are the paired lateral chambers of the brain which contain two blood vessel clumps or tufts, choroid plexuses, which secrete a clear, watery substance, called the cerebrospinal fluid, as noted previously. This fluid flows from the lateral ventricles through two small holes (the foramina of Monro), one in each lateral ventricle, into a single midline reservoir—the third ventricle. Another blood vessel tuft, a choroid plexus, contributes further cerebrospinal fluid which drains downward and backward through a narrow communication, the aqueduct of Sylvius, into another midline chamber—the fourth ventricle (5). This ventricle contains still another blood vessel tuft, or choroid plexus. In the roof of this chamber is a fine membrane which contains several holes, the foramina of Luschka and Magendie, through which the cerebrospinal fluid escapes into the subarachnoid space, where it courses down the spinal canal, along the base of the brain, and upward over the top or convexity of the brain. Here partial absorption is believed to occur into the bridging blood vessels and Pacchionian granulations, which traverse the subarachnoid space and eventually the subdural space, and drain into the large venous channels or sinuses. In the fourth venticle floor the highly vital medullary centers for cardiac and respiratory control are located.

At the base of the brain lie its important blood vessels, the paired carotid arteries and their branches, which are united frontally by the anterior communicating arteries and caudally by the posterior communicating arteries, the posterior cerebral arteries, and the basilar artery to form the circle of Willis (2). From this complex arise the smaller blood vessels which extend into the brain substance and provide its nourishment as tiny perforating arteries.

References

1. Crosby, E. C., Humphrey, T. and Lauer, E. W.: *Correlative Anatomy of the Nervous System*. The Macmillan Company, New York, 1962.
2. Kaplan, H. A. and Ford, D. H.: *The Brain Vascular System*. Elsevier Publishing Company, Amsterdam, 1966.
3. Pernkopf, E.: *Atlas of Topographical and Applied Human Anatomy*, Vol. 1, Head and Neck. W. B. Saunders Company, Philadelphia, 1963.
4. Spalteholz, W.: *Hand-Atlas of Human Anatomy*. J. B. Lippincott Company, Philadelphia, One Volume Edition.
5. Strong, O. S. and Elwyn, A.: *Human Neuroanatomy*, 4th ed., edited by R. C. Truex. The Williams & Wilkins Company, Baltimore, 1959.

chapter three

Classifications of Craniocerebral Lesions

In this five year football survey, 1959 to 1964 seasons, all minor craniocerebral injuries were excluded. Therefore cerebral concussion will be discussed under "First Aid" (Chapter 11). Although scalp lacerations and contusions may be painful and unsightly if present, they are not ordinarily a source of any grave disability.

Cerebral Contusion and Lacerations

Cerebral contusion is a pathologic condition, that is, an ecchymosis (a black and blue mark) on the surface of the brain. This may cause some brain damage from which the patient apparently may recover completely (2) or have partial return of function, or have some severe residual neurological disability (3). The semi-solid brain is supported on its brain stem in watery cerebrospinal fluid within the intracranial cavity. If the player falls striking the back of his head and the brain rebounds forward impinging and bruising the tips of the frontal and temporal lobes upon the bony protuberances or the frontotemporal junction against the sharp sphenoid ridge of the skull, he may sustain a contusion or laceration of the brain (1, 6, 7). *Such a lesion in the frontotemporal junction of the brain at the superior temporal gyrus, vestibular projection (7, 8, 10) and association areas, may be responsible for the dizziness which is so frequently complained of in "concussions" or contusions of the brain (10, 11).* A prolonged interval may elapse before such symptoms subside.

In this series of cases which were followed up over a five year period there were 17 football players who were listed as having contusions or lacerations. This diagnosis was made on the basis of a severe head injury followed by a neurologic deficit such as severe personality change, hemiparesis, aphasia, memory loss, combativeness (6), prolonged convulsive seizure patterns, or other neurologic abnormalities without the presence of any of the expanding intracranial lesions such as hematomas on the membranes of the brain or within the brain proper. If the abnormal neurologic findings described above were present with a clear cerebrospinal fluid on lumbar puncture and these symptoms persisted, a diagnosis of cerebral contusion was made. If a bloody cerebrospinal fluid was obtained then a diagnosis of a probable cerebral laceration was made. Clinically these patients cannot be differentiated from those having petechial hemorrhages and intracerebral clots the diagnosis of which is all too frequently made on pathologic specimens (5, 9). An example of a severe type of contusion, and probably multiple petechial hemorrhages, is described in Case 6. There were, of course, many thousands of cases of contusion and lacerations which were not reported in the survey.

Skull Fractures

A skull fracture is a break of the cranium resulting from trauma. Such fractures may be classified as:

a) Closed (or simple) fractures are ones with intact scalp and/or mucous membranes overlying the fracture.

b) Open (or compound) fractures are ones with a laceration of the scalp and/or the mucous membranes over the site of the fracture.

A further subdivision of this classification is recorded below.

A skull fracture is indicative of the sudden application of a physical force, i.e., trauma. The symptoms depend upon the site and type of fracture and the degree of involvement of the underlying meninges and brain. Pain, headache, anosmia (loss of sense of smell), blurred or double vision, dizziness, tinnitus (ringing in the ears), nausea, vomiting, and/or memory impairment may occur. On the other hand, the patient may be completely asymptomatic.

The signs of a skull fracture may be an alteration of the state of consciousness. A laceration, swelling, or discoloration of the scalp may be present. There may be hemorrhage from the nose, watery discharge (cerebrospinal fluid) from the nose (rhinorrhea) or ears (otorrhea). A contusion behind the ear, i.e., a "black and blue mark" (Battle's sign), is due to a disruption of the mastoid emissary vein. There may be associated neurologic findings which may indicate the presence of an expanding lesion requiring surgical intervention.

Although the x-rays of the skull demonstrate the type and extent of the fracture, they do not indicate the amount of underlying brain damage. *Some of the most serious brain injuries occur without any evidence of skull fracture.* Since the skull is relatively non-resilient, there is a direct transmission of force to the intracranial contents causing contusions, petechial hemorrhages, and intracerebral hematomas of the brain. If skull fracture occurs there is a dissipation of the blow with less transmission of energy to the brain. This may produce less severe intracranial damage than if the skull had not been broken (Fig. 5A).

Football Survey. There were only 11 skull fractures in our series resulting in four deaths (Fig. 5B). Two of the players who succumbed had worn full equipment; one of these had an associated extradural hematoma and died within 36

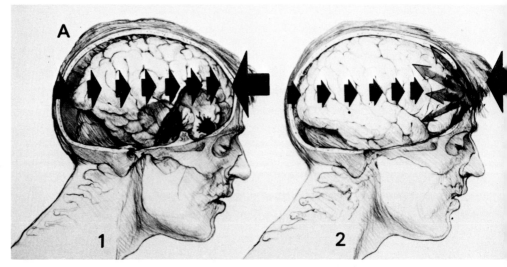

SKULL FRACTURES: 11 CASES WITH 4 DEATHS

Fig. 5A. The differences in effect between a closed head injury 1) without and 2) with fracture following blows of equal magnitude are illustrated. 1. The blow to the frontal region causes the brain to move posteriorly and strike the occipital lobes against the skull and on the rebound the frontotemporal region of the brain impinges upon the sphenoid ridge causing laceration, contusion of the brain, or/and an intracerebral blood clot. This mechanism is defined as a contrecoup injury. 2. If skull fracture occurs, there is an initial dissipation of the force of the blow when the fracture occurs with less rebound phenomenon and diminished injury to the frontotemporal junction at the sphenoid ridge as indicated by the arrows.

B

Equipment	No Neurological Deficit	Neurological Deficit	Seen by Neurosurgeon	Operation Performed	Time Interval: Injury to Operation	Associated Injury*	Interval: Injury to Death	Prognosis	Death
F	No	Yes	Yes	No	-	-	-	Fair	No
?	Yes	No	Yes	No	-	-	-	Excellent	No
P	No	Yes	Yes	No	-	-	-	Fair	No
0	No	P.W.	Yes	No	-	-	-	Poor	No
?	No	P.W.	Yes	No	-	IC	-	Hopeless	No
?	NP.W.	No	Yes	Yes	4	-	-	Excellent	No
0	No	Yes	Yes	No	-	SD	2	-	Yes
F	Yes	No	Yes	No	-	-	-	Excellent	No
F	No	Yes	Yes	Yes	6 1/2	ED	36	-	Yes
F	No	Yes	No	No	-	-	2	-	Yes
0	No	Yes	No	No	-	ED	8	-	Yes

*Abbreviations used are: IC, intracerebral clot; SD, subdural hematoma; ED, extradural hemotoma; NP.W, non-penetrating wound; P.W., penetrating wound; F, full; P, partial.

Fig. 5B. The incidence of skull fractures in the survey is shown. (Reprinted from Schneider, R. C.: Serious and Fatal Neurosurgical Football Injuries. *Clin. Neurosurg., 12:* 226, 1966, by permission of The Congress of Neurological Surgeons.)

hours. Two of the other players who died had worn no equipment; one of these had an associated acute subdural hematoma, which was not operated upon, and he died within 2 hours after injury; the second boy with a concomitant extradural hemorrhage also remained unoperated upon and died 8 hours after injury. Eighty-two percent of these patients with skull fractures were seen by neurosurgeons. Two of the patients were operated upon with survival of one player; the second one had the extradural hematoma noted above. The two of the seven survivors who were graded as "poor" or "hopeless" had sustained associated penetrating wounds of the brain. The other five players who recovered from their injury were graded as having had an "excellent" or "fair" outcome.

For the purposes of further definition it must be stated that a) a linear fracture is one in which there is no displacement of the bones of the skull whereas the term b) depressed skull fracture indicates a fracture with inward bending of a part of the calvarium. Two examples are given in football players; Case 1 is a linear skull fracture and Case 2 is a depressed skull fracture.

Case 1: An 11 year old, right-handed, sandlot football player was running down the field for a pass when he ran into a tree striking his left temporal region. He was not unconscious but remained confused for a few minutes and vomited twice. Upon examination at the hospital he was found to be neurologically negative; since he had a small bruise of the scalp, x-rays were taken showing a linear fracture in the left temporal area (Fig. 6). The patient was hospitalized for 24 hours and, since his blood pressure, pulse, and respirations were normal and he was asymptomatic, he was discharged on the following day. The boy made a complete recovery.

Comment. Linear fractures are only of importance in that they indicate the severity of the blow which the patient received and their location may suggest damage to the underlying intracranial structures. For example, fractures in the temporal area traversing the groove of the middle meningeal artery suggest transection of the vessel may have occurred and the patient should be observed carefully for an extradural hemorrhage. (This is the only case used in this monograph where injury has been sustained indirectly, i.e., where the individual has not been injured directly in playing the football game itself but by running into an inanimate object.)

Case 2. A 14 year old, sandlot football player who was *not* wearing a helmet was kicked in the left parietal area of the head. He was not rendered unconscious, but on his way to the hospital he had a convulsive seizure with the head and eyes turned toward the right side. His left pupil was slightly larger than the right one and there was a fine nystagmus on right lateral gaze. Otherwise there was no neurologic abnormality. The patient responded to anticonvulsant therapy administered intravenously, and subsequent x-ray examination showed a depressed skull fracture of the left parietal area (Fig. 7). The patient was taken to the operating room where a horseshoe-shaped scalp flap was reflected and a burr hole was made. The 5 cm. in diameter depressed skull fracture was elevated. There had been no penetration of the dura. The wound was closed, and the patient recovered very nicely without any neurologic sequelae.

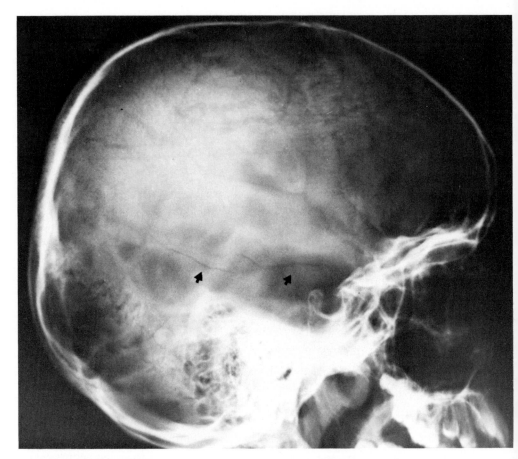

Fig. 6. Case 1. The skull x-ray shows a linear fracture in the temporal-occipital region (arrows).
     The presence of the fracture line at this site traversing the posterior branch of the middle meningeal artery should provide the suspicion that the patient may be developing an extradural hemorrhage. Fracture lines at other areas may alert the observer to similar underlying lesions. A linear fracture in the posterior part of the skull which extends across the lateral or transverse (dural or venous) sinus or runs downward into the foramen magnum should lead one to consider a posterior fossa extradural hematoma. If at the superior sagittal or longitudinal (dural or venous) sinus near the vertex of the skull a bridging cerebral vein may be torn resulting in a subdural hemorrhage.

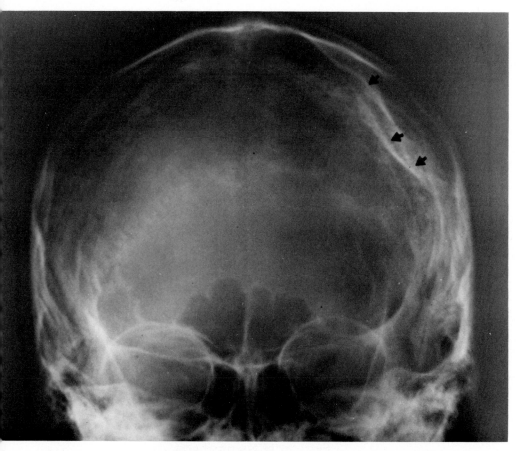

Fig. 7. Case 2. The arrows indicate the depressed fracture of the inner and outer tables of the skull in the left parietal region. Although the fragments were displaced intracranial for nearly an inch there was no penetration of the dura.

If such a depressed fracture of the skull is permitted to remain without elevation of or removal of the bone fragments, particularly over the motor area of the brain, the chances of post-traumatic convulsions are great. In those instances where the depressed fracture involves the posterior wall of the frontal sinus and there is dural penetration there may be a clear, colorless cerebrospinal fluid leakage through the nose signifying a tear in the dura and the arachnoid membrances thus providing a direct pathway for infection through this communication from the environment to the space around the brain. It is therefore a compound fracture which must be operated upon with elevation of the bone fragments and sealing off of this fistula thus preventing meningitis, cerebritis, brain abscess, and death.

Comment. This patient had no dural penetration and yet he had a convulsive episode perhaps due to slight brain contusion or subarachnoid bleeding. From numerous studies on head injury patients it is well documented that if the dura is penetrated the chance of the patient having late recurrent convulsive seizures is markedly increased (17).

It may be concluded from our present series that if the football player sustained a skull fracture without dural penetration or an associated lesion such as an extradural, subdural, or intracerebral hemorrhage, he had a relatively good chance of survival without residual neurologic symptoms or signs.

Further definition of numerous skull fractures as listed by the Committee on Nomenclature of Trauma of the Congress of Neurological Surgeons are listed for the sake of completeness: a) Fracture, basal, skull: fracture involving the base of the cranium; b) Fracture, comminuted, skull: fracture with fragmentation of bone; c) Fracture, diastatic, skull: 1) separation of cranial bones at a suture; 2) fracture with a marked separation of bone fragments; d) Fracture, expressed, skull: fracture with outward displacement of part of the cranium; e) Fracture, stellate, skull: multiple radiating linear fractures.

Using stresscoat patterns Gurdjian et al. (12) showed that a low velocity blow caused an inbending of an area of impact and an outbowing of adjacent bone. In their work the linear fracture started at the outwardly bowed area and extended both toward and away from the point of impact (13, 14). These lines may extend in a basilar direction proceeding into the internal auditory meatus or the cribriform plate and if associated with otorrhea or rhinorrhea, may result in acute or chronic recurrent bouts of meningitis (15, 16). Fortunately neither this type of fracture nor extensive compound depressed skull fractures have been a problem in the football players; the helmet appears to have afforded adequate protection.

Extradural Hemorrhage

An extradural hemorrhage is one which lies between the inner table of the skull and the dura, one of the three membranes between the skull and the brain. The most common source for such bleeding is the middle meningeal artery which in the adolescent or adult becomes incorporated in a groove in the inner table of the skull (Fig. 8, A and B). A fractured skull in this region may cause a transection of the artery resulting in a brisk arterial hemorrhage. Within an interval of only minutes to a few hours, death may occur unless surgical intervention is performed. Another less common source of bleeding may be the laceration of the dura with tearing of the arachnoidal (Pacchionian) granulations or bridging superior cerebral veins entering the longitudinal or lateral sinuses, or more commonly, a laceration of one of the sinuses itself. Since such hemorrhage is venous in origin and therefore under much less pressure than in the middle meningeal hemorrhages, there is usually a greater latent period between injury and the presentation of the

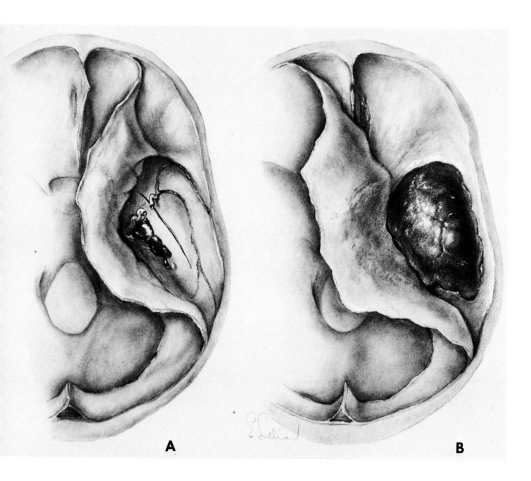

Fig. 8A. The dura has been reflected from the bone of the middle fossa showing the fracture line transecting the middle meningeal artery causing the onset of hemorrhage.

Fig. 8B. The extradural clot almost fills the middle fossa in this instance.

For further orientation of the figure, the nose and orbits lie toward the top of the page and the occipital region is located just above the legend. As the hemorrhage increases in size it dissects away more extradural vessels causing them to rupture and the hematoma often expands rapidly with compression of the brain stem and a fatal outcome. This site is usual for approximately 85% of all extradural hemorrhages.

patient for surgical treatment (26). Jackson and Speakman (20) recorded such a case operated upon 36 days after the initial symptoms.

Extradural hemorrhage is relatively uncommon for it comprises between only 1 and 3% of the head injury cases (30). The mortality rate for patients with this serious complication, according to Spurling in 1946 (36), varied between 30 to 50% in the largest centers in this country. This rate has been lowered significantly in the succeeding 25 years. Jamieson and Yelland (21) in 1968 reported reducing their mortality rate of 26.7% in their first 60 cases to 8% in their last 60 patients. The mortality figure still is particularly appalling when one considers that the successful removal of such a lesion so frequently results in recovery with no neurologic deficit.

Football Survey. In the five year interval of the football survey, there were five players who were diagnosed as having extradural hemorrhages (Fig. 9). Three of the players wore helmets, one had no helmet, and it was not known whether the fifth player had any equipment. Two of the players had sustained skull fractures. One of these patients had worn a helmet and the other had not. Eighty percent of these football players had been seen by neurosurgeons but apparently were beyond the point of recovery when first seen. One had been operated upon within 6½ hours after injury. The other two players succumbed in 2 and 3 days after injury, respectively.

Case 3. A 14 year old, high school boy was engaged in a tackle drill when one player struck him in the temporal area. He did not lose consciousness, but within 30 minutes had a convulsive seizure, remained unconscious, progressed into deep coma, and then became apneic. The patient was transported to the local hospital where he remained with a respirator controlling his breathing for an hour. A right temporal craniectomy was performed with evacuation of a 300 cc. extradural hematoma, but the patient had severe hypotension and an obviously irreversible neurologic state. He was taken to a medical center while still on the respirator where it was recorded that his pupils were dilated and fixed, and he was totally unresponsive. The patient was treated by supportive measures. From the time of injury to death was approximately 36 hours. No autopsy was obtained.

Comment. This patient had a rapidly progressive extradural hemorrhage which required immediate attention by the local physician who courageously made a burr hole to endeavor to save the patient's life. The fact that he had a 300 cc. hemorrhage in a short period of time suggested that bleeding was arterial and very brisk. Since there was no autopsy, one cannot be sure whether there were other associated lesions. Once there had been a respiratory failure with fixed, dilated pupils, the patient more than likely had reached the point of no return. The neurosurgeon had nothing further to offer from a surgical standpoint; the situation was hopeless.

EXTRADURAL HEMATOMAS: FIVE CASES WITH FOUR DEATHS

Equipment	Fract.	Seen by Neuro-surgeon	Operation Performed	Time Inter-val-Injury to Operation	Prognosis	Time Interval: Injury to Death	Post-mortem
F	No	Yes	No	-	Poor	-	No
F	Yes	Yes	Yes	6 1/2 hrs	-	36 hrs	Yes
?	No	Yes	No	-	-	2 days	?
0	Yes	No	No	-	-	8 hrs	Yes
F	No	Yes	No	-	-	5 days	Yes

Fig. 9. The data on the patients who had extradural hematomas in this survey are given. The mortality rate was 80% in spite of the fact there was an 8 hour to 5 day interval from the injury until death. (Reprinted from Schneider, R. C.: Serious and Fatal Neurosurgical Football Injuries. *Clin. Neurosurg., 12:* 226, 1966, by permission of The Congress of Neurological Surgeons.)

Extradural hemorrhage is the only type of traumatic intracranial football lesion for which a photograph was not available in this survey. However, because of its lethal quality, a drawing of such a lesion has been presented (Fig. 8, A and B).

Neurologic Data. The patient sustains a blow upon the head which may or may not cause unconsciousness. A cardinal symptom of extradural hemorrhage has been said to be the occurrence of a lucid interval, i.e., the presence of a period of clinical improvement between an initial unconscious episode and a relapse into a semi-comatose state. This period may be of a relatively few minutes or hours duration if the bleeding is arterial or of several days duration if there is venous hemorrhage (26). The above statement must be tempered somewhat since Rowbotham (30) cites the fact that in about one-quarter of the cases of extradural hemorrhage, there is no initial unconsciousness. Headache usually becomes progressively severe over the side of the lesion and is frequently associated with increased irritability and projectile vomiting. A dilated pupil may be found for as the hemorrhage spreads it presses upon the ipsilateral oculomotor nerve catching it between the posterior cerebral and anterior superior cerebellar arteries (23, 35). As further bleeding occurs there is pressure upon the lateral corticospinal (pyramidal) tract in the brain stem ipsilaterally with the appearance of one extensor plantar reflex (a Babinski sign), and with further displacement of the brain stem against the contralateral margin of the skull or rigid tentorium, the opposite lateral corticospinal (pyramidal) tract is compressed causing the second extensor plantar reflex (Fig. 10, A and B). *This is the classical temporal lobe or tentorial pressure cone syndrome,* which may be present initially without any shift in vital signs, i.e., blood pressure, pulse, or respirations, to suggest an increased intracranial pressure. A patient with such a lesion may be conscious and talking and yet 5

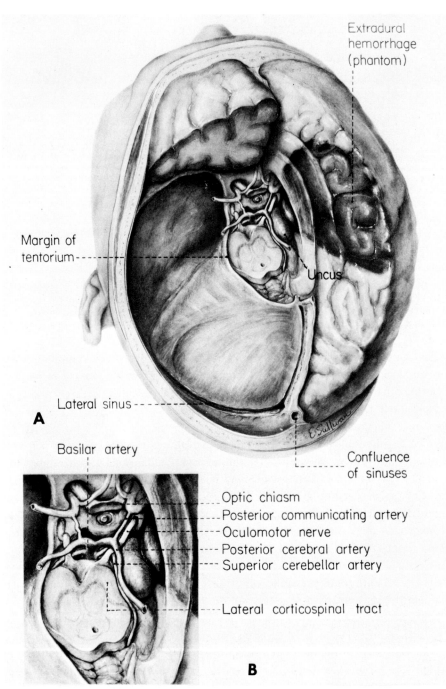

Extradural
hemorrhage
(phantom)

Margin of
tentorium

Uncus

Lateral sinus

A

Basilar artery

Confluence
of sinuses

Optic chiasm
Posterior communicating artery
Oculomotor nerve
Posterior cerebral artery
Superior cerebellar artery

Lateral corticospinal tract

B

Fig. 10. The mechanism responsible for the temporal lobe or tentorial pressure cone is shown. [Reprinted from Schneider and Tytus (34), by permission of J. B. Lippincott Company.]

Fig. 10A. The major portion of the left cerebral hemisphere has been removed showing the tentorium, the midbrain, adjacent structures, and the expanding right phantom extradural hemorrhage.

Fig. 10B. The right uncus compresses the third nerve, the latter being caught between the posterior cerebral and the superior cerebellar arteries. The right lateral corticospinal tract is pressed upon directly by the uncus; contralaterally, the left corticospinal tract is compressed against the free margin of the tentorium.

minutes later may be found dead (35). Emphasis often has been placed upon compression of the posterior cerebral and superior cerebellar arteries causing hypoxia (43), but too little note has been made of the possibility of sudden occlusion of the dural sinuses which occurs much more rapidly due to the relatively less musculature in the walls of these venous channels than in arterial ones. Aphasia and paresis or paralysis of the contralateral extremities usually do not occur for brain stem decompensation occurs too rapidly. There may be an intracranial hypertension and bradycardia suggesting increased intracranial pressure but with a tentorial pressure cone this appears very late. Skull x-rays often show a fracture line traversing the groove of the middle meningeal artery in the temporal or parietal area. *To spend valuable time in resorting to neuroradiologic studies in these patients with extradural hematomas, as a rule, is to court disaster.* The sense of urgency and simple trephination are the most important factors in cutting down the mortality rate (21, 35). In the rare case angiography may be justifiable if time permits the use of the procedure for localizing lesions in unusual places (18, 21, 26, 28). Carotid arteriography was used in only 26 of Jamieson's series of 167 cases. More recently Alexander (18) has stressed the importance of diagnosing vertex extradural hematomas by angiography. Such lesions compress the sagittal sinus at the vertex and occlude the venous lacunae causing some degree of cerebral hemisphere edema. In this acute lesion the urgency of the situation seldom permits time for a brain scan.

Extradural hematoma of the posterior fossa presumably is a rare entity but an increasing number of reports are appearing sporadically in the literature. No such lesion has been recorded in our football survey, but for the sake of completeness, a brief resume concerning this lesion is recorded here. Coleman and Thomson (19), in presenting the first case of closed extradural cerebellar hematoma reported in the literature, suggested the following diagnostic criteria for such a lesion.

> "There is a history of a blow to the back of the head severe enough to produce a fracture of the skull which may or may not cause unconsciousness. This is followed by headache of gradual increasing severity and is usually accompanied by nausea and vomiting. Drowsiness and restlessness appear and progress until the patient lapses into unconsciousness. However, during the drowsy state, several things may be noted. The patient prefers to lie on one side and will promptly return to the same side when placed upon his back. Nuchal rigidity develops, nystagmus may or may not be present, and the deep reflexes disappear. As unconsciousness deepens, generalized hypotonia develops, the pulse and respirations become irregular and death is imminent unless there is prompt surgical intervention with removal of the clot."

It has been this author's (25, 31, 34) experience that there is no definite clinical picture common to all cases of extradural hematoma of the posterior fossa. In addition to Coleman and Thomson's criteria (19), the author would add that the important significance of an abrasion or laceration of the scalp in the occipital region with concomitant suture line separation or fracture over the transverse sinus or through the foramen magnum should be re-emphasized. In the majority of cases the state of consciousness varies from lucidity to varying degrees of coma with minimal neurologic findings referable to the posterior fossa. In most instances there is little or no change in the vital signs to indicate a rapidly expanding intracranial lesion, and if such a transition is awaited, the patient may succumb before operation is performed (33).

Although the occurrence of contrecoup lesions has been known since the days of Hippocrates and Galen, they are often forgotten. Even if the posterior fossa exploration is positive for an extradural hematoma, there may be contrecoup either contusion, extradural, or subdural hematomas (29) or destruction of the frontotemporal junction causing symptoms referable to that location (33). *Whether the extradural hemorrhage is supratentorial or infratentorial the dura should always be opened to exclude an associated underlying surgical lesion.*

Schneider and Tytus (34) have summarized the reasons for the high mortality rate in extradural hemorrhage. They are:

1. The failure to alert *all* physicians to the problems involved.

2. Failure to suspect extradural hemorrhage in the presence of an apparently minor injury.

3. Failure to understand the significance of a temporal lobe or tentorial pressure cone and too great reliance on changes in vital signs and state of consciousness (22, 37).

4. Failure to realize that the gradual progressive development of a decerebrate rigidity pattern may result from an extradural hemorrhage (22).

5. Failure to consider that massive and fatal extradural hemorrhage may occur without significant change in vital signs because of continuous profuse cerebrospinal fluid otorrhea or rhinorrhea (34).

6. Failure to suspect an extradural hematoma of the posterior fossa (24, 25, 31).

7. Failure to detect an extension of a supratentorial extradural hematoma below the lateral sinus into the posterior fossa (27).

8. Failure to treat the extradural hemorrhage properly at the time of operation.

9. Failure to anticipate contrecoup associated injuries such as subdural, subarachnoid, and/or intracerebral hematomas (29).

10. Failure to realize that extradural hemorrhage may occur as a complication to otologic and rhinologic infections (32).

Subdural Hemorrhage

Subdural hemorrhage occurs in the subdural space, the potential area between the dura and the arachnoid, the second innermost of the three membranes between the skull and the brain. This space, similar to the extradural one, is traversed by bridging superior cerebral veins, extending from the cerebral cortex of the brain to the larger venous channels, the dural sinuses (62). The majority of these vessels are found at the vertex or top of the brain as they drain into the superior longitudinal or sagittal sinuses which lie enclosed within the dural layers (Fig. 11) (63). In addition, there are arachnoidal (Pacchionian) granulations that are tuft-like collections of highly folded arachnoid which project through the dura mater at the lateral margins of the superior sagittal sinus as well as the other dural sinuses. It is through these membranes that part of the cerebrospinal fluid (which is contained in the subarachnoid space) is returned into the blood stream. A greater number of bridging cerebral veins may be found in the frontal and

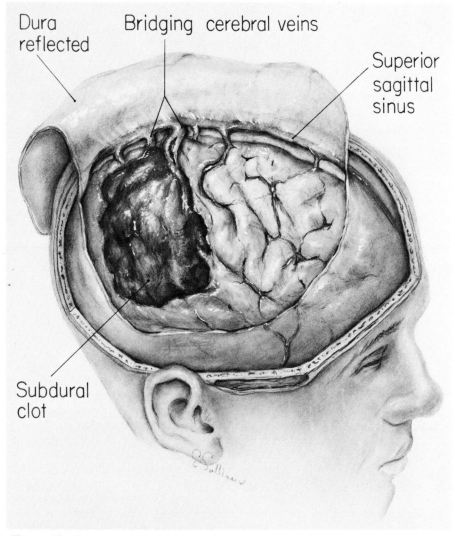

Fig. 11. The diagram shows the dura incised and reflected upward to expose the right cerebral hemisphere, the longitudinal sinus lying within the falx, and the bridging cortical veins entering the sinus. The latter, when torn, are the most frequent sources for subdural hemorrhages.

parietal areas with fewer ones located in the occipital, temporal, and fronto-temporal regions draining into the lateral and sphenoidal sinuses from their respective areas (39, 41, 55, 65). Disruption of any of these vessels may be responsible for the development of an acute subdural hemorrhage· or the more gradual subacute and chronic subdural hematomas.

Acute Subdural Hemorrhage

An acute localized primary subdural hemorrhage had been regarded as a relatively rare lesion (68). Various authors have defined this acute lesion as a subdural hemorrhage which occurs within a 24 hour period after injury (47, 54); others have suggested that a hemorrhage which occurs within a 3 day period should be regarded as an acute one (44, 48, 61). McLaurin and Tutor believed that a lesion should be designated as an acute one if the time interval was within 24 hours of injury (56).

Football Survey. Unfortunately, in this series of 69 cases of subdural hematoma, the time interval between injury and operation or death could not be ascertained in one-quarter of them (Fig. 12A). By far the most alarming figure in this study was the number of very acute subdural hematomas, 24, which had occurred, where the interval between injury and operation or injury and death was only 6 hours. Six of these patients died without operation. Eighteen players were operated upon with five survivals, two of whom had hopeless brain damage, but fortunately the three others had excellent results. Thirteen players with acute subdural hematomas died following operation with an operative mortality rate of 71%. *However, it should be emphasized that many of these players sustained their injury and shortly thereafter, within 30 to 60 minutes, became deeply comatose and arrived at a hospital in an agonal state with the pupils dilated and fixed.* Operation was resorted to very frequently as a desperation measure where there was nothing to lose and the emotional pressures associated with the situation dictated to the surgeon this apparently fruitless procedure was the necessary course of action.

An example of acute subdural hemorrhage is presented.

> **Case 4.** A 17 year old, high school football player, wearing full equipment, including a rigid plastic helmet, had blocked a hard driving opponent. The boy staggered because of marked dizziness, approached the sidelines where he complained of headache, and within minutes lost consciousness. The team physician described a posture of decerebrate rigidity with bilateral muscular twitching of his body and extremities. Upon the player's arrival at a local hospital, he was deeply comatose with dilated pupils, which responded minimally to light. Peculiarly enough, his condition was essentially the same as it had been when he was admitted to the hospital a year previously. On that occasion he was taken to the x-ray department where he began to respond and soon made a rapid and uneventful recovery. Because of his previous injury an electroencephalogram (EEG) had been made just a week before this, his second injury, and was found to be normal and, after neurologic and physical examination, he was given permission to play football.

SUBDURAL HEMATOMAS: 69 CASES WITH 28 DEATHS

A

Time Interval*	Operated, Recovered					Operated, Died	Unoperated, Died
	Excellent	Fair	Poor	Guarded	Hopeless		
6 hours (18)**	3				2	13	6
7 to 24 hours (2)	1					1	1
25 to 48 hours (3)	2					1	1
49 hours to 1 week (2)	1			1			
Over 1 week (9)	5	2		1		1	3
Over 1 month (6)	6						1
Time unknown (17)	5	2	6	2	2		
Total	23	4	6	4	4	16	12

* Time between injury and operation, or injury and death.
** Numbers in parentheses represent total number of cases operated upon.

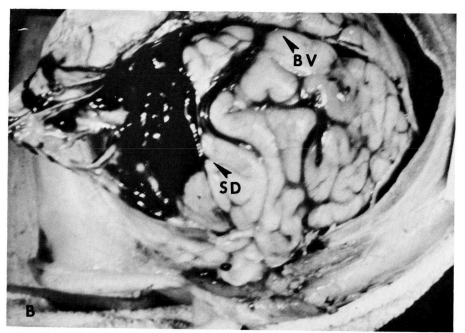

Fig. 12A. The incidence of subdural hematomas, the most devastating and yet occasionally operable lesions. (Reprinted from Schneider, R. C.: Serious and Fatal Neurosurgical Football Injuries. *Clin. Neurosurg.*, *12:* 226, 1966, by permission of The Congress of Neurological Surgeons.)

Fig. 12B. Case 4. The autopsy specimen demonstrates the residual acute subdural hematomas (SD) overlying the right parietal region with engorgement of the large bridging cerebral veins (BV), the probable source of the lesion. (compare this figure with Fig. 11.)

Immediately after this, his second injury, the patient's systolic blood pressure was 170 mm. initially and his pulse was rapid but the pressure finally stabilized at 130/70. While x-rays were being taken his respirations ceased and mouth to mouth respirations were administered. A tracheostomy was performed and he was placed on a respirator. Burr holes were made in the right frontal, right parietal, and left posterior frontal regions. A massive acute right subdural hematoma was evacuated and a large anteriorly bleeding bridging vein, the source of the hemorrhage, was coagulated. The patient never regained consciousness and succumbed 9 hours after injury.

The autopsy revealed massive cerebral edema with some residual subdural hematoma over the right frontoparietal and temporal regions with extension along the midline of the falx (Fig. 12B). Examination of the brain after fixation showed some necrotic right temporal cortex with acute petechial hemorrhages in the right temporal and parietal lobes and in the tegmentum and the base of the pons. There were bilateral tentorial and cerebellar pressure cones.

Comment. One of the interesting and tragic points about this case is that the player had had a good physical and neurologic examination only a week before this catastrophe and was believed to be in good condition. Even the additional precaution of an EEG had been made and his status was found to be normal. (This problem will be discussed later.) This boy was moribund at the time of admission to the hospital after his second injury. The surgeon raised the question whether direct admission to the operating room would have saved his life. This is problematical but the patient already seemed to have progressed beyond the point of recovery.

Such is the characteristic pattern of any number of these acute subdural hematomas in football players. The mortality rate for this lesion in this group is comparable to that listed in the literature: 83%, Laudig et al. (54), 90%, Ecklin et al. (44), 80% Gurdjian and Webster (47), and 73% McLaurin and Tutor (56).

As a contrast, a second case of acute subdural hematoma, which was successfully treated, is presented (Case 46) which was *not* included in our statistical survey since this injury occurred after the compilation of this data.

Subacute Subdural Hematomas

These subacute lesions are part of the same process, but their designation depends merely on the length of time between the injury and the occurrence of symptoms, a thing which artificially separates the lesions into different categories. The author has categorized any case in which the symptoms occurred after 48 hours or 3 days and less than 1 month after injury as a subacute subdural hematoma. If this pattern is followed, a review of Figure 12A shows that there were 14 players who fell into this classification. Of this group 43% who were operated upon had excellent results, four others had fair or guarded recovery, and death was the result for two players. Four of these 14 players died without the benefit of operation.

Chronic Subdural Hematomas

If one arbitrarily defines a chronic subdural hematoma (63) as occurring a month or more after injury, there were seven players in this group. Because of the gradual readjustment of the brain to changes in slowly increasing intracranial pressure, postoperative results are much better in these cases than in either the acute or subacute phases of such lesions. Six of these football players with this injury were operated upon with excellent results. Unfortunately there was one additional patient with a chronic subdural hematoma who succumbed without the benefit of a surgical procedure.

A case illustrating such a chronic lesion is presented.

> **Case 5.** A 17 year old, right-handed, high school player sustained a head injury August 17, 1963. He was not rendered unconscious and could play for a few more minutes. By the following day he complained of pain over the right eye and in the back of his neck which was accentuated by walking, running, flexing the neck, and rotation of his head. The pain subsided during September 1963, but on October 24 he had episodic spells of vomiting for 24 hours. He had no convulsive seizures or fainting spells. A lumbar puncture revealed the pressure was 440 mm. of water. His blood pressure was 130/70 and the pulse was 48 per minute. He had blurred optic discs. The patient was alert and oriented, and the remainder of his neurologic examination was normal. His EEG showed a suppression of right-sided voltage and the brain wave pattern, a diffuse right-sided abnormality. The right internal carotid arteriogram exhibited a displacement of the right anterior cerebral artery across the midline and an area devoid of blood vessels between the cortex of the brain and the skull in the right parietal area (Fig. 13A). On November 1, 1963, burr holes were made in the right coronal, posterior parietal, and temporal areas, with through and through drainage of the chronic subdural hematoma. The thickened inner and outer membranes were removed as completely as possible through these holes and drains were left in situ. After 36 hours these drains were removed and the patient appeared markedly improved (Fig. 13B). A pneumoencephalogram made on November 11, 1963, still showed some shift of the ventricular system, but the patient's clinical condition was satisfactory and he was discharged on November 14, 1963. The patient made a complete recovery and returned to high school. Nine years later he was still well.

Comment. This patient represents the typical pattern of a head injury with transient symptoms, followed by a symptom-free interval with the subsequent recurrence of symptoms 3 months later. In spite of the large subdural hematoma it is interesting to observe that there were only subtle changes in the EEG. The right internal carotid arteriogram demonstrated the characteristic displacement of the vessels downward from the skull in the right parietal area. Multiple trephines were made to drain this subdural hematoma and this was accomplished successfully. Fifty percent of these cases may be treated in this way. The others may require that a bone flap be reflected for the removal of the membranes.

In summary there were 41 patients with subdural hematomas who were saved

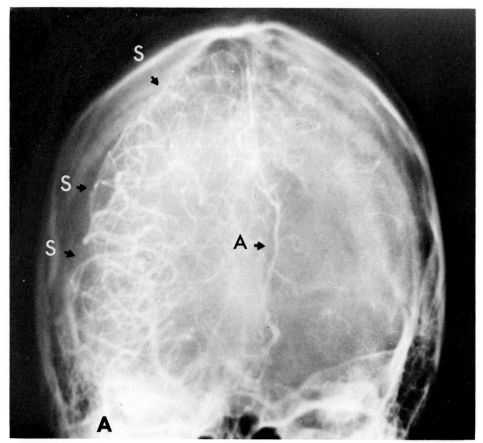

Fig. 13A. Case 5. The arteriogram made by injecting the right internal carotid artery exhibits inward displacement of the surface vessels (arrows-S) from the skull and the anterior cerebral artery across the midline (arrow-A) by the subdural hemorrhage. The pattern is that of a typical chronic subdural hematoma.

by operative procedures, and 27 of these patients, two-thirds of them, either had "excellent" or "fair" results. As one might anticipate, the results shown on the chart indicate that the greater number of good results occurred the longer the interval was between injury and operation.

In this series of cases there were 69 patients with subdural hematoma with only one skull fracture in the group suggesting that the direct transmission of force from the blow to the head may be responsible for a shearing effect on the cerebral bridging veins at the superior or lateral sinuses resulting in subdural hemorrhage.

Neurosurgical Data. In 1857 Virchow (66) made a diagnosis of pachymeningitis hemorrhagica interna in some patients who really had subdural hemorrhages. Trotter (64) in 1914 has been credited with describing the subdural collection of blood which has come to be regarded as a chronic subdural hematoma. A paper by Putnam and Cushing (60) further clarified the problem and related one of the early experiences with an acute subdural hemorrhage. There have been many subsequent publications on this topic which provide good general discussions (46, 49, 51, 53, 57, 58). One of the most interesting was by Gardner (45) who presented the theory that a membrane is formed around the blood clot from the inner layer of the meninges. As the blood disintegrates within this semi-permeable structure, there is an increased osmotic pressure with a further uptake of fluid in the sac with enlargement of the clot. Ecklin (44), Monro (57), Voris (67), and others emphasized that the pathogenesis of subdural hemorrhage or hematoma was

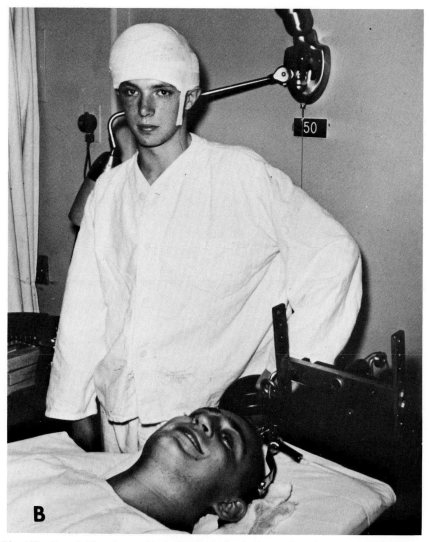

Fig. 13B. Case 5. The player with the head dressing is shown after the removal of a chronic subdural hematoma. He made a complete recovery.

Case 30. The second player with the Vinke skeletal tong traction had the next hospital registration number. He sustained a fracture-dislocation of the cervical spine was operated upon immediately after his companion shown in the picture. He, too, made a good recovery.

merely a lesion which was following its transition from an acute to subacute and finally chronic phase.

Rowbotham (62) stressed the fact that there is no clinical syndrome which can be attributed to acute subdural hemorrhage. Associated diffuse neuronal or intrinsic cerebral damage was believed to be responsible in many cases for the symptoms of this acute lesion and the subdural hematoma was merely coincidental. This is true in high speed vehicular accidents. McLaurin and Tutor (56) also have suggested that venous bleeding alone probably does not cause early symptoms unless accompanied by severe cerebral contusion or laceration. As a result of the high mortality figures in the surgical treatment of acute subdural hemorrhage quoted previously, a certain sense of futility had been engendered with the concept that operative procedure is of no practical value and perhaps may not even be worth the effort (39, 40, 52, 67). However, Chambers (41) has emphasized the fact that not all of these patients have had intrinsic cerebral damage and that immediate surgical intervention may result in recovery. He indicated that the deepening of the state of consciousness alone demanded surgical intervention and that to await changes in blood pressure, pulse rate, respirations, or other altered neurologic sequelae was to court disaster. In 1949 Whalley (68) had supported this thesis by publishing a paper describing the evacuation of an acute subdural hematoma with good recovery. Case 4 reported above supports the belief that although the surgical mortality rate is high in acute post-traumatic subdural hemorrhage, the salvage of a number of such individuals may be accomplished. However, in contrast to vehicular accidents, the forces involved in football head contact are usually of a much lesser degree with mere shearing of bridging cerebral veins and often there is slight or no brain damage. Since the lesion is rather frequent in football players, the keynote to survival lies in the aggressive surgical approach suggested by Chambers (41) and subsequently shown by Jamieson and Yelland (21).

Subacute and chronic subdural hematomas may show a much more benign course often manifested by headache, nausea, vomiting, blurred vision, and diplopia. There may be the gradual onset of convulsions, anisocoria, hemiparesis, aphasia, or other symptoms of increased intracranial pressure. A rising blood pressure and a diminution in pulse rate may occur. A slowly developing tentorial pressure cone with a dilated ipsilateral pupil and bilateral extensor plantar reflexes is not uncommon as has been described for the extradural hemorrhages. By definition, these symptoms may occur from 3 days to a few weeks after injury. There may be a lucid interval, i.e., a period of clarity between an unconscious state and the development of a secondary comatose one. Because of the slow rate of appearance of symptoms and signs, it is usually possible to procure preliminary studies which may aid in the planning of the operative approach. Skull x-rays may show a calcified pineal gland displaced away from the side of the lesion or possibly a fracture of the skull. The EEG occasionally may show the presence of slow waves over a localized area or perhaps over an entire hemisphere.

The brain scan may be of value in demonstrating an area of increased radioactive uptake over the region of the blood clot. In 1952 Peyton et al. (59) first showed the value of a brain scan in a chronic subdural hematoma. Subsequently numerous other series of scans have been reported with results showing 75 to 91% accuracy (38, 42, 50). Cowan et al. (42) recorded the highest degree of accuracy in scans of lesions which were 10 days or more after an injury. The diagnostic value of the arteriogram is quite evident as is seen by the displacement of the blood vessels from their normal vascular pattern in the demonstration of Case 5 in this series of football players. If there is any lingering doubt after performing these diagnostic procedures, or if the latter diagnostic methods are not available, a pneumoencephalogram, performed by removing cerebrospinal fluid and replacing it by air or oxygen, may fill the ventricular system showing displacement or abnormal filling of the ventricles of the brain. The latter procedure is used much less frequently than in by-gone days for it is often unnecessary or uncomfortable and there is some slight degree of risk because of air embolism or alteration of pressures within the intracranial cavity due to a shift of its contents.

The modes of surgical therapy will be discussed in Chapter 11.

Subdural Hydroma

Peet (58) described this lesion as a subdural collection of clear, colorless, or xanthochromic fluid not associated with a hematoma. It is believed to be due to a traumatic tear of the arachnoid with a small ball-valve flap which permits fluid to enter the subdural space but not to drain from it. The symptoms and signs are similar to those seen in subdural hematoma but are usually less severe. The surgical therapy is identical except that it is usually confined to burr hole drainage alone and the response to treatment carries a much more favorable prognosis.

Intracerebral and Intraventricular Hemorrhage

Intracerebral Hemorrhage

The hemorrhages previously mentioned lie upon or beneath the membranes enveloping the brain and are not within the brain substance. Intracerebral bleeding refers to hemorrhage within the brain itself, and consequently may present with a much more serious prognosis with either permanent neurologic disability or loss of life (Fig. 14). Such intracerebral hemorrhages occurring in the pons or brain stem purposely have been placed in a separate category for there may be multiple factors involved in their etiology.

Petechial Hemorrhages

When intracerebral hemorrhages are mentioned, massive intracerebral bleeding is the type of lesion which comes to mind. Actually petechial hemorrhages measuring from 1 to 5 mm. frequently occur in various areas throughout the brain. These may be manifested by transient lapses of memory, personality changes, or

INTRACEREBRAL HEMORRHAGE: 11 CASES WITH 6 DEATHS. INTRAVENTRICULAR
HEMORRHAGE: 3 CASES WITH 2 DEATHS

Lesion	Unoperated		Operated	
	Survival	Post-mortem	Survival	Post-mortem
Intracerebral clot (5)*	1 hopeless	1	1 hopeless, 1 guarded	1
Intracerebral clot plus subdural (4)			2 hopeless	2
Intracerebral clot plus subdural plus pontine hemorrhage (2)				2
Intraventricular clot (3)		2	1 poor	
Total	1 hopeless	3	1 guarded 1 poor 3 hopeless	5

*Numbers in parentheses represent total number of patients in each group.

Fig. 14. The data on intracerebral and intraventricular hemorrhages found in the football survey are given. (Reprinted from Schneider, R. C.: Serious and Fatal Neurosurgical Football Injuries. *Clin. Neurosurg.*, *12:* 226, 1966, by permission of The Congress of Neurological Surgeons.)

impairment in judgment, if they are present in the frontal region. If healing occurs with scarcely any scar formation, there may be little or no demonstrable neurologic deficit. In other instances recovery may not be quite so fortuitous. An example is reported as Case 28; the football player had severe brain damage probably with multiple petechial hemorrhages no doubt not only in the frontal lobes but also in the deeper underlying structures of the brain. He continued to have a glassy stare, impaired recollection of events, slight tremor, unstable gait, and visual problems even 2½ years following his injury (5). After this length of time such residual neurologic symptoms are probably permanent for the most part (89). This is the pattern of symptoms that has given rise to the term of "punch drunk," a pattern frequently seen in old boxers who have sustained many severe blows to the head (85). Petechial hemorrhages usually are not demonstrated by brain wave tests (EEG) (except as a generalized cerebral dysrhythmia) or other laboratory tests and they are only seen at the autopsy table (Fig. 15). These small lesions are formed by pressure gradients in various portions of the brain. They may occur in the brain stem at the time of impact (84).

Massive Intracerebral Hemorrhage

This type of bleeding is often seen in closed head injuries. It may be associated with a blow to one side of the head which causes brain injury on the opposite side as the brain strikes the firm unyielding skull. Occasionally there will be an injury to the occipital region with damage occurring to the opposite frontotemporal area as the brain impinges against the sharp sphenoid ridge, causing laceration of the brain and tearing of the Sylvian veins followed by the formation of an intracerebral clot (71). Injuries in which the head is struck on one side and there is associated brain damage on the opposite side are known as "contrecoup" injuries (87). The patient may have a seemingly minor injury, may lose consciousness only transiently, or may remain in a comatose state. He may develop a dilated pupil, a paralysis of the extremities on the opposite side of the body, a rising blood pressure, and diminished pulse rate and, if not treated surgically, will succumb in a relatively short interval. Occasionally the tapping of a subacute frontotemporal liquid hematoma may result in a major degree of recovery. On the contrary, the patient may remain alive for years in a vegetative state owing his life to the triumphs of our modern medicine.

Intraventricular Hemorrhages

In these cases the patient may suffer a shearing blow tearing the brain and the choroid plexuses (small "bean-shaped" structures which partially contribute to the formation of the cerebrospinal fluid). The associated blood supply (the artery of the choroid plexus) is disrupted and/or laceration of the brain occurs causing acute hemorrhage within the ventricles (the chambers of the brain) so that death usually occurs very shortly after injury (Fig. 15, Case 6).

Football Survey. There was a total of 14 of these lesions with eight deaths (Fig. 14). [This group, of course, excludes any of the intrapontine (brain stem) lesions.] Obviously, these are among the most severe injuries, for there has been damage in the depths of the brain. Four players in this category remained unoperated upon; one survived as a hopeless case and the other three died. Only one of the 14 players had an associated skull fracture. Five of the patients with these injuries were operated upon and survived, but none did well. One player had a guarded prognosis, one was in a poor condition postoperatively, and three others were hopeless. Five players who were operated upon died.

An example of a player sustaining such a tragic injury is presented.

> **Case 6.** A 16 year old, right-handed, high school football player, wearing full equipment, sustained a blow to his nose by an opponent's elbow which entered directly between the face guard and the top of the helmet. He was not unconscious immediately, but lapsed into coma 20 or 30 minutes later. When taken to the hospital and seen by the neurosurgeon three hours after injury, he had fixed, dilated pupils and was moribund. He died shortly thereafter. At postmortem examination there was no skull fracture, but he had bilateral acute subdural hematomas, multiple petechial hemorrhages and a large intraventricular blood clot with adjacent subependymal necrosis (Fig. 15).

Comment. In this instance there was no skull fracture and yet the intracranial structures had sustained severe damage. The boy had been wearing full equip-

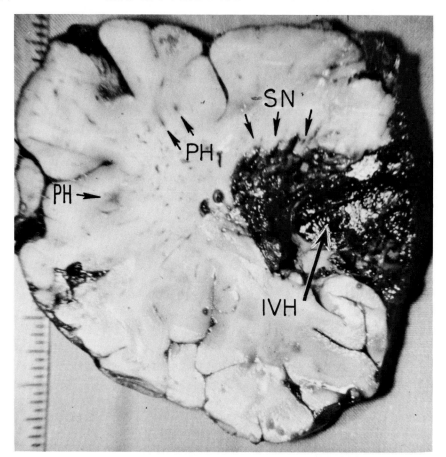

Fig. 15. Case 6. The postmortem specimen shows only a cross section of the right cerebral hemisphere demonstrating multiple petechial hemorrhages in the cerebral substance (PH), intraventricular hemorrhage (IVH), and subependymal necrosis (SN).

ment. Unfortunately, in some instances, such as this one, a blow from the elbow, which ordinarily may glance off of the helmet, was guided by the face guard into the gap between the face guard and helmet. A midline vertical bar on the face guard might have prevented the penetration of such a blow. The interval from initial trauma to coma and a critical condition probably was less than half an hour. Operation would not have saved the patient. In such cases the sharp border of the falx may cut directly into the corpus callosum causing laceration of this structure, subependymal hemorrhage, and necrosis with intraventricular hemorrhage. Another possible mechanism for such an injury is that the falx may have a lacerating effect by a combination of sudden stretching and downward shifting of force which produces corpus callosum lesions (81).

Pontine Lesions

Intrapontine hemorrhage or edema is extremely difficult to assess, diagnose accurately, or treat. These lesions must be divided into the primary ones which occur immediately upon impact at the time of injury and the secondary ones which appear later due to the compression of the arteries and veins near the base of the brain (83).

From the clinical standpoint, if the patient is admitted to the hospital with immediate decerebrate rigidity, i.e., the arms and legs in rigid extension and the hands turned ulnarward in a "flipper" position, one assumes the presence of midbrain concussion, contusion, or primary hemorrhage. If this pattern were to develop a few hours after injury, it is often believed that there has been a progression of neurologic signs and the possibility exists of an expanding supratentorial intracranial lesion such as an extradural, subdural, or intracerebral hemorrhage. The primary brain stem hemorrhage should be treated conservatively by supportive measures, such as steroids, whereas the latter type of lesion requires further procedures to confirm the diagnosis of a supratentorial lesion and provide the opportunity to proceed with surgical therapy.

Football Survey. An example of primary contusion and hemorrhage into the brain stem is described.

> **Case 7.** A 16 year old high school senior wearing full equipment made a tackle in a football game with his head meeting the thigh of the oncoming ball carrier. He never regained consciousness. Immediately after the injury he was taken to a local hospital where he was found to have bilaterally fixed, dilated pupils, and he was immediately transferred to a medical center. His blood pressure was 290/170, pulse was 120 per minute, and his temperature was 101.4 degrees. He was non-responsive. On admission to the hospital his pupils were dilated and fixed, he had no corneal reflexes, and his respirations were shallow and irregular. The remainder of his neurologic examination was normal. Within five minutes his respirations ceased and he was intubated and maintained on supported respirations. A lumbar puncture revealed a grossly bloody cerebrospinal fluid with a pressure of 460 mm. of water. Twenty cc of normal saline solution were injected rapidly into the subarachnoid space, but there was no change in the vital signs. After a discussion of the extremely poor prognosis with his parents 3½ hours after injury, the patient was taken to the operating room where bilateral parietal burr holes were made. These revealed a diffuse, very thin, insignificant subdural hematoma. Both hemispheres were explored by needling them, but there was no large supratentorial hemorrhage or intracerebral clot. The patient died 8 hours after injury.
>
> The postmortem examination demonstrated a right hemispheric cerebral edema (swelling) and traumatic hemorrhages in the brain stem with subpial and subependymal hemorrhages in the region of the third and fourth ventricles (Fig. 16A).

Comment. The subdural hematomas in this case were minimal, diffuse, and negligible as the source of this patient's neurologic deficit. It would appear that there had been a direct transmission of force to the brain stem causing primary brain stem hemorrhage which traversed the entire extent of the stem.

Another case report is presented and from the pathologic specimen it would

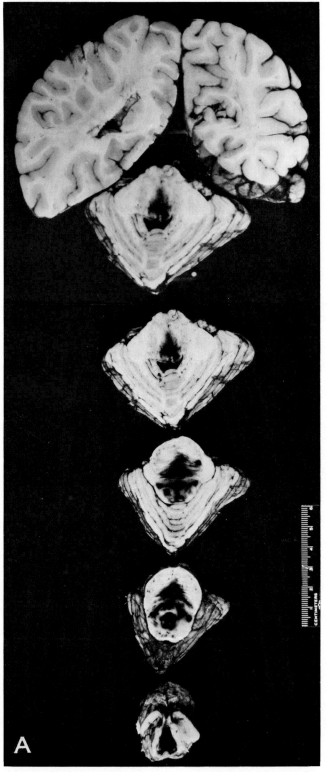

Fig. 16A. Case 7. The postmortem specimen shows the right cerebral hemisphere edema and the hemorrhage in the brain stem, suggesting a primary brain stem lesion occurring immediately at the time of injury. (However, there is distortion of the hemispheres due to the brain being sectioned on a bias.)

appear the injured football player had not only had a primary hemorrhage in the pons immediately at the time of impact but also sustained a progressively expanding supratentorial intracranial lesion with a secondary intrapontine one.

Case 8. This college football player was noted to be confused and walked the wrong way from the line in an intercollegiate game. He was wearing full equipment, and the mechanism of injury was unknown, for he continued to play for a few plays before he collapsed and became unconscious and died within 24 hours. Although he had had a previous head injury, it apparently had not been a severe one. At postmortem examination both the primary hemorrhage in the brain stem and secondary pressure effects with a red cerebral infarct were observed (Fig. 16B).

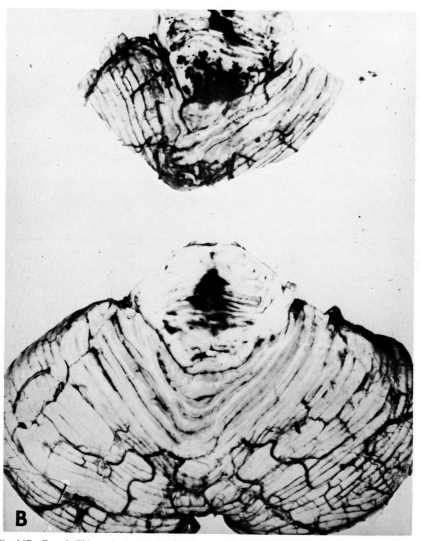

Fig. 16B. Case 8. This patient shows both primary and secondary hemorrhages in the brain stem.

Comment. The mechanism of injury was sought in movies of the game, but unfortunately they merely showed the player was confused and walking in the wrong direction. There had been some previous history of cerebral trauma, which was never defined clearly, and attempts actually had been made to conceal it deliberately prior to his participation in this sport. Apparently it had no relationship to his more recent injury.

This problem is so important that a third case is presented in which the football player sustained a head injury resulting in a primary supratentorial lesion which was evacuated, but the player developed a secondary brain stem lesion due to impairment of the blood supply resulting in infarction and brain stem destruction.

> **Case 9.** At 4 P.M. on September 5, 1962, a 17 year old high school player wearing full equipment tackled another player and their heads collided. This occurred at football practice. The player stood up, walked 30 feet, and finally collapsed. He remained unconscious and was transported to the local hospital where he had widely dilated, fixed pupils, and Cheyne-Stokes respirations. Burr holes were made at 9:00 P.M. that evening, and an acute subdural hematoma was evacuated from the left anterior and posterior parietal areas. Nevertheless, the patient's respirations became labored and ceased so that intermittent positive pressure breathing was instituted. He died at 3:30 P.M. on September 8, 1962.
>
> At postmortem examination there were wide areas of degenerative changes and cerebral edema. Hemorrhages were noted in the midbrain (Fig. 16C) and between the two layers of the right tentorium.

Comment. It would appear the hemorrhage in the midbrain was secondary to increased intracranial pressure from the acute subdural hematoma occurring initially with massive brain swelling and infarction. The lesion is in the characteristic place near the base. In the previous pages the high mortality rate in acute subdural hematomas has been noted. Perhaps more prompt removal of the acute subdural lesion might have saved this football player's life.

Finally one further interesting case report of midbrain injury in a football player has come to the attention of the author. *It is of great importance for it demonstrates that early aggressive medical therapy may save an occasional patient with a midbrain injury.*

> **Case 10.*** A 17 year old high school football player had been complaining of a headache for a week. In a football game on October 11, 1958, he dove headlong at a player who was running away from him. He immediately complained of a severe headache, and about five minutes later collapsed in a huddle. He was supported and walked to the sidelines with his companions holding his head. When he reached the bench he again collapsed and the team physician noted anisocoria, Cheyne-Stokes respirations, and the patient developed an ashen color. The neurosurgeon saw him ½ hour later, noted the patient's pupillary inequality with the left pupil definitely larger than the right and the left eye turned downward and outward. The patient now ex-

---

* This case does not fall within the five year interval of our survey.

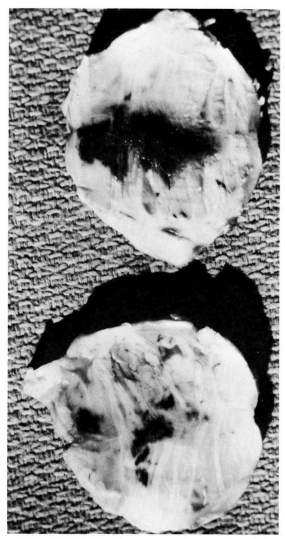

Fig. 16C. Case 9. The specimen demonstrates possible secondary midbrain hemorrhage, although the suddenness of onset of symptoms and early fixed dilated pupils might indicate early primary trauma to this region.

hibited decerebrate rigidity, the pupils did not react to light, and he had bilateral extensor plantar reflexes. Nevertheless, he had excellent venous pulsations in the left retina. A diagnosis of severe brain stem injury was made by the neurosurgeon, and the boy was considered to be critical. Massive doses of hydrocortisone were started, and 2 to 3 hours later he was able to answer questions coherently. Two or three weeks later his mental state cleared remarkably, but the left eye still tended to turn downward and outward and he "saw double." His skull and cervical spine x-rays were normal. A month after his discharge from the hospital he was found to have no neurologic abnormality.

Comment. Subsequently the patient became interested in neurosurgery, but his grades were unsatisfactory and he developed a serious neuropsychiatric difficulty necessitating neuropsychiatric treatment for 4 years after which he was lost to follow-up reports. This lad had a remarkable case of midbrain concussion or edema, with what seemed to be a transient temporal lobe pressure cone, a pattern of decerebrate rigidity, and anisocoria which cleared on massive steroid therapy. Unfortunately, this is too rare a sequela and such recovery from an apparent moribund state is remarkable. The rapid administration of steroid therapy probably saved this boy's life by preventing a secondary devastating midbrain lesion due to vascular ischemia following supratentorial cerebral edema.

In summary these 17 pontine injuries were the most lethal group of lesions occurring without any fracture of the skull. A number of them suggested there was a direct transmission of force directly through the non-resilient helmet to the brain stem and pons or shearing of the bridging cerebral veins causing subdural hematomas or intracerebral clots and secondary lesions due to vascular compression.

A study of the chart (Fig. 17) shows the number of pontine hemorrhages which were associated with an epidural (extradural) hemorrhage: 1, subdural hematoma: 12, or subdural hemorrhage and an associated intracerebral clot: 2. Only two patients seemed to have isolated pontine lesions.

There was a 100% mortality rate among seven patients who were not operated upon, but it should be emphasized that *primary* pontine hemorrhages are not surgical lesions. Of the remaining nine players who were treated surgically, one survived in poor condition. He had had a decerebrate pattern with an associated subdural hematoma which had been removed.

Neurosurgical Considerations. It is of extreme importance to observe that in none of these 17 patients with pontine hemorrhage was there any evidence of skull fracture and that only one of the players who sustained intracerebral and intraventricular hemorrhages had an associated skull fracture. There is an old axiom which has been known to neurosurgeons for many years and bears repetition: "The most severe brain injuries are found in patients who have closed head injuries without skull fracture." The earliest reference to this statement is attributed to Morgagni (86) who described it as follows: "cerebrum, agitatum versus caput durum et retropulsum per illud, subit uno momento duos notos contrarios; su

PONTINE LESIONS: 17 CASES WITH 16 DEATHS

Lesion	Unoperated			Operated		
	Survival	No Post-mortem	Post-mortem	Survival	No Post-mortem	Post-mortem
Pontine hemorrhage (2)*..........	0		1			1
Pontine hemorrhage plus epidural (1).........................	0		1			
Pontine hemorrhage plus subdural (12).........................	0	1	4	1 Poor	1	5
Pontine hemorrhage plus subdural plus intracerebral clot (2).......	0					2
Total......................	0	1	6	1 Poor	1	8

*Numbers in parentheses represent total number of patients in each group.

Fig. 17. The incidence of pontine lesions as noted in the football survey is given. (Reprinted from Schneider, R. C.: Serious and Fatal Neurosurgical Football Injuries. *Clin. Neurosurg.*, *12:* 226, 1966, by permission of The Congress of Neurological Surgeons.)

cranium non frangitur, totus impetus percussionis dirgitur in cerebrum." ("The brain driven against the skull and repelled by it, is thus subjected, within a moment, to two motions in opposite directions; if the skull is not fractured, the whole force of the percussion is directed against the brain itself.")

In his experimental traumatic work on the dog's brain, Duret (74) observed petechial hemorrhages within the brain stem particularly in the subependymal region of the fourth ventricle. These were thought to be due to a shock-like wave of cerebrospinal fluid as it was ejected with force from the aqueduct of Sylvius, destroying blood vessels and causing subependymal hemorrhages and necrosis. Cassasa (72) reported five patients who had a lucid interval from 3 to 24 hours who subsequently died of traumatic intracerebral hemorrhage. These lesions consisted of multiple punctate petechial hemorrhages scattered throughout the brain parenchyma (there had been no associated lacerations, scalp lesions, or fractures of the skull). It was Cassasa's theory that these lesions were caused by a sudden overfilling of the perivascular lymph spaces with cerebrospinal fluid, causing a laceration of the vessel by tearing of its wall in the vicinity of such a fibrillar attachment. In more chronic cases Martland and Beling (85) emphasized the presence of multiple minute punctate hemorrhages which were distributed primarily in the regions supplied by the terminal branches of "central ganglionic system of blood vessels."

In 1891 Bollinger (70) described five patients, each of whom had a relatively minor head injury and 3 days to 3 or 4 weeks later developed small areas of softening of the brain. These were regarded as due to an injury of the arterial walls with an eventual necrosis and rupture of the vessel resulting in an intracerebral hemorrhage. Bollinger has designated this as "traumatic spätapoplexie" and the terminology remains in the literature. In 1940 Symonds (88) presented such a case who had suffered a head injury and 10 weeks supervened between the injury and the onset of symptoms of his intracerebral hemorrhage.

Dill and Isenhour (73) produced intrapontine hemorrhages experimentally by inflating balloons intracranially over the parietal area of the dog's brain causing the midbrain, pons, and medulla to be compressed downward and into the foramen magnum. Such herniation caused lateral compression of the pontine structures and an elongation of the pons in its longitudinal axis. This change in configuration of the pons effected a stress on the smaller vessels in the pons and particularly at some of the long central branches of the basilar artery with tension placed at points of fixation of these vessels. These authors believed anoxia of the tissue played no part in the lesions which developed.

Attwater (69) in 1911 reviewed 67 cases of pontine hemorrhages and concluded there were two main causes of hemorrhage into the pons: 1) any large intracranial hemorrhage which might cause a rise in intracranial tension and a secondary pontine lesion or 2) a severe blow to the head sufficiently violent to fracture the base of the skull and cause the pontine hemorrhage "due to sudden change in the tension set up in the neighborhood of the pons." In 1925 Wilson and Winkelman (90) in discussing 129 cases of postmortem examinations, 13 of which had pontine hemorrhages, thought the pontine hemorrhage was due to compression of this structure against the clivus resulting in embarrassment of the perforating paramedian and circumferential mesencephalic arteries. In recent years Kaplan (78) and Kaplan and Ford (79) have beautifully demonstrated these vessels in very concise publications. Lindenberg and his associates (76, 80, 84) in a series of papers have discussed extensively the mechanisms of contusion in blunt injuries with special attention to the part played by the compression of certain arteries at the base of the brain and the role of the tentorium in this mechanism. If blunt forces are involved in closed head injuries, the distribution of contusions in the deeper cerebral substance is due to the relationship of the brain to the tentorium. Primary involvement of the brain stem, pons, and medulla occurs if the force is in the direction of the tentorium and if the head strikes a stationary object so that impact is imparted to the forehead, convexity, and low occipital region. Secondary lesions are developed in the midbrain and pons as a result of a compression of the arteries about the incisura of the tentorium. Lindenberg (83) has stressed that, as the supertentorial contents are displaced towards and into the incisura, the extra-arterial pressure becomes greater than the intra-arterial pressure during transient falls in the systemic blood pressure. It is these secondary lesions which may occur a half hour after injury and very abruptly result in a catastrophe. The reader is referred to a concise monograph by Finney and Walker (75) in which the mechanisms of transtentorial herniations are reviewed giving a comprehensive understanding of many of these related problems.

Extraneous Brain Tumors, Congenital Craniocerebral and Traumatic Extracranial Vascular Lesions

The importance of this group of lesions stems from the fact that on numerous occasions attempts have been made to implicate them as the major cause of death in football injuries, thus removing the onus of trauma as the primary source for most of the fatalities.

Football Survey. There were four football players that fell into this special category and all four of the men died (Fig. 18). One patient had a hopeless infiltrating brain tumor, an astrocytoma. Three congenital lesions were recorded; two were arteriovenous anomalies of the brain and one was a congenital skull deformity. *It should be emphasized that only 1.7% of this series of football injury cases had primary skull or brain abnormalities which could be regarded as contributing to the patient's demise rather than attributable to the traumatic insult itself.*

An example of a sandlot football player who died of one of these arteriovenous anomalies is given.

Case 11. An 18 year old college student was playing touch football without any equipment when he attempted to catch a forward pass sustaining a mid-air collision without any blow to the head. Shortly thereafter the patient complained of pain in his right shoulder and arm. Twenty-four hours later he had headache with numbness of the right arm and a generalized convulsive seizure. He was admitted to a hospital and an arteriogram demonstrated an arteriovenous abnormality in the left parietal area (Fig. 19, A and B). Four days after the onset of his symptoms a left posterior parietal craniotomy was performed. The brain was found to be under very severely increased pressure. A 2 cm. incision was made in the brain to the depth of 1 cm. and black, clotted

MISCELLANEOUS LESIONS: 23 CASES WITH 5 DEATHS

Lesion	Injury	Deaths
Cerebral contusions and lacerations..................	17	
Arterial anomalies...................................	2	2
Astrocytoma...	1	1
Congenital deformity of skull.......................	1	1
Basilar artery thrombosis...........................	1	1
Internal carotid artery thrombosis..................	1	
Total..	23	5

Fig. 18. In the football survey there were 23 miscellaneous lesions. The two arterial anomalies, one astrocytoma (brain tumor), and one congenital deformity of the skull all succumbed. They comprise only 1.7% of the cases in the series, implicating trauma as cause for the fatalities and serious injury. (Reprinted from Schneider, R. C.: Serious and Fatal Neurosurgical Football Injuries. *Clin. Neurosurg., 12:* 226, 1966, by permission of The Congress of Neurological Surgeons.)

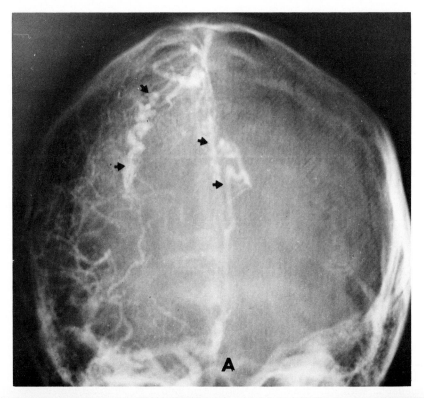

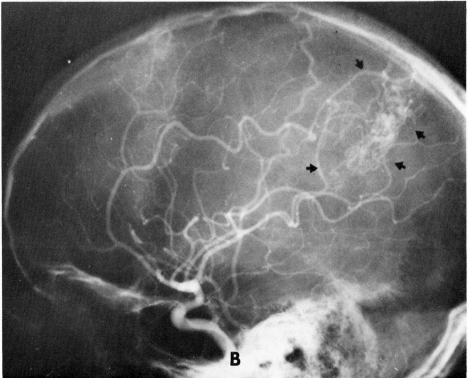

Fig. 19A. Case 11. The marked arteriovenous anomaly of the left parietal area is demonstrated with a shift of the anterior cerebral artery across the midline (arrows).

Fig. 19B. Case 11. The intracerebral clot with the anomaly is outlined (arrows).

blood was extruded under great pressure producing a cystic cavity 6 cm. in diameter. The hemorrhage also had penetrated into the left lateral ventricle forming a complete cast of this cavity. All bleeding was controlled and the wound was closed. The patient succumbed 14 days after injury.

At autopsy there was a left subdural hematoma and a left parietal arteriovenous anomaly with associated brain destruction.

Comment. Such an arteriovenous anomaly was present at birth (congenital). The arterial blood drained directly into large venous channels instead of first flowing through the normal web-like capillary network prior to emptying into the finer veins and gradually progressing into larger venous channels. The abnormal veins in such anomalies may be readily torn when exposed to slight trauma. If this action occurs in the depths of the brain, a massive intracerebral hemorrhage may form rapidly as has been described above. This is a tragic case for currently with the use of steroids, tracheostomy, blood gas determinations, improved neuroradiologic techniques, and a more aggressive surgical approach complete excision of the clot and the anomaly might have been accomplished probably with neurologic deficit but with the preservation of life.

Traumatic Extracranial Vascular Lesions Causing Intracranial Damage

Although protection is provided as adequately as possible to the head and neck, soft tissue injuries in the cervical region do occur and are frequently overlooked. Trauma to the neck in some football players may result either in transient spasm or actual permanent occlusion of the internal carotid or vertebral arteries in the neck leading to spasm or thrombosis with the deprivation of blood to the brain.

Anatomical Considerations. A simple diagram is provided for those readers who are unfamiliar with the relationships of these structures (Fig. 20). The common carotid artery extends upward in the soft tissues of the neck within the carotid sheath bifurcating at the superior horn of the thyroid cartilage into the internal and external carotid arteries. In the upper neck region it closely approximates the cervical spine, enters the carotid canal, and penetrates the skull through the foramen lacerum. It is then kinked somewhat in a carotid siphon and, after passing laterally and superior to the optic nerves, bifurcates into its anterior and middle cerebral artery branches. The vertebral arteries enter the foramina transversaria of the spine at the C6 vertebra and then proceed upward to the C1 vertebra where they curve medially over the C1 laminae passing directly under the occipital condyles of the skull. The vertebral vessels then enter the cranium through the foramen magnum anterolateral to the medulla joining on the clivus to form the basilar artery.

The primary factors related to injury of these vessels are (110): 1) their proximity to bone against which vascular compression may occur, 2) the close anatomical relationship between an artery and a vein so that an arteriovenous fistula may occur (98), and the anatomical site where a rotational or torsional force may be exerted upon a vessel at the junction between a relatively fixed portion and a more freely mobile segment (110).

Football Survey. There were two football players who sustained serious blunt vascular injury, i.e., injury to the internal carotid and the vertebral arteries in the neck (Fig. 18).

Internal Carotid Artery Thrombosis

The common carotid artery with its external and internal branches lies for the most part loosely within the carotid sheath. With most movements of the head and neck the vessel is readily mobile in its soft tissue bed. However, Boldrey et al. (91) have shown that with rotation of the head toward the contralateral side, the internal carotid artery may become compressed firmly against the tubercle of the C1 vertebra resulting in thrombus formation. In other instances direct blows to the neck may compress the vessel or contuse it acutely against the relatively resistant cervical spine causing acute spasm or thrombosis. This is one basis for the most effectively disabling karate maneuver when the neck is struck with the lateral border of the extended hand. A similar injury may be incurred by the football player when a firm slashing blow is delivered to the neck when attempting to tackle. It occasionally may follow in the maneuver known as "clotheslining."

The following case report illustrates this type of injury (Fig. 18).

> **Case 12.** While being tackled, a high school football player was struck directly in the neck causing a contusion to the carotid artery with the gradual development of aphasia, a right hemiplegia, and a Horner's syndrome. Ten days after the injury a left carotid angiogram was performed showing a complete occlusion of the internal carotid artery at the base of the skull. The patient was treated with supportive measures. Gradually he improved but had a final residual neurologic deficit of difficulty in concentration, a lack of initiative, impairment of the fine movements of the right hand, and retardation of performance of some skilled or complicated acts with his right extremities.

Comment. This patient was seen 8 years ago when neurosurgeons were not nearly as well informed or equipped to perform angiography and possibly subsequent acute thromboendarterectomy (the removal of a blood clot from the occluded blood vessel) (97). Early diagnosis might have demonstrated the fresh thrombus in the lower extent of the internal carotid artery and under special circumstances excision of it *might have been* feasible with more complete recovery. Such an injury calls for emergency action if permanent neurologic damage is to be avoided. If late extension of the thrombus to the base of the skull has occurred, then surgical intervention is probably to no avail for back-flow of the blood from the distal portion of the vessel is not likely.

Neurosurgical Data. There still have been relatively few publications concerning carotid artery thrombosis following blunt trauma to the neck. In 1952 when this author and an associate (108) reported two cases of internal carotid artery thrombosis following non-penetrating wounds of the neck sustained in vehicular acci-

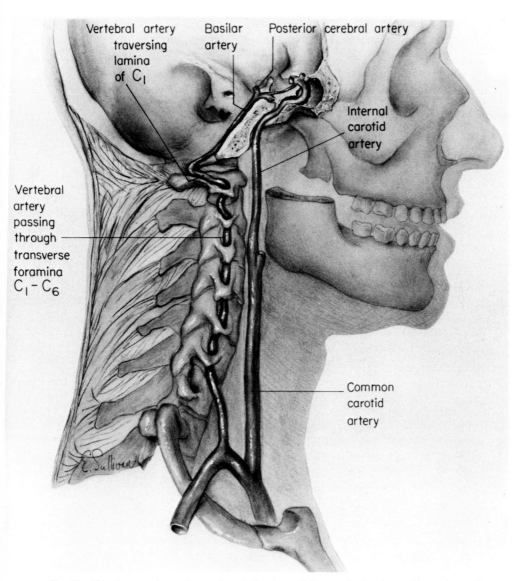

Fig. 20. This diagram demonstrates the relationships of the vertebral and carotid arteries to the bony spine, skull, and soft tissues of the neck. The site of bifurcation of the common carotid artery is slightly higher than normal.

dents, six previous papers treating this topic could be found (92, 93, 95, 102, 105, 112). The first recorded case of such a lesion was probably that of Vernueil's in 1872 (112). This patient was found under a railroad car with multiple injuries. He had developed a right hemiplegia and coma and died 5 days later. At autopsy a thrombus was found in the left internal carotid artery about 2 cm. distal to the bifurcation of the common carotid vessel. Vernueil (112) indicated that the etiology was a direct sudden wrenching of the neck with no blow to the artery itself.

When Schneider and Lemmen in 1952 (108) reported their two cases of blunt traumatic internal carotid artery thrombosis, emphasis was placed upon the fact that *the patient was much more alert and oriented for the rather extensive degree of neurologic impairment than from a traumatic intracranial lesion.* In a subsequent report Olafson and Christoferson (107) confirmed this observation in two of their patients and suggested that this was a syndrome in patients who have sustained internal carotid artery thrombosis after minor episodes of cervical trauma. Higazi (99), in reporting the youngest case with this type of lesion recorded in the literature, a boy 10 years of age, noted this disproportionate degree of alertness and orientation compared to his aphasia and hemiparesis which led to angiography and confirmation of the diagnosis.

Boldrey et al. (91) had observed that in non-traumatic cases of thrombosis of the internal carotid artery a common site for occlusion was at the C1 level. Rotation of the head frequently caused compression of the vessel by the atlantal tubercle. Such a mechanism of sudden traumatic wrenching of the neck without direct impact at the site of the occlusion is consistent with Verneuil's (112) original concept of the mechanism which is responsible for the lesion. There are numerous other recent interesting reports presented in the literature but it is impossible to amplify this discussion here (94, 96, 97, 103, 104, 106, 110, 111, 113). It is most significant that the lesion be recognized in its acute phase (111) and be treated sufficiently early so that if thromboendarterectomy were performed it would not worsen the situation by the development of a "red" infarct of the brain at the time of revascularization of the involved cerebral area.

Basilar-Vertebral Arterial Thrombosis

Because of the direct relationship of the basilar and vertebral arteries to the skull (100, 101) and spine, they are more readily subject to severe damage than the more freely mobile common carotid arteries and their internal and external carotid branches.

Football Survey. There was but one basilar artery thrombosis case in the series of football players studied. In this instance there was an acute onset of the symptoms resulting in the basilar artery thrombosis. One other case of delayed thrombosis of the vertebral artery is presented as a contrast problem.

Acute Onset with Basilar Thrombosis

Case 13. A semi-professional football player, wearing full equipment, was tackled and found unconscious under the pile of players. On admission to the hospital an hour later his vital signs were normal; he vomited several times. The right pupil was slightly larger than the left one but both reacted to light. Although semi-comatose he responded to painful stimuli bilaterally. There were purposeful motions of the left upper extremity with withdrawal movement of the left lower one. Minimal movements of the right arm were elicited on painful stimuli with decerebrate posturing of the right leg, with right hyperreflexia and a right extensor plantar reflex. X-rays of the skull and cervical spine, including the odontoid process, were normal. The patient was deliberately dehydrated. Dilantin was given and oxygen was administered. A lumbar puncture revealed a pressure of 120 mm. of water and the markedly bloody spinal fluid suggested a probable cerebral laceration. Five hours after his injury decerebrate spasms still continued and the patient was treated with a hypothermic blanket. On the following day gastric suction was instituted.

Forty-eight hours after injury bilateral frontal burr holes were made followed by a ventriculogram. This procedure revealed a right ventricle displaced away from the midline with no evidence of an epidural or subdural hematoma. The patient's blood pressure initially was 120/70 and upon tapping the ventricles his pressure dropped to 40/0. Neo-Synephrine was given without any initial effect, but by the end of the operation his blood pressure was 120/70. His temperature was 100 degrees and attempts were made to lower it to 90 degrees with the aid of the hypothermic blanket. His electrolytes were balanced gradually but he developed oliguria and a progressively declining blood pressure. Death occurred 7 days after his injury.

At autopsy the case of death was basilar artery thrombosis with infarction of the pons and aspiration pneumonia.

Comment. There was no evidence of a skull fracture or a cervical spine fracture or fracture-dislocation to account for his autopsy findings.

Delayed Occlusion of Both Vertebral Arteries with Thrombosis of Basilar Artery

In rare instances delayed thrombosis of both vertebral arteries may occur with severe residual neurologic deficit or death. The following case was not recorded in the football survey since the accident had transpired after its completion.

Case 14.* A 14 year old boy was injured in a football accident. Although he was unconscious for a short time he walked home following his recovery. He consulted an orthopedic surgeon because of a left clavicular fracture. That evening at dinner he had two vomiting episodes. On the following day the patient was found unresponsive and tetraplegic. He was taken to the hospital where his temperature rose to 107 degrees. A tracheotomy was performed because of an apneic episode. Subsequently he was transferred to a second hospital where a lumbar puncture, bilateral carotid angiography, and spine and skull x-rays were unremarkable.

When examined the patient was mute but had an alert and very apprehensive appearance. He was unable to follow commands. Some spontaneous weak and nonpurposeful movements were noted in his arms. He had a left Horner's syndrome, and could not protrude the tongue. There was an incomplete tetraparesis with the legs spastic and the arms flaccid. He had a complete sensory loss of all modalities below the C6 dermatome bilaterally. There were hyperactive patellar, Achilles, and biceps reflexes with absent triceps reflexes bilaterally. Extensor plantar reflexes were noted on both sides, but no pyramidal tract signs were found in the arms. The abdominal reflexes were absent.

The patient was placed on a Stryker frame with indwelling catheter drainage and given prophylactic antibiotic therapy. Although there was no frac-

---

* Reprinted from Schneider et al. (109) by permission of the *Journal of Neurosurgery.*

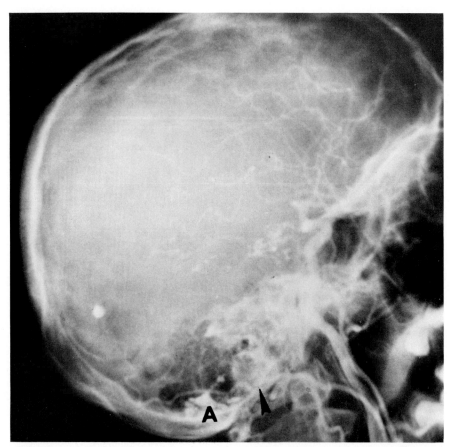

Fig. 21A. Case 14. A right retrograde brachial arteriogram revealed obstruction of the right vertebral artery at the foramen magnum (arrow). The right carotid artery filled intracranially. [Reprinted
from Schneider et al. (109), by permission of the *Journal of Neurosurgery*.]

ture-dislocation on the cervical spine x-rays skeletal traction was instituted.
The state of consciousness gradually improved from complete lethargy to a
more alert condition but he remained mute throughout the entire period of
hospitalization. Myelography failed to reveal an obstruction of the subarachnoid space throughout the cervical spine or at the level of the foramen
mangum. A right retrograde brachial cerebral arteriogram demonstrated
obstruction of the right vertebral artery near the foramen magnum (Fig. 21A).
Three days later a left retrograde brachial arteriogram showed a thrombosis
of the left vertebral artery at the same level (Fig. 21B). After another 3 days
elapsed a left carotid arteriogram demonstrated good filling bilaterally of
the posterior cerebral arteries but no flow was seen in the basilar artery.

    When transferred to a rehabilitation institute 3 months later he was still
mute; he had, however, a weak grasp with the right hand, a flexion of the
forearm, and a weak extension of both legs. Gradually he developed control
of his tongue and a gag reflex. The patient's grasp with the right hand improved slowly so he could work an electric typewriter, but his left hand was

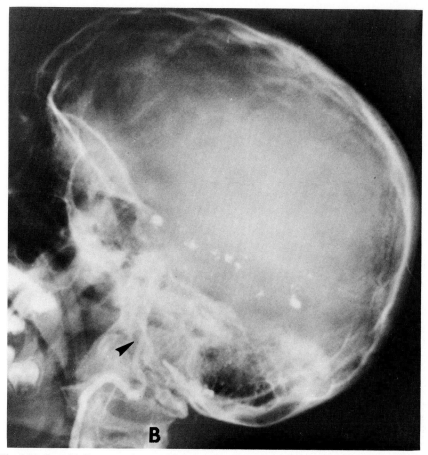

Fig. 21B. Case 14. Four days later a left retrograde brachial arteriogram demonstrated thrombosis of the left vertebral artery (arrow) at the level of the foramen magnum on the lateral view (20). [Reprinted from Schneider et al. (109), by permission of the *Journal of Neurosurgery*.]

not nearly as functional. The generalized spasticity in his extremities seemed to be increasing when last examined.

Comment. The mechanism is unknown but there could have been an acute cervical hyperextension injury with spasm and *delayed* thrombosis of the basilar artery.

Neurosurgical Data. It is rather amazing how little attention has been directed to the literature on blunt injuries to the neck with or without fracture-dislocation of the spine which have resulted in spasm or thrombosis of the vertebral or basilar arteries causing neurologic sequelae and death (Fig. 18) (110).

The reason for spending so much time on reviewing these problems with injury to the vessels in the neck by blunt trauma is twofold. 1) Foremost is the fact that the early recognition of the condition and proper diagnosis by angiography is important if these patients are to have the opportunity for good surgical therapy.

These lesions probably occur more frequently in football players than has been previously suspected. It is very easy for the physician to attribute the neurologic deficit which is found to intracranial trauma. There is a need for a high index of suspicion that such a lesion may exist. 2) The discussion also provides an explanation of why certain types of tackling, such as "clotheslining," should be banned.

For a further discussion of trauma to the arterial system the reader is referred to "Mechanisms of Injury" (Chapter 6).

References

Cerebral Contusion

1. Calhoun, H. D., Crosby, E. C., Kooi, K. A. and Schneider, R. C.: Cortical and Subcortical Lesions Evoking Vestibular Symptoms. *Clin. EEG, 3:* 6, 1972.
2. Gurdjian, E. S., Webster, J. E., Latimer, F. R. and Haddad, B. F.: Studies on Experimental Concussion: Relation of Physiological Pressure Increase at Impact. *Neurology, 4:* 674, 1954.
3. Kahn, E. A., Crosby, E. C., Schneider, R. C. and Taren, J. A., Editors: *Correlative Neurosurgery.* Charles C Thomas, Publisher, Springfield, Ill., 1969.
4. Kaplan, H. A. and Browder, J.: Observations on the Clinical and Brain Wave Patterns of Professional Boxers. *J.A.M.A., 156:* 1138, 1954.
5. Kaplan, H. A.: Chronic Residua of Head Trauma. *Clin. Neurosurg., 12:* 266, 1966.
6. McLaurin, R. L. and Helmer, F.: The Syndrome of Temporal Lobe Contusion. *J. Neurosurg., 23:* 296, 1965.
7. Penfield, W. P. and Kristiansen, K.: *Epileptic Seizure Patterns.* Charles C Thomas, Publisher, Springfield, Ill., 1951.
8. Penfield, W. P.: Vestibular Sensation and the Cerebral Cortex. *Ann. Otol. Rhinol. Laryngol., 66:* 691, 1957.
9. Rowbotham, G. F.: *Acute Injuries of the Head.* 4th ed. E. & S. Livingstone, Ltd., Edinburgh, 1964.
10. Schneider, R. C., Calhoun, H. D. and Crosby, E. C.: Vertigo and Rotational Movement in Cortical and Subcortical Lesions. *J. Neurol. Sci., 6:* 493, 1968.
11. Schneider, R. C., Calhoun, H. D. and Kooi, K. A.: Rotational and Circling Automatisms Secondary to Cortical and Subcortical Lesions of the Frontotemporal Junction. *J. Neurosurg., 35:* 554, 1971.

Skull Fractures

12. Gurdjian, E. S., Webster, J. E. and Lissner, H. R.: Observations on the Mechanism of Brain Concussion, Contusion and Laceration. *Surg. Gynecol. Obstet., 101:* 680, 1955.
13. Gurdjian, E. S. and Webster, J. E.: *Head Injuries.* Little, Brown & Company, Boston, 1958.
14. LeCount, E. R. and Apfelbach, C. W.: Pathologic Anatomy of Traumatic Fractures of Cranial Bones and Concomitant Brain Injuries. *J.A.M.A., 74:* 501, 1920.
15. Schneider, R. C. and Thompson, J. M.: Chronic and Delayed Traumatic Cerebrospinal Fluid Rhinorrhea as a Source of Recurrent Attacks of Meningitis. *Ann. Surg., 145:* 517, 1957.
16. Vance, B. M.: Fractures of the Skull. Complications and Cause of Death. A Review of 512 Necropsies and 61 Cases Studied Clinically. *Arch. Surg., 14:* 1023, 1927.
17. Walker, A. E.: *Post-traumatic Epilepsy.* Charles C Thomas, Publisher, Springfield, Ill., 1949.

Extradural Hemorrhage

18. Alexander, G. L.: Extradural Hematoma at the Vertex. *J. Neurol. Neurosurg. Psychiatry, 24:* 381, 1961.
19. Coleman, C. C. and Thomson, J. L.: Extradural Hemorrhage in the Posterior Fossa. *Surgery, 10:* 985, 1941.
20. Jackson, I. J. and Speakman, T. J.: Chronic Extradural Hemorrhage. *J. Neurosurg., 7:* 444, 1950.

21. Jamieson, K. G. and Yelland, J. D. N.: Extradural Hematoma. Report of 167 Cases. *J. Neurosurg.*, *29:* 13, 1968.
22. Jefferson, G.: Bilateral Rigidity in Middle Meningeal Hemorrhage. *Br. Med. J.*, *2:* 683, 1921.
23. Jefferson, G.: Tentorial Pressure Cone. *Arch. Neurol. Psychiatry*, *40:* 857, 1938.
24. LeCount, E. R. and Apfelbach, C. W.: Pathologic Anatomy of Traumatic Fractures of the Cranial Bones and Concomitant Brain Injuries. *J.A.M.A.*, *74:* 501, 1920.
25. Lemmen, L. J. and Schneider, R. C.: Extradural Hematomas of the Posterior Fossa. *J. Neurosurg.*, *9:* 245, 1952.
26. McLaurin, R. L. and Ford, L. E.: Extradural Hematoma. Statistical Survey of Forty-seven Cases. *J. Neurosurg.*, *21:* 364, 1964.
27. McKenzie, K. G.: Extradural Hemorrhage. *Brit. J. Surg.*, *26:* 346, 1938.
28. Perot, P., Ethier, R. and Wong, A.: An Arterial Posterior Fossa Extradural Hematoma Demonstrated by Vertebral Angiography. Case Report. *J. Neurosurg.*, *26:* 255, 1967.
29. Reigh, E. E. and O'Connell, T. J.: Extradural Hematoma of the Posterior Fossa with Concomitant Supratentorial Subdural Hematoma. Report of Case and Review of Literature. *J. Neurosurg.*, *19:* 359, 1962.
30. Rowbotham, G. F.: *Acute Injuries of the Head.* 4th ed. E. & S. Livingstone Ltd., Edinburgh, 1964.
31. Schneider, R. C. Kahn, E. A. and Crosby, E. C.: Extradural Hematomas of the Posterior Fossa. *Neurology*, *1:* 386, 1951.
32. Schneider, R. C. and Hegarty, W. M.: Extradural Hemorrhage as a Complication of Otologic and Rhinological Infections. *Ann. Oto. Rhinol. Laryngol.*, *60:* 197, 1951.
33. Schneider, R. C., Lemmen, L. J. and Bagchi, B. K.: The Syndrome of Traumatic Intracerebellar Hematoma with Contrecoup Supratentorial Complications. *J. Neurosurg.*, *10:* 122, 1953.
34. Schneider, R. C. and Tytus, J. S.: Extradural Hemorrhage: Factors Responsible for the High Mortality Rate. *Ann. Surg.*, *142:* 938, 1955.
35. Schneider, R. C.: Craniocerebral Trauma. In *Correlative Neurosurgery*, 2nd ed., edited by E. A. Kahn, E. C. Crosby, R. C. Schneider and J. A. Taren, Chap. 25. Charles C Thomas, Publisher, Springfield, Ill., 1969.
36. Spurling, R. G.: In *Craniocerebral Trauma in Surgical Treatment of the Nervous System*, edited by F. W. Bancroft and C. Pilcher. J. B. Lippincott Company, Philadelphia, 1946. pp. 27–62.
37. Sunderland, S.: The Tentorial Notch and Complications Produced by Herniations of the Brain Through the Aperture. *Br. J. Surg.*, *45:* 422, 1958.

Subdural Hemorrhage and Subdural Hydroma

38. Brinkman, C. A., Wegst, A. V. and Kahn, E. A.: Brain Scanning with Mercury 203 Labelled Neohydrin. *J. Neurosurg.*, *19:* 644, 1962.
39. Browder, J.: A Resume of the Principle Diagnostic Features of Subdural Hematoma. *Bull. N.Y. Acad. Med.*, *19:* 168, 1943.
40. Bucy, P. C.: Subdural Hematoma. *Ill. Med. J.*, *82:* 300, 1942.
41. Chambers, J. W.: Acute Subdural Hematomas. *J. Neurosurg.*, *8:* 263, 1951.
42. Cowan, R. J., Maynard, C. D. and Lassiter, K. R.: Technetium-99$_m$Pertechnetate Brain Scans in the Detection of Subdural Hematoma: A Study of the Age of the Lesion as Related to the Development of the Positive Scan. *J. Neurosurg.*, *32:* 30, 1970.
43. Dott, N. M., Alexander, G. L. and Ascroft, P. B.: Injuries of the Brain and Skull. In *Surgery of Modern Warfare*, 3rd ed., chap. 65, ed. by M. B. Hamilton. E. & S. Livingstone, Ltd., Edinburgh, 1944.
44. Ecklin, F. A., Sordillo, S. V. R. and Garvey, T. Q., Jr.: Acute, Subacute, and Chronic Subdural Hematoma. *J.A.M.A.*, *161:* 1345, 1956.
45. Gardner, W. J.: Traumatic Subdural Hematoma with Particular Reference to the Latent Interval. *Arch. Neurol. Psychiatry*, *27:* 847, 1932.
46. Groff, R. A. and Grant, F. C.: Chronic Subdural Hematoma. *Int. Abst. Surg.*, *74:* 9, 1942.
47. Gurdjian, E. S. and Webster, J. E.: *Head Injuries, Mechanisms, Diagnosis and Management.* Little, Brown & Company, Boston, 1958.

48. Gurdjian, E. S. and Thomas, L. M.: Surgical Management of the Patient with Head Injury. *Clin. Neurosurg.*, *12:* 56, 1966.
49. Horrax, G. and Poppen, J. L.: The Frequency, Recognition and Treatment of Chronic Subdural Hematomas. *N. Engl. J. Med.*, *216:* 381, 1937.
50. Kahn, E. A., Crosby, E. C., Schneider, R. C. and Taren, J. A., Editors: *Correlative Neurosurgery*, 2nd ed., Charles C Thomas, Publisher, Springfield, Ill., 1969.
51. Kaplan, A.: Chronic Subdural Hematoma. *Brain*, *54:* 430, 1931.
52. Kaplan, A.: Subdural Hematoma, Acute and Chronic, with Some Remarks About Treatment. *Surgery*, *4:* 211, 1938.
53. Kennedy, F. and Wortis, H.: "Acute" Subdural Hematoma and Acute Epidural Hemorrhage. A Study of Seventy-two Cases of Hematoma and Seventeen Cases of Hemorrhage. *Surg., Gynecol. Obstet.*, *63:* 732, 1936.
54. Laudig, G. H., Browder, E. J. and Watson, R. A.: Subdural Hematoma. A Study of One Hundred Forty-Three Cases Encountered During a Five Year Period. *Ann. Surg.*, *113:* 170, 1941.
55. Leary, T.: Subdural Hemorrhages. *J.A.M.A.*, *103:* 897, 1934.
56. McLaurin, R. L. and Tutor, F. T.: Acute Subdural Hematoma. Review of Ninety Cases. *J. Neurosurg.*, *18:* 61, 1961.
57. Munro, D.: Cerebral Subdural Hematomas. A Study of Three Hundred and Ten Verified Cases. *N. Engl. J. Med.*, *227:* 87, 1942.
58. Peet, M. M.: Extradural Hematoma, Subdural Hematoma, Subdural Hydroma. In *Injuries of the Skull, Brain and Spinal Cord*, 2nd ed., edited by S. Brock, Chap. 7. The Williams & Wilkins Company, Baltimore, 1943.
59. Peyton, W. T., Moore, G. E., French, L. A. and Chou, S. N.: Localization of Intracranial Lesions by Radioactive Isotopes. *J. Neurosurg.*, *9:* 432, 1952.
60. Putnam, T. J. and Cushing, H.: Chronic Subdural Hematoma; Its Pathology, Its Relation to Pachymeningitis Hemorrhagica and Its Surgical Management. *Arch. Surg.*, *11:* 329, 1925.
61. Rosenbluth, P. R., Arias, B., Quantetti, E. V. and Carney, A. L.: Current Management of Subdural Hematoma. Analysis of 100 Consecutive Cases. *J.A.M.A.*, *179:* 759, 1962.
62. Rowbotham, G. F.: *Acute Injuries of the Head*, 4th ed., E. & S. Livingstone, Ltd., Edinburgh, 1964.
63. Schneider, R. C.: Craniocerebral Trauma. In *Correlative Neurosurgery*, 2nd ed., edited by E. A. Kahn, E. C. Crosby, R. C. Schneider and J. A. Taren. Chap. 25. Charles C Thomas, Publisher, Springfield, Ill., 1969.
64. Trotter, W.: Chronic Subdural Hemorrhage of Traumatic Origin and Its Relation to Pachymeningitis Hemorrhagica Interna. *Br. J. Surg.*, *2:* 271, 1914.
65. Vance, B. M.: Ruptures of Surface Blood Vessels on Cerebral Hemispheres as a Cause of Subdural Hemorrhage. *Arch. Surg.*, *61:* 992, 1950.
66. Virchow, R.: Hematoma durae matris. *Verhandl. Dtsch. Phys. Med. Gesselsch.*, *7:* 134, 1857.
67. Voris, H. C.: The Diagnosis and Treatment of Subdural Hematomas. *Surgery*, *10:* 447, 1941.
68. Whalley, N.: Acute Subdural Hematoma Amenable to Surgical Treatment. *Lancet*, *1:* 213, 1948.

Intracerebral and Intraventricular Hemorrhage

69. Attwater, H. L.: Pontine Hemorrhages. *Guy's Hosp. Rep.*, *65:* 339, 1911.
70. Bollinger, O.: Uber traumatische Spätapoplexie. Ein Beitrag zur Lehre der Hirnerschutterung. *Int. Beitr. Wiss. Med. Festchr. Rudolph Virchow, Berlin. 2:* 457, 1891.
71. Browder, J. and Turney, M. F.: Intracerebral Hemorrhage of Traumatic Origin: Its Surgical Treatment. *N.Y. State J. Med.*, *42:* 2230, 1942.
72. Cassasa, C. B.: Multiple Traumatic Cerebral Hemorrhages. *Proc. N.Y. Pathol. Soc.*, *24:* 101, 1924.
73. Dill, L. V. and Isenhour, C. E.: Etiologic Factors in Experimentally Produced Pontile Hemorrhages. *A.M.A. Arch. Neurol. Psychiatry*, *41:* 1146, 1939.
74. Duret, H.: *Études expérimentales et cliniques sur les traumatismes craneocérébraux*, V. Adrien Delahaye, Paris, 1878.
75. Finney, L. A. and Walker, A. E.: *Transtentorial Herniation*. Charles C Thomas, Publisher, Springfield, Ill., 1962.

76. Freytag, E.: Autopsy Findings in Head Injuries from Blunt Forces. Statistical Evaluation of 1,367 Cases. *Arch. Pathol. 75:* 402, 1963.
77. Gurdjian, E. S., Lissner, E. R., Hodgson, V. R. and Patrick, L. M.: Mechanism of Head Injury. *Clin. Neurosurg., 12:* 112, 1966.
78. Kaplan, H.: Arteries of the Brain. An Anatomic Study. *Acta Radiol., 46:* 364, 1956.
79. Kaplan, H. and Ford, D. H.: *The Brain Vascular System*. Elsevier Publishing Company, Amsterdam, 1966.
80. Lindenberg, R.: Compression of Brain Arteries as Pathologic Factor for Tissue Necroses and Their Areas of Predilection. *J. Neuropathol. Exp. Neurol., 14:* 223, 1955.
81. Lindenberg, R., Fisher, R. S., Durlacher, S. H., Lovitt, W. F., Jr. and Freytag, E.: Lesions of the Corpus Callosum Following Blunt Mechanical Trauma to the Head. *Amer. J. Pathol., 31:* 297, 1955.
82. Lindenberg, R. and Freytag, E.: The Mechanisms of Cranial Contusions. A Pathologic-anatomic Study. *A.M.A. Arch. Pathol., 69:* 440, 1960.
83. Lindenberg, R.: Significance of the Tentorium in Head Injuries, from Blunt Forces. *Clin. Neurosurg., 12:* 129, 1966.
84. Lindenberg, R. and Freytag, E.: Brain Stem Lesions Characteristic of Traumatic Hyperextension of the Head. *Arch. Pathol., 90:* 509, 1970.
85. Martland, H. S. and Beling, C.: Traumatic Cerebral Hemorrhage. *Arch. Neurol. Psychiatry, 22:* 1001, 1929.
86. Morgagni: As cited by Martland, H. S. and Beling, C. (Ref. 85).
87. Schneider, R. C., Lemmen, L. J. and Bagchi, B. K.: The Syndrome of Traumatic Cerebellar Hematoma with Contrecoup Supratentorial Complications. *J. Neurosurg., 10:* 122, 1953.
88. Symonds, C. P.: Cerebral Thrombophlebitis. *Br. Med. J., 2:* 348, 1940.
89. Ünterharnscheidt, F. and Seiler, K.: Vom Boken Mechanik, Pathomorphologic und Klinik der traumatischen. Schäden des Zns bei Boxern. *Fortschr. Neurol. Psychiat., 39:* 109, 1971.
90. Wilson, G. and Winkelman, N. W.: Gross Pontile Bleeding in Traumatic and Nontraumatic Cerebral Lesions. *A.M.A. Arch. Neurol. Psychiat., 15:* 455, 1926.

Extraneous Brain Tumors, Congenital Craniocerebral, and Traumatic Extracranial Vascular Lesions

91. Boldrey, E., Maas, L. and Miller, R. R.: Role of Atlantoid Compression in Etiology of Internal Carotid Artery Thrombosis. *J. Neurosurg., 13:* 127, 1956.
92. Caldwell, H. W. and Hadden, F. C.: Carotid Artery Thrombosis: Report of Eight Cases Due to Trauma. *Ann. Intern. Med., 28:* 1132, 1948.
93. Elvidge, A. R. and Werner, A.: Hemiplegia and Thrombosis of the Internal Carotid System. *Arch. Neurol. Psychiat. 66:* 752, 1951.
94. Flora, G. and Hilbe, G.: (Die Posttraumatische Karotisthrombose) Post-traumatic Carotid Artery Thrombosis. *Z. Allgemeinmed., 46:* 1487, 1970.
95. Greco, T.: Le trombosi post-traumatische della carotide. *Arch. Ital. Chir., 39:* 757, 1935.
96. Gruss, P.: Occlusion of the Internal Carotid Artery Following Dull Blows to the Head and Neck. *Munch. Med. Wochenschr., 113:* 177, 1971.
97. Gurdjian, E. S., Hardy, W. G., Lindner, D. W. and Thomas, L. M.: Closed Cervical Trauma Associated with Involvement of the Carotid and Vertebral Arteries. *J. Neurosurg., 20:* 418, 1963.
98. Hamby, W. B.: *Carotid-Cavernous Fistula*. Charles C Thomas, Publisher, Springfield, Ill., 1966.
99. Higazi, I.: Posttraumatic Internal Carotid Artery Thrombosis. *J. Neurosurg., 20:* 354, 1963.
100. Lindenberg, R.: Incarceration of a Vertebral Artery in the Cleft of a Longitudinal Fracture of the Skull. *J. Neurosurg., 24:* 908, 1966.
101. Loop, J. W., White, L. E., Jr. and Shaw, F. M.: Traumatic Occlusion of Basilar Artery Within a Clival Fracture. *Radiology, 83:* 38, 1964.
102. Moniz, E., Lima, A. and de Lacerda, R.: Hémiplégies per thrombose de la carotide inferne. *Presse Med. 45:* 977, 1937.
103. Murray, D. S.: Posttraumatic Thrombosis of the Internal and Carotid Arteries After Non-penetrating Injuries of the Neck. *Br. J. Surg., 44:* 556, 1957.

104. New, P. F. and Momose, K. J.: Traumatic Dissection of the Internal Carotid Artery at the Atlanto-axial Level, Secondary to Non-penetrating Injury. *Radiology*, *93:* 41, 1969.

105. Northcroft, G. B. and Morgan, A. D.: A Fatal Case of Traumatic Thrombosis of the Internal Carotid Artery. *Br. J. Surg.*, *32:* 105, 1944.

106. Ojemann, R. G. and Hoser, H. W.: Acute Bilateral Internal Carotid Artery Occlusion. Report of a Case Following a Parachute Jump. *Neurology*, *14:* 565, 1964.

107. Olafson, R. A. and Christoferson, L. A.: The Syndrome of Carotid Occlusion Following Minor Craniocerebral Trauma. *J. Neurosurg.*, *33:* 636, 1970.

108. Schneider, R. C. and Lemmen, L. J.: Traumatic Internal Carotid Artery Thrombosis Secondary to Non-penetrating Injuries to the Neck. A Problem in the Differential Diagnosis of Craniocerebral Trauma. *J. Neurosurg.*, *9:* 495, 1952.

109. Schneider, R. C., Gosch, H. H., Norrell, H., Jerva, M., Combs, L. and Smith, R. A.: Vascular Insufficiency and Differential Distortion of Brain and Cord Caused by Cervicomedullary Football Injuries. *J. Neurosurg.*, *33:* 363, 1970.

110. Schneider, R. C., Gosch, H. H., Taren, J. A., Ferry, D. J., Jr. and Jerva, M.: Blood Vessel Trauma Following Head and Neck Injuries. *Clin. Neurosurg.*, *19:* 312, 1972.

111. Toakley, G. and McCaffery, J.: Traumatic Thrombosis of the Internal Carotid Artery. *Aust. N.Z. J. Surg.*, *34:* 261, 1965.

112. Verneuil: Thrombose de l'artere carotide. *Bull. Acad. Med. (Paris)*, *1:* 46, 1872.

113. Yamada, S., Kindt, G. W. and Youmans, J. R.: Carotid Artery Occlusion Due to Nonpenetrating Injury. *J. Trauma*, *7:* 333, 1967.

chapter four

Anatomy of the Spine and Spinal Cord

Spine

Usually the spine is composed of 24 mobile vertebral bodies, 7 of which are in the cervical region, 12 in the thoracic area, and 5 in the lumbar portion (Fig. 22A). The sacrum usually has five bony segments and the coccyx, an indeterminate number; they are fused together making these two portions of the spine fairly immobile. In the cervical and lumbar areas there is a lordotic curve (i.e., with the convexity of the curve bulging forward) whereas in the thoracic or sacral regions there is a kyphotic curvature (i.e., the convexity of the spine is posteriorly or toward the rear).

In the cervical, thoracic, and lumbar regions, an intervertebral disc is present between each pair of vertebral bodies. The disc consists of a semi-solid or gelatinous center, the nucleus pulposus, which lies in the middle of a firm annulus fibrosis. Both superiorly and inferiorly, the disc space is bounded by thin cartilaginous plates which are a part of the vertebral bodies. Anterior and posterior longitudinal ligaments tend to help bind these vertebrae together and lend support to the intervertebral discs throughout the entire length of the spine (7).

In general most of the vertebral bodies and their various projecting portions have a similarity throughout the length of the spine. Two of the greatest exceptions are the first and second cervical vertebrae (see Fig. 22, B and C). The first cervical vertebra, or atlas, has no body but merely has both an anterior and posterior arch. On either side, separating the arches are the two lateral masses from which extend the superior and inferior articular facets. The occipital bone of the skull is attached to the first cervical vertebra by firm fibrous anterior and posterior atlanto-occipital ligaments. (12). The second cervical vertebra, or the axis, has the usual anatomical vertebral construction except anteriorly and centrally on the body where there is the prominent odontoid process which fits tightly behind the anterior arch of the atlas, being held solidly in place by the firm transverse ligaments of the axis, which

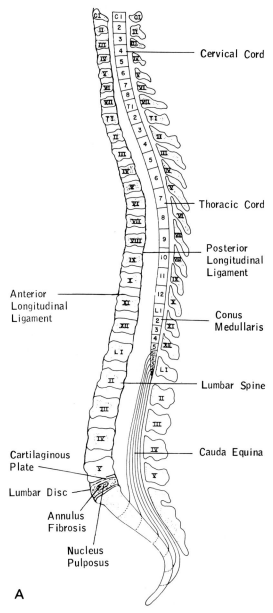

Fig. 22A. A few of the fundamental anatomical relationships of the spine and spinal cord are shown.

pass behind the odontoid process. The cruciform ligament is formed primarily by the transverse and alar ligaments, the latter extending from the odontoid process to the occipital condyle, providing added stabilization to the odontoid process, but also permitting considerable movement (5). Laterally are the superior and inferior articular facets of each vertebra, forming the foramina which are traversed by the spinal nerves. The transverse processes are peculiar in the cervical region for they

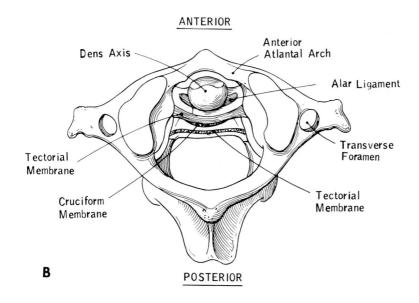

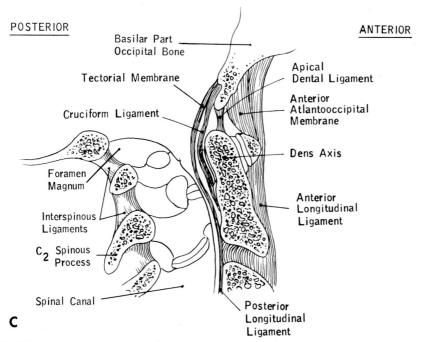

Fig. 22B. The anatomical relationships in the region of the atlanto-axial joint between the C1 and the C2 vertebrae are very different than those in other parts of the spine. This diagram shows the important peculiarities from a superior view looking downward on the joint.

Fig. 22C. The lateral view of this joint shows the normal approximation of the anterior ring of the atlas to the odontoid process (dens-axis) of C2 vertebra with the important ligamentous structures.

have foramina transversaria through which the vertebral arteries pass. The spinous processes protrude from the posterior portion of the laminar arches. The interspinous ligaments, the ligamentum flavum, and the capsular ligaments join with the previously mentioned anterior and posterior longitudinal ligaments to stabilize the spine throughout its length (10). In the thoracic area there is another region of special anatomical structures. Posterolaterally on the vertebral body there are articular facets for the heads of the ribs, which lend great stabilization to the thoracic spine. The lumbar spine, of course, does not have any rib articulations, but the structure of the body, the bony contours, and the muscles and ligaments are all considerably larger in this region. The five sacral vertebrae are fused together as a solid structure and have foramina both anteriorly and posteriorly through which the sacral nerves pass.

The paraspinous muscles extend from the skull caudally along the spinous processes and upon the laminae downward to insert on the ilium and the sacrum, primarily serving to maintain the spine in extension. The intercostal and the abdominal muscles are largely the ones which effect flexion of the spine.

Spinal Cord

The spinal cord is a continuation of the pathways to and from the brain (Fig. 22A). It achieves its widest diameter in the midcervical region, narrows in the tho-

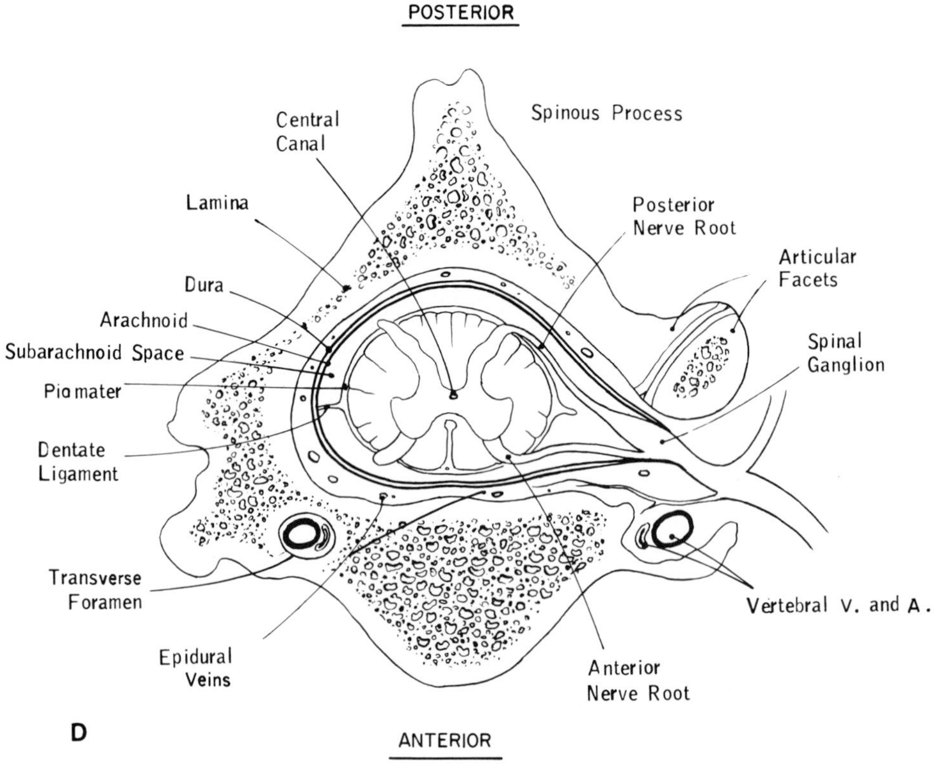

Fig. 22D. A cross section of spine and spinal cord is shown. This diagram exhibits the relationships between the bony spine, meninges, spinal cord, and nerve roots.

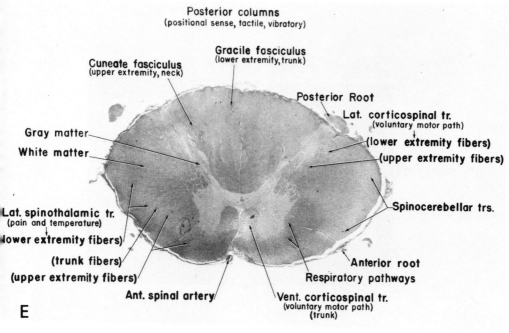

Fig. 22E. A cross section of the cervical spinal cord illustrating only a few of the major pathways and the functions which they transmit is shown.

racic area, and tapers to a conus medullaris (the end of the spinal cord) at the L1-L2 intervertebral space. From this point the cauda equina (nerve roots) spread diffusely downward into the lumbar and sacral regions.

The spinal cord and cauda equina are surrounded by the continuation of the same membranes—the dura, the arachnoid and the pia mater—which envelop the brain (Fig. 22D). The cerebrospinal fluid is contained in the subarachnoid space, bathing the intraspinal contents similar to the way it does the intracranial contents.

On cross section of the spinal cord, the dura, arachnoid, and pia are shown encompassing it (13). The longitudinal fibers of the outer part of the pia form the dentate ligaments which extend the length of the cord to the first lumbar nerve root midway between the dorsal and the ventral nerve roots. There are 21 tapered projections of these dentate ligaments which insert in the dura laterally between the point of emergence of the nerve roots (3) and tend to support the cord. These ligaments definitely restrict movement of the cord in a cephalad and caudal direction (2) and occasionally they restrain posterior displacement of the cord.

The posterior nerve roots bearing the afferent (incoming) sensory fibers of the nerves and the anterior nerve roots carrying the efferent (outgoing) motor fibers are demonstrated. The butterfly pattern of the gray matter (the cellular component within the cord) with its central canal is shown surrounded by the white matter with its grouped fiber tracts (Fig. 22E). The posterior columns of the spinal cord include the pathways which convey a part of motion, position, and vibration sensa-

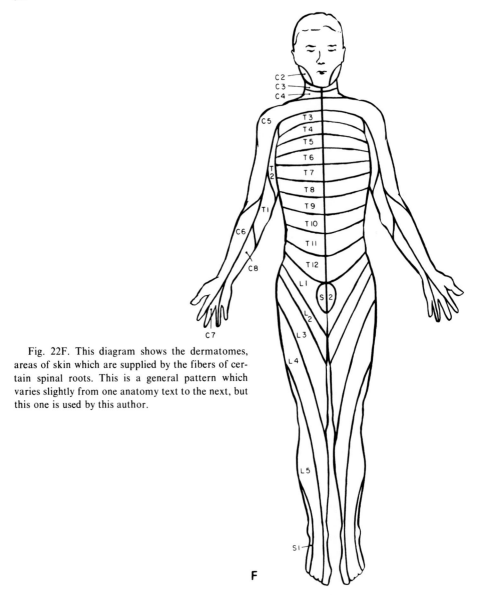

Fig. 22F. This diagram shows the dermatomes, areas of skin which are supplied by the fibers of certain spinal roots. This is a general pattern which varies slightly from one anatomy text to the next, but this one is used by this author.

F

tion to the brain. The lateral portions of the spinal cord contain the lateral corticospinal tracts which are the motor pathways leading to the motor neurons, axons of which innervate the muscles of the trunk and extremities and supply the various parts of the body. In the more ventral portions of the spinal cord anterior to the level of the dentate ligaments are the lateral spinothalamic tracts which carry pain, temperature, and part of touch sensation to the brain. The modalities of sensation noted above are transmitted from various segmental zones of the body [the dermatomes (Fig. 22F)] to the sensory pathways by the sensory roots. The anterior nerve roots carry the impulses from the motor pathways to the specific muscles or groups of muscles (the myotomes).

The major part of the blood supply to the cord is from the paired vertebral arteries which, shortly after entering the foramen magnum, give off prebasilar branches that unite in the midline to form the anterior spinal artery. This vessel extends downward along the anterior surface of the cord supplying branches almost segmentally, the sulcal arteries (9), which project, usually alternately, upward into the cord supplying the central portion of the cord (Fig. 34G). To a major degree arm, hand, and trunk areas and the medial portion of the lateral corticospinal tract are supplied by this vessel (14). On the periphery of the cord the pial arterial plexus is formed primarily from the usually paired posterior spinal arteries and the anterior and posterior radicular arteries. From this pial meshwork arterioles perfuse the periphery of the cord generally supplying the sensory fibers of the posterior columns (the pathways for motion, position, and vibration sense), and the lateral spinothalamic tract (the fiber tract for superficial pain and temperature), and the leg fibers of the lateral corticospinal tract (the motor pathway). Turnbull (16) has shown by microangiographic studies that terminal arterioles do not connect within the spinal cord but enter an extensive interlocking network which forms an intermediate zone between the peripheral pial arterial mesh, and the central, sulcal artery, distributions. There is great variability. Gillilan (6) has emphasized the importance of the venous drainage of the spinal cord. The veins of the spinal cord usually accompany arteries as the central and anterior veins but otherwise may take individual courses not related to the arteries. In about 15% of anatomical dissections there are zones of poor arterial overlap or collateral circulation in the region of the T4 and L1 segments which may have some clinical significance. In such instances the cervical and the upper thoracic regions are supplied by the anterior spinal artery. In the middle thoracic area the middle and lower thoracic cords are nourished by the greater radicular artery of Adamkiewicz (1) entering at some point between the T9 and T12 levels. A similar radicular vessel of lesser importance supplies the conus medullaris. Considerable variations occur in different areas of the cord (11), and these are occasionally of clinical significance in spinal injuries (14).

This is a very superficial discussion of the major anatomical features with which the less informed group of readers probably may be concerned; the many other more intricate anatomical studies may be consulted for complete details. A few are appended here for reference material (3, 4, 8, 12, 15, 16).

References

1. Adamkiewicz, A. W.: Die Blutgefässe des menschlichen Rückenmarkes. II Die Gefässe Rückenmarkes oberfläche. *S. B. Akad. Wiss. Wien, Klabt. III, 85:* 101, 1882.
2. Brieg, A.: *Biomechanics of the Central Nervous System. Some Basic Normal and Pathologic Phenomena.* Almqvist and Wiksells, Stockholm, 1960.
3. Crosby, E. C., Humphrey, T. and Lauer, E. W.: *Correlative Anatomy of the Nervous System.* the Macmillan Company, New York, 1962.
4. Djindjian, R., Hurth, M. and Houdart, R.: In *Angiography of the Spinal Cord.* L'angiographie de la Moelle Epiniere. University Press, Baltimore, 1970.
5. Fielding, J. W.: Cineroentgenography of the Normal Cervical Spine. *J. Bone Joint Surg., 39-A:* 1280, 1957.

6. Gillilan, L. A.: Veins of the Spinal Cord. Anatomic Details; Suggested Clinical Applications. *Neurology, 20:* 860, 1970.

7. Hadler, L. B.: *The Spine*, Charles C Thomas, Publisher, Springfield, Ill., 1956.

8. Hassler, O.: Blood Supply to the Human Spinal Cord: A Microangiographic Study. *Arch. Neurol., 15:* 302, 1966.

9. Herren, R. Y. and Alexander, L.: Sulcal and Intrinsic Blood Vessels of the Human Spinal Cord. *Arch. Neurol. Psychiatry, 4:* 678, 1939.

10. Howorth, M. B. and Petrie, J. G.: *Injuries of the Spine*. The Williams & Wilkins Company, Baltimore, 1964.

11. Kadyi, H.: *Über die Blutegefässe des menschlichen Rückenmarkes*. Gubrynowicz & Schmidt, Lemberg, 1889.

12. Pernkopf, E.: *Atlas of Topographical and Applied Anatomy*, vol. I, Head and Neck. W. B. Saunders Company, Philadelphia, 1963.

13. Pierson, G. A.: Anatomy of the Spine and Spinal Cord. In *Surgery of the Spine and Spinal Cord*, edited by C. H. Frazier and A. R. D. Allen, Appleton-Century-Crofts, New York, 1918.

14. Schneider, R. C.: Trauma to the Spine and Spinal Cord. In *Correlative Neurosurgery*, 2nd ed., edited by E. A. Kahn, E. C. Crosby, R. C. Schneider and J. A. Taren, Chap. 26. Charles C Thomas, Publisher, Springfield, Ill., 1969.

15. Suh, T. H. and Alexander, L.: Vascular System of the Human Spinal Cord. *Arch. Neurol. Psychiatry, 41:* 659, 1939.

16. Turnbull, I. M.: Microvasculature of the Human Spinal Cord. *J. Neurosurg., 35:* 141, 1971.

chapter five

Classification of Spine and Spinal Cord Data

Fortunately, or unfortunately, man is unaware of the complex organism that he is and adapts to his environment without much thought or knowledge of the anatomical features which make it possible for him to survive in a well balanced state of health. He forgets that the cervical spinal cord, a structure approximately the diameter of a man's finger is a rather durable cable transmitting the impulses to and from the brain which provide sensation and motor power for the body and extremities. The pathways for respiration, bladder, bowel, and other functions also traverse it. In a sense the cervical spinal cord is fairly well protected by its tough dura, the bony cover (the spine), and the associated paraspinal musculature. On the other hand, the flexible cervical spine must be regarded as a firm structure which holds the relatively fragile spinal cord as a captive within its canal. Severe flexion or hyperextension of the cervical spine without fracture or dislocation may result in irreparable damage to the cord. With fracture dislocation of the cervical spine the chances of such cord injury occurring are substantially increased. Since the football players "lead" with their heads, the cervical injuries are practically the only cord injuries. Although there is comparatively less room for the thoracic cord in its narrower spinal canal than the cervical one, there are no recorded injuries to this area in our series. The thoracic spine receives added support from the rib cage. In the lumbar area there is proportionately more room for the conus medullaris (or the end of the cord) which extends into the upper one or two lumbar segments, and the remainder of the lumbar contains the cauda equina (the cord "frayed out" into nerve roots).

If the spinal cord is slightly concussed or contused, the patient may recover completely or have partial to complete neurologic deficit depending on the degree of injury. If the cauda equina is damaged by squeezing but remains in continuity, recovery of motor function may occur by regeneration because the roots of the cauda equina resemble peripheral nerves.

It is the responsibility of the neurosurgeon to counsel the physician, coach, and trainer, to portray for them some of the tragedies of spinal cord injuries and to suggest methods of avoiding such catastrophies.

Football Survey. In this series only the very serious and fatal spinal cord injuries were completely investigated. There was a total of 78 cervical spine and spinal cord injuries in this category (Fig. 23) (44). Sixteen players sustained fracture-dislocations without neurologic deficit and fortunately made a complete recovery. Ten more had such lesions with transient or permanent neurologic disabilities. *The tragic group of 30 players sustaining complete transverse myelitis, that is, with complete loss of all motor power, sensation, bladder and bowel control, are listed with 16 deaths.* Perhaps the latter players were the fortunate ones when one considers the long life of disability, heartbreak, and misery for the young men who survived. Lesser degrees of cervical injury are listed. There was no doubt many other players with cervical disc injuries were not regarded to be as spectacular and they were not reported by the neurosurgeon. It should also be emphasized that the vast majority of the neck injuries without neurologic involvement are seen by the orthopedic surgeon and these, of course, have not been recorded in this survey.

Football has provided this author, as a neurosurgeon, with an unusual opportunity to study trauma to the spine and spinal cord, making observations which have proven to be of value in arriving at diagnoses and providing the proper type of therapy. This author treated a football player who had a crush fracture of the cervical vertebra which he first described as a *"tear-drop" fracture* of the cervical spine in 1948 (38). [Later the author added to the literature several more cases with Dr. E. A. Kahn (39).] It was this same patient, who displayed one of the first

SPINE AND SPINAL CORD INJURIES: 78 CASES WITH 16 DEATHS

	Injury	Deaths
Cervical fracture-dislocation		
Complete recovery.............................	16	
Complete deficit..............................	30	16
Partial deficit................................	8	
Contusion....................................	2	
Cervical compound fracture.......................	2	
Cervical cord contusion...........................	8	
Cervical vascular insufficiency....................	3	
Cervical disc....................................	8	
Cervical injury with CSF* Leak....................	1	
Totals....................................	78	16

*Abbreviation used is: CSF, cerebrospinal fluid.

Fig. 23. The cervical spine and spinal cord injuries recorded in the neurosurgical football survey are given. [Reprinted from Schneider (44) by permission of The Congress of Neurological Surgeons.]

two patterns of the *acute anterior cervical spinal cord injury syndrome*, a then new indication for operative intervention (36). The careful neurologic evaluation of another football player which initiated the studies responsible for this monograph resulted in a further understanding of the impairment of blood supply with vascular insufficiency to the spinal cord as one of the mechanisms responsible for *the syndrome of acute central cervical cord injury*, a pattern (37) which suggested that surgery was contraindicated in such cases. These three clinical entities have received general acceptance in the literature (18, 48) and have been of considerable practical importance in the diagnosis and treatment of spine and spinal cord injuries. These features will be presented in further detail in association with the specific case reports.

Cervical Fracture and/or Dislocation

Cases have been selected to illustrate the type of lesions. In some instances (which have been so designated), they are not selected from this survey because the x-rays or autopsy material may not be clear for publication purposes. Under certain circumstances, although the case was from the football survey, it may be more appropriate to list it in the discussion of other sections in this book. A few examples which tend to follow the survey will be presented. Not all categories will be listed because of reduplication or the similarity of lesions.

Combined Head and Spinal Injuries—Complete Recovery

Since many of the blows to the football player may involve both the head and spinal cord, it is surprising that with the many individuals playing the game more combined lesions are not seen. Examples of such chronic and acute injuries are included below.

Atlanto-axial Dislocation

At the uppermost part of the cervical spine there is proportionately more room for the cervical spinal cord within its bony canal than in the lower portion.

Atlanto-axial lesions of this type more frequently occur in hyperflexion than in hyperextension. They may be due to tears of the transverse portion of the cruciform alar, and other check ligaments or occur with fracture of the odontoid process (Fig. 22, B and C), (1, 25).

> Case 15.* While leaping to catch a pass this professional football player was tackled from the rear, landing on his back and striking his occiput. Although dazed and dizzy he did not lose consciousness. He had pain in the back of the head, neck, and between the scapulae. The unremitting headache finally subsided after 2 weeks. Approximately 2 months later he sustained an identical type of injury. Thereafter his symptoms progressed so that he missed two games but was able to complete the season. Whenever he bent over or flexed his neck he experienced dizziness and blurred vision. At no time did he lose consciousness. When lying down with both hands behind his head he

---

* Reprinted from Schneider et al. (46), courtesy of the *Journal of Neurosurgery*. It was not in the survey.

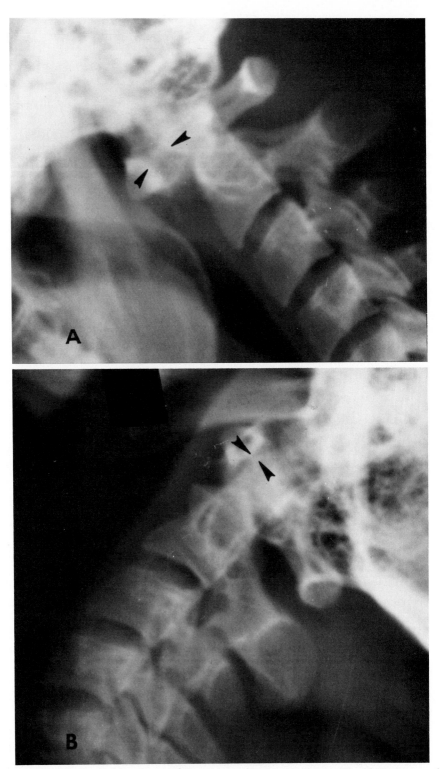

Fig. 24. Case 15. Lateral x-ray views of the cervical spine show the degree of instability between the atlas and axis. (Open mouth views excluded any fracture of the odontoid process.) [Reprinted from Schneider et al. (46), by permission of the *Journal of Neurosurgery*.]

Fig. 24A. In flexion there is a 7 to 8 mm. dislocation as noted between the arrows.

Fig. 24B. In hyperextension the anterior ring of the atlas fits firmly against the odontoid process.

noted tingling in his arms which disappeared when he placed his arms beside his body. After starting football practice again during the following summer his symptoms recurred with greater severity and led to medical consultation.

On examination he had a fairly full range of motion of his neck except for pain and partial limitation of cervical flexion. The cervical spine x-ray films showed an 8 mm. atlanto-axial dislocation on forward flexion of the neck (Fig. 24A), which was corrected by hyperextension (Fig. 24B). A fracture of the odontoid process had been excluded and it was believed that the dislocation was secondary to a disruption of the transverse portion of the cruciform ligament (Fig. 22, B and C). A stabilization procedure was performed with wiring of the laminae of C1 and C2 so that the spine was maintained in correct position.

Comment. The mechanisms of injury in this player were quite clear. He initially fell on his back striking his head throwing the spine into cervical hyperflexion with disruption of the check ligaments. There was moderate acute cerebral concussion with dizziness and headache but no unconsciousness. The chronic symptoms of tingling in the hands and arms should have led to an earlier cervical spine x-ray examination. Open mouth views are always included to demonstrate a fractured odontoid process. The importance of flexion-hyperextension views is well demonstrated in this case. The chronicity of this type of lesion as noted here is not uncommon and is often seen in vehicular accidents. Obviously the diagnosis should have been made and the patient's spine should have been fused earlier. The player could have died readily from vascular insufficiency as judged by the visual blurring manifestations. After spinal fusion he made a complete recovery.

Complete Deficit—With Death

There were 30 patients who sustained immediate complete paralysis. As noted above, 16 of these players succumbed. The following case illustrates such an acute cervical fracture-dislocation.

Case 16. A professional football player received a head injury, had transient unconsciousness and a cervical spine flexion injury with a fracture-dislocation at the C5-C6 level and complete transverse myelitis. He died shortly thereafter. The autopsy demonstrated almost a two-thirds transection of the cervical spinal cord at the C5-C6 level (Fig. 25B). In addition there were subarachnoid and subpial hemorrhages over the cerebellar hemispheres as though there had been bleeding from torn bridging cerebral veins which enter the lateral sinuses (Fig. 25A). There was no associated extradural, subdural, or intracerebral hemorrhage which might have been a surgical lesion.

Comment. The latter case is presented to emphasize the fact that both the head and neck may be injured and extreme care must be taken in moving the football player after injury. Both the skull and the cervical spine should be x-rayed in serious neurosurgical injuries.

Partial Deficit

Occasionally fracture-dislocation of the spine occurs with a partial lesion to the spinal cord yet a subsequent amazing degree of recovery. There are a few specific

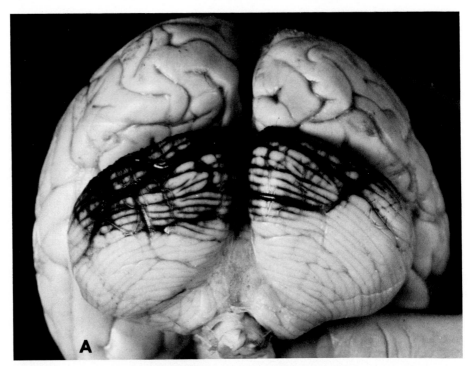

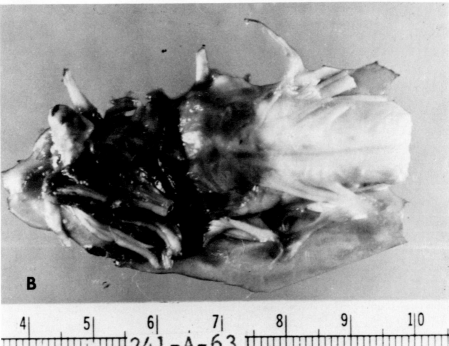

Fig. 25A. Case 16. Non-surgical subpial and subarachnoid hemorrhages were found over both cerebellar hemispheres.

Fig. 25B. Case 16. The anterior surface of the cervical spinal cord displays the marked hemorrhage at the C5-C6 level, with almost complete transection of the cord.

types of fractures in certain areas of the spine which may be related to definite clinical syndromes.

The "Tear-Drop" Fracture-Dislocation Associated with the Acute Anterior Cervical Spinal Cord Syndrome

This is a fracture of the cervical spine which the author designated as a "tear-drop" fracture in 1948 (36). It was so designated because the fracture was a crushing one with the anterior portion of the body "dripping" anteriorly like a drop of water, and since there was a strong emotional component frequently associated with such lesions, this author called it a "tear-drop" fracture-dislocation. The important part of such a fracture is not the anterior fragment of bone but the posterior margin of the vertebral body which is displaced into the spinal canal often causing a spinal cord injury. The lesion may be one of anterior cervical spinal cord contusion or compression, as occurred in the case reported below, or one of cord destruction. The fracture itself occurs with an acute flexion injury so that the inferior body of the upper vertebral body actually cleaves away the anterior margin of the inferior vertebra and the posterior portion projects into the spinal canal presenting a characteristic lesion. It is the posterior fragment of bone displaced into the bony canal which causes compression or destruction. These fractures are extremely unstable ones and if spinal fusion is not performed a nidus of new bone will be laid down posteriorly over the vertebral bodies, eventually causing chronic anterior cervical spinal cord compression.

The first example of such a "tear-drop" fracture, which this author described by this term was seen in the football player whose case report is presented.

Case 17.* A college football player sustained an injury to his neck during a game on November 13, 1948. He had an immediate complete areflexic paralysis of all four extremities but had preservation of motion, position and touch sensations with a loss of pain and temperature of the C6 dermatome. Upon arrival at the hospital cervical spine x-rays demonstrated a "tear-drop" fracture-dislocation of the C5 vertebra (Fig. 26A). The lumbar puncture showed no block on the Queckenstedt test, and a clear colorless cerebrospinal fluid was obtained. Myelography was not performed for fear of causing further spinal cord damage. Skeletal traction was applied.

A diagnosis of acute anterior cervical spinal cord injury was made and a laminectomy of C4-C5 and C6 vertebrae was performed 20 hours after injury. There had been a bilateral fracture of the C5 lamina; on the right side this bone had been depressed 4 mm. The dura was opened, and the dentate ligaments, which were very taut, were sectioned. A mass was palpated anterior to the cord. The overlying dura was incised and an extruded disc and a few pieces of bone were removed from the C5-C6 interspace. The interspace was thoroughly curetted out, the dura left open, and the remainder of the wound closed in layers.

Postoperatively the patient gradually improved. Slight voluntary movement occurred in the lower extremities by December 7, 1948 and 4 months later he could walk short distances without support. Eventually he graduated

* Not included in football survey. [Reprinted from Schneider (36), by permission of the *Journal of Neurosurgery.*]

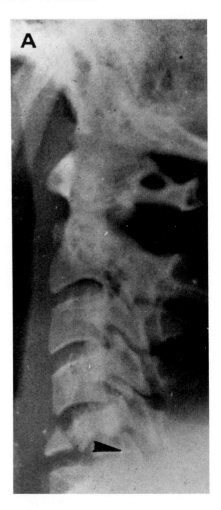

Fig. 26A. Cervical spine film shows the typical "tear-drop" fracture of C5 vertebral body. The anterior border of the C4 vertebral body descends downward on acute flexion injury cutting through the body causing the "tear-drop" fracture of C6 vertebral body anteriorly. The most important part of such a fracture is the posterior inferior part of the vertebral body which is displaced into the spinal canal (arrow) causing an acute anterior cervical spinal cord injury syndrome. [Reprinted from Schneider (36), by permission of the *Journal of Neurosurgery.*]

from college as an education major and was able to continue his work in physical education in spite of the fact that he had some slightly increased tonus in the lower extremities and bilateral extensor plantar reflexes. Currently he might be decompressed and fused posteriorly or stabilized by an anterior fusion.

Comment. This patient did not have a progression of neurologic signs, a block on the Queckenstedt test (jugular vein compression), or a compound fracture, the three commonly accepted criteria for operation at that time. He was operated upon on the basis of the anterior cervical cord injury syndrome, a pattern which had first been noted by this author in a cervical disc case two months previously.

The Acute Anterior Cervical Spinal Cord Injury Syndrome

In 1947 Kahn (26) first described the role of the dentate ligaments in chronic cases of anterior cervical spinal cord compression. He reported that in chronic calcified cervical discs which compressed the spinal cord primarily anteriorly,

B HERNIATED DISK
(Diagram of Stress Analysis)

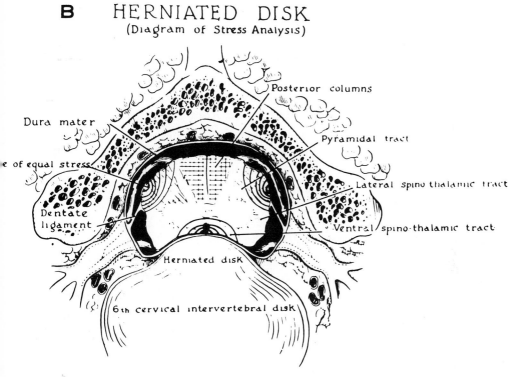

Fig. 26B. "Showing lines of stress in anterior spinal cord compression. Greatest stress is anterior on tracts disturbance of which would not be demonstrable by clinical tests. Secondary stress is directly on pyramidal tracts. The leg is most lateral in pyramidal tracts, while the hand area is most medial, explaining usual sparing of the hands." [Reprinted from Kahn (26), by permission of the *Journal of Neurosurgery.*]

there was a second area of stress caused by the dentate ligaments pulling downward on the cord resulting in traction at the site of the lateral corticospinal tracts (Fig. 26B). When the dentate ligaments were sectioned in these chronic cases, the cord was permitted to move freely in a posterior direction removing the primary site of pressure anteriorly and relieving the secondary stress on the lateral corticospinal tracts. For a few of these patients there was postoperative improvement and fair recovery.

This football player's case was regarded as an *acute phase* of what has become known as the chronic dentate ligament syndrome (26). *The acute anterior cervical spinal cord injury syndrome may be characterized as an immediate acute paralysis of all four extremities with a loss of pain and temperature to the level of the lesion, but with preservation of posterior column sensation of motion, position, vibration, and part of touch (36, 38).*

Such patients have had their immediate neurologic deficit. There is no progression of neurologic signs nor is there any block on the jugular vein compression test. Since the neurosurgeon is unable to distinguish between anterior spinal cord compression or irreparable cord destruction, operation is indicated.

Thus the "tear-drop" fracture may become an indication for operation on two counts: 1) the instability of the lesion requires spinal fusion to prevent chronic deformity and subsequent neurologic deficit; and 2) the "tear-drop" fracture may have an associated anterior cervical cord injury syndrome which may require a decompressive laminectomy (39).

Combined Cervical Spinal Cord Concussion or Contusion and Cervical Nerve Root Injury

Concussion of the spinal cord is similar to cerebral concussion in that the patient has transient tetraplegia perhaps due to a protruded or ruptured disc as noted in the case report. The symptoms are transitory with complete recovery or with recurrence upon further injury. Contusion of the cord usually suggests a bruise to the cord with or without recovery.

There were eight players with cervical cord contusion and an additional eight individuals with a diagnosis of cervical disc in the football survey. This case is presented to show a probable relationship of both lesions. The cervical disc problem will be discussed under "Diagnosis and Treatment" (Chapter 13).

> **Case 18.*** Early one fall the patient was in a football scrimmage when he was struck and fell to the ground, conscious and able to talk, but totally tetraplegic with generalized paresthesias in the extremities. He was carried from the field and recovered promptly except for some generalized tingling throughout his body and his lower extremities. However, he was "able to re-enter the game and continued to play in subsequent games." Later he fractured a leg and recovered after 7 weeks to return to football. His trainer and the attending physician were informed about the transient paresthesias which he began to have in his upper and lower extremities, but they did not force him to abandon the game.
>
> During the *next summer* while playing football, he again developed tetraplegia similar to the initial episode in the preceding year. Following this he could stand only for a short period of time without help. The cervical spine x-rays appeared normal and he resumed playing professional football the rest of that fall. Finally after his third episode of tetraplegia he was released by the professional team. The player was seen by a neurosurgeon who had another set of cervical spine x-rays taken which were normal, and he was started on a program of cervical traction. He now had paresthesias in his left thumb, index, and third fingers, with these symptoms being most noticeable at the tip of the left index finger. The player was a well developed muscular man who had full movement of his cervical spine in all directions. There was hypalgesia in the left thumb, index, and third fingers. The brachioradialis reflex was slightly diminished on the left and normal on the right. The biceps and triceps reflexes and all other deep reflexes, sensory modalities, motor, and coordination examinations were within normal limits throughout the body. He had no extensor plantar reflexes or Hoffman's signs. An electromyogram revealed a left C6 nerve root involvement. The neurosurgeon diagnosed a cervical spine strain and a protrusion of the C5-C6 intervertebral disc with transient cervical cord compression. At this time the patient showed only residual nerve root

---

* Not included in football survey.

injury. The player was treated conservatively with cervical traction and advised to give up football. His recovery has been good.

Comment. This player was extremely fortunate to have *survived three episodes of tetraplegia* and made a good recovery; any one of them might have resulted in a lifetime of complete paralysis. Since complete recovery occurred, the diagnosis of concussion should be made here instead of contusion. If the anatomical diagram (Fig. 22D) is examined, it may be seen that the C6 dermatome is represented on the thumb and index finger and likewise on the radial portion of the forearm whereas the C7 dermatome is portrayed as being primarily in the middle finger. All neurologists and neurosurgeons will agree there is some degree of variation in dermatomes and there is occasional anatomical overlap which accounts for inclusion of the middle finger in the sensory pattern in this patient's C6 dermatome loss. The diagnosis of C6 nerve root injury was confirmed by the electromyogram. This patient made a good recovery on a regime of conservative management demonstrating that surgery is not always necessary in the treatment of such lesions. Such a patient should not be operated upon with the hope of returning to the game, a treatment which has been requested of this author on several occasions. Such a course of action would be too dangerous for fear of reinjury and tetraplegia.

The remaining cervical lesions which are listed in Figure 23, namely, two cervical compound fractures and one cervical injury with cerebrospinal fluid leak, are relatively rare and merely require recognition of the fact that they exist.

Lumbar Spine Lesions

Football Survey. Since the neurologic sequelae are usually neither quite as spectacular following a lumbar intervertebral disc rupture or a lumbar fracture-dislocation nor quite as devastating as the result of many cervical spine injuries in football players, it is presumed that the neurosurgeons failed to report these injuries.

Lumbar Discs

It is interesting that only one player with a ruptured disc (44) was noted in this survey (Fig. 27). This patient was operated upon and made an excellent recovery.

	Injury	Deaths
LUMBAR DISC	1	0
LUMBAR FRACTURE PARTIAL DEFICIT	1	(1)
BRACHIAL PLEXUS	1	0
	3	(1)

( ) = Death

Fig. 27. Tabulation of miscellaneous lumbar and brachial plexus injuries in the football survey is shown. [Reprinted from Schneider (44) by permission of the Congress of Neurological Surgeons.]

Many players with these lesions were unreported. For example, this author forgot to include two of his own cases, no doubt because they were chronic lumbar nerve root compression cases and not acute problems. Many such football players first see other groups of physicians and chiropractors, often not being referred to the neurosurgeons until they develop problems or complications which have arisen during their treatment. A football player with a history of a ruptured disc will be discussed under "Diagnosis and Treatment" (Chapter 13).

Lumbar Fracture

Lumbar fractures of the spine are extremely rare in football players for in this recorded series only one player had such an injury with partial neurologic deficit (Fig. 27). In this instance the player died months after injury following a chronic urinary infection, which is relatively rare in these days of remarkable control of most urinary tract infections with the excellent antibiotic armamentarium which is available to the physician.

There are several reasons why the incidence of lumbar injuries is so low in these athletes. The lumbar spine is supported by extremely powerful muscles with the added fixation of the thoracic cage stabilizing above and the support of the pelvic structures below. The fine physical conditioning prevents many potential injuries in this area. Usually compression fractures or fracture-dislocations occur at the thoracolumbar junction. They often are due to acute flexion but more commonly are caused by a fall directly or flat upon the buttocks or on the heels with the legs extended. The latter two types of blows are rare in football; most frequently there is a direct blow to the thoracolumbar or lumbosacral spine the force of which can be satisfactorily withstood. Finally, and most important, on contact the football player doesn't lead with his buttocks like he does with his head and cervical spine, the latter being less well muscled and much more fragile may be easily fractured.

Brachial Plexus

In the football survey there was one brachial plexus injury reported (Fig. 27) (44). Like the player with the protruded or ruptured cervical disc the lesion is less spectacular and forgotten. The topic will be discussed further in the differential diagnosis of cervical "pinched nerve" lesions.

References

To avoid repetition, these have been included with the references in Chapter 6, "Mechanisms of Injury."

chapter six

Mechanisms of Injury

There is probably no better experimental or research laboratory for human trauma in the world than the football fields of our nation. A football player may sustain a serious or fatal injury in a scrimmage or game and the mechanism be faithfully recorded by the photographic or television camera. A careful and exacting study of many thousand feet of film which were reviewed with numerous football coaches, particularly the fine group at the University of Michigan, have provided some very enlightening material regarding the mechanisms of neurosurgical injuries. It was often difficult to identify the injured player and visualize the action clearly. Some of the films were slightly blurred since they are excerpts from movies taken by amateur photographers or necessarily have been selected from third generation films. Currently it is becoming increasingly difficult to procure such data for the institutions fear the ever increasing problem of personal liability litigation which the legal profession has been introducing into sports, tarnishing athletics and cluttering up the agenda in the courts.

The mechanisms of injury fall primarily into broad categories and in some instances have been alluded to in terms used by the coach, player, and trainer.

"Piling On"

This infraction of the rules is frequently a menace to the player, but in the past few years more vigorous penalization by officials has done much to combat deliberate viciousness and brutal assaults on key players.

Case 19 (Fig. 28, A–C). This professional halfback was tackled throwing him out of the field of play. As he fell, one of the opposing players doubled up both arms into flexion raking the downed player with his elbows, hitting him in the left loin with his left knee and striking his head with the right foot. The ball carrier was not rendered unconscious, but was severely dazed, dizzy, and staggered markedly as he was led from the field to the bench by two trainers. He sat there until the end of the half time intermission. As he walked to the locker room, he was apparently still confused and unstable for he fell, striking his head again. He was not instructed to lie down, nor was he sent to the hospital, but was permitted to dress and rejoin the squad on the bench for the

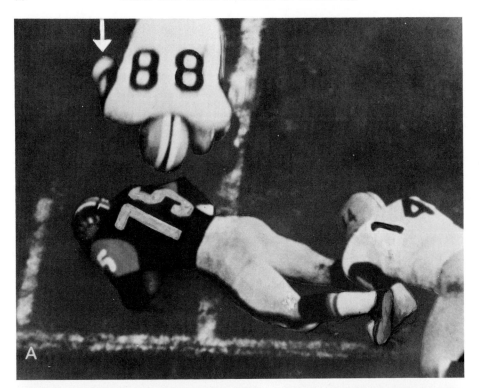

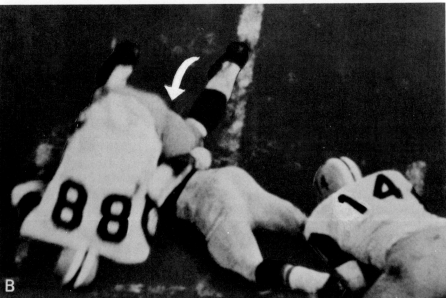

Fig. 28A. Case 19. The ball carrier (75) has already been downed by one tackler (14) so the ball carrier is definitely across the sideline and outside of the field of play. Another tackler (88) deliberately drew both upper extremities into flexion as he fell upon the ball carrier, contusing the latter's back as he was gliding over him (arrow indicates direction of motion).

Fig. 28B. Case 19. This view demonstrates the tackler's (88) left knee striking directly in the left loin of the ball carrier (arrow).

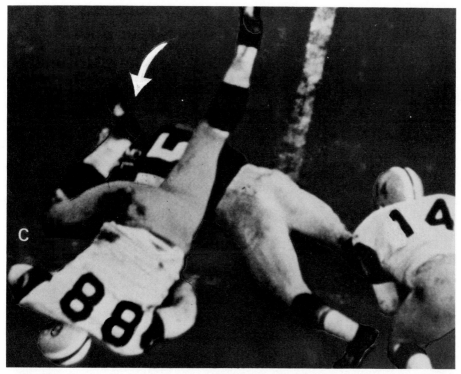

Fig. 28C. Case 19. The final picture shows the tackler's (88) right knee now flexed so the right foot strikes the ball carrier (75) directly upon the head (arrow).

second half of the game. That evening he was hospitalized for observation and a diagnosis of cerebral contusion was made. A neurosurgeon was not called in consultation although one was available on 10 minutes' notice. Fortunately this patient's condition improved so that he could be discharged on the following day.

Comment. This sort of conduct warrants the imposition of a personal foul upon the opposing player and at the discretion of the official may justifiably result in the expulsion of the offending player from the game. The failure to evoke such action frequently results in certain reprisals by the injured player, if he can continue, or by his teammates, resulting in a very much rougher game with an increase in the potential number of serious injuries.

"Knee-to-Head Injury"

This is the classical mechanism responsible for the most serious or fatal injuries in football. It is most frequently the cause of broken necks on kick-offs and punt returns usually occurring with excessive flexion of the cervical spine. The players should be taught to tackle around the opponents' thighs and hips with the head up and off center to avoid the high driving knees of a fast moving ball carrier. Failure to do this may result in a solid impact of the knee of the offensive player against the head of the tackler or blocker resulting in cerebral concussion, contusion, blood clot formation, or most frequently, a broken neck.

Case 20 (Fig. 29, A–C). This college tackler, visualized in the series of plays, put his head downward, and the ball carrier went directly over his head so the knee of one of the tackler's own teammates struck him on the head. The injured man was not rendered unconscious but required hospitalization for a day until his headache had disappeared. The period of hospitalization reassured the physician and the coach that the player was not developing an expanding intracranial blood clot.

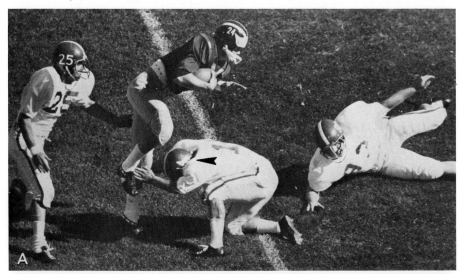

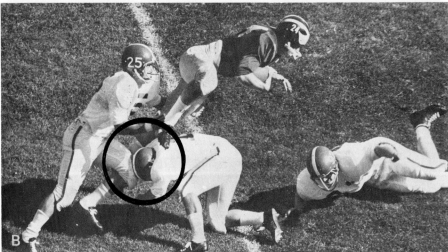

Fig. 29A. Case 20. The white shirted player (arrow) has his head down and is about to tackle the dark shirted ball player (24), who is leaping high into the air.

Fig. 29B. Case 20. The ball carrier vaults over the would-be tackler who has flexed his spine and put his head downward so his own teammate's knee has struck him directly on the head.

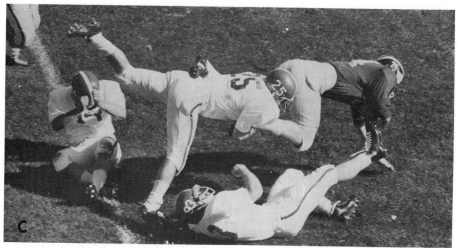

Fig. 29C. Case 20. The play is completed as the player makes the tackle, but the original tackler falls in a sitting position holding his head with both hands.

"Knee-to-Face Guard" Mechanism with Hyperextension Injuries

In this instance a blow of the ball carrier's knee to the face guard of a tackler was responsible for an upward and backward thrust of the latter's head resulting in the posterior rim of the helmet driving into the cervical spine. This caused a cervical fracture-dislocation with immediate complete transection of the cord and death.

    Case 21. An 18 year old football player was injured in a man-to-man college football scrimmage at 5:00 P.M. on October 9, 1959. While attempting to make a tackle, the opposing player's knee struck his face guard, forcing his cervical spine into hyperextension, causing a C4-C5 fracture-dislocation with an immediate complete tetraplegia and a sensory level to the C5 dermatome. The player was not moved but was made comfortable on the field, examined by the school physician, and finally lifted under the supervision of medical attendants onto a stretcher and conveyed by ambulance to the hospital. Within two hours of the accident he was x-rayed. His films showed a C4-C5 vertebral fracture-dislocation (Fig. 30A). Crutchfield tongs were inserted by an orthopedic surgeon and the dislocation was reduced with the aid of traction. The reduction was confirmed by x-ray and he was placed on a Stryker frame with continuous skeletal traction. In spite of good nursing care and supportive therapy, the patient developed respiratory difficulty and died 16 days after his injury.

    A post mortem examination revealed the fracture-dislocation of C4 on C5 vertebral body with complete transection of the cervical spinal cord. There was vascular engorgement of the lungs and pulmonary edema as is commonly seen in the patients who have required respirator treatment.

Comment. In his report to the Committee on Injuries and Fatalities of the American Football Coaches Association, the athletic director stated the mechanism of injury was clearly visible. "There was no pile-up since only two men were involved.

At the moment of contact the ball carrier jumped into the air and his knee struck the face guard of the tackler, snapped his head back, and resulted in a dislocated vertebra in the neck, which mangled the spinal cord." (43).

It would be well to heed this thoughtful observer's comments. "This face guard protruded three and one-half inches (3½ in.) from the base of the helmet. It is my thinking this type of injury would not have occurred without the protruding face guard which is made of a plastic-like material which does not give and acted as a lever in causing the injury." This type of helmet was specified. The mechanism involved in this case was one of sudden hyperextension of the head when the face guard was hit and the sharp firm posterior margin of the helmet struck the cervical spine resulting in fracture-dislocation and spinal cord destruction.

Dr. Edward Reifel (43), while still a neurosurgical resident at the University of Michigan Medical Center, provided an ingenious method to demonstrate this mechanism. If fine steel wires are applied to the chin strap, face guard, outer shell of the helmet, and the suspension and an x-ray is taken (Fig. 30B), one can see readily the potential mechanical advantage which may be generated by the lever arm of the face guard, using C1 vertebra as a fulcrum, being displaced upward and backward and the posterior margin of the rigid helmet being driven downward and forward into the cervical cord. The site of the spinal injury may vary according to the internal distance between the crown of the internal suspension of the helmet and its rigid outer shell which might result in either a raising or a lowering of the posterior margin of the helmet. Action pictures are shown to demonstrate this mechanism as a potential danger (Fig. 30, C and D). Although the helmet manufacturer was informed of the importance of cutting the headgear higher posteriorly, the design remains the same 10 years later (Fig. 30B).

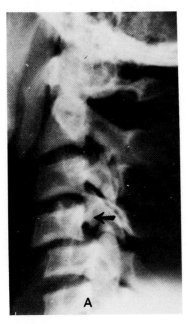

Fig. 30A. Case 21. Lateral x-ray view of the spine shows the cervical fracture-dislocation of the C4 vertebral body anteriorly on the C5 vertebra.

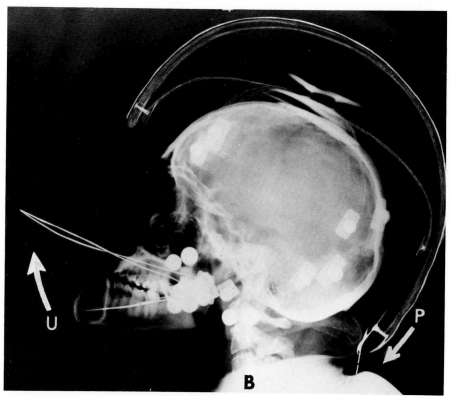

Fig. 30B. This lateral x-ray shows a helmet on a head with steel wires attached to the chin strap, the face guard, the inner web support, and the outer rigid shell. The helmet is firmly held on the head by the chin strap. If C1 vertebra is regarded as the fulcrum, the upward sweep of a long lever arm, the face guard (arrow, U.), causes the development of marked mechanical advantage as the posterior rim of the rigid helment (arrow, P.) guillotines the cervical cord. [Reprinted from Schneider et al. (43) by permission of the *Journal of the American Medical Association.*]

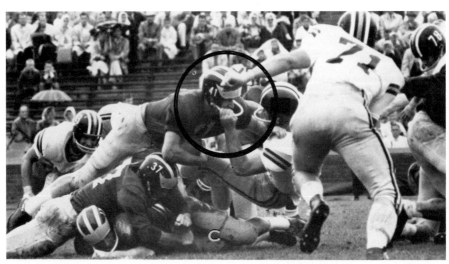

Fig. 30C. "Action picture showing the firm plastic face guard grasped by a tackler serving as an effective lever for sudden severe hyperextension of the ball carrier's head on the cervical spine." [Reprinted from Schneider et al. (43) by permission of the *Journal of the American Medical Association*.]

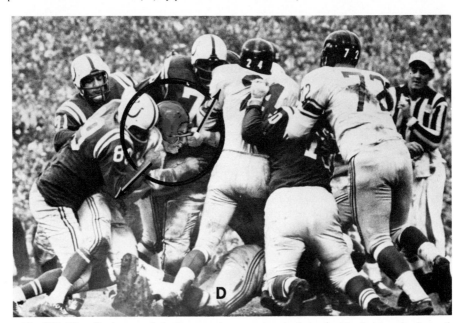

Fig. 30D. The effective use of the face guard as a weapon is shown in this photograph of a professional football player. One opponent is exerting counter traction by holding the player down by the shoulders (arrow). Another opponent is pulling upward with the face guard as a handle (arrow). Fortunately the helmet's chin strap has slipped permitting the helmet to slide upward (Retouched.) (Reprinted from Riger, R. and Maule, T.: *The Pros*. Simon and Schuster, New York, 1960.)

Hyperextension Injuries of the Cervical Spine with Vascular Insufficiency to the Brain Stem and Cervical Spinal Cord

Brain Stem Arterial Insufficiency Secondary to Atlanto-Axial Dislocation (45)

Occasionally one injury may lead to another problem starting a chain reaction which results in death. This is well illustrated in the next case in which a marked cervical hyperextension injury eventually caused a fatality.

Case 22.* (Fig. 31A). A 25 year old, 245 pound, professional football player was removed to the sidelines in the third-quarter of the game because of severe fatigue. He sat on the bench until 3 or 4 minutes before the end of the game, at which time he was told by the coach he would not be needed again and was sent to the locker room. He took a shower, drank a cold drink, and ate two salt tablets. While leaning backward on the bench he began to stamp his feet because of "pins and needles sensation." He arose, walked about, became confused, disoriented, belligerent, and was hostile. Within the space of a few minutes he was again lucid for a short time only to have a recurrence of confusion followed by a loss of consciousness. The player was placed supine on a bench. His head turned to the left slightly and his eyes looked toward the left and upward. The pupils became fixed, his respirations were labored, and he developed a decorticate rigidity with the arms in a semiflexed position and the lower extremities in severe extension bilaterally. He was placed in an ambulance and was sent to the hospital where upon arrival it was necessary to assist him with a respirator. By this time there was laking in the retinal vessels and his respirations ceased at 6:10 P.M. approximately 2 hours after his injury.

At autopsy he had a superficial abrasion of the nose. There was no fracture of the skull. The brain had marked hyperemia and flattening of the cerebral convolutions, and there was a moderate cerebellar pressure cone with no evidence of epidural, subdural, subarachnoid, or intracerebral hemorrhage. "There was a fracture and anterior-dislocation of the first cervical vertebra on the ondontoid process of the second cervical vertebra; the adjacent spinal muscles were hemorrhagic. The cervical spinal cord at this level was crushed and lacerated, anteriorly, almost in two."

Comment. A review of the moving pictures of the game showed that the "player was hit about the face and head thrown forcibly backward." Upon rechecking the movies this author found that the fatally injured player sustained two severe cervical "deceleration hyperextension" injuries by blows on the plastic face guard in successive plays. He continued playing and Figure 31A shows the player diving to make a tackle. He was first struck head-on by one of the ball carrier's knees and then the other knee dropped him to the ground where he lay supine for a few moments. In the next play he was apparently dazed and ineffectual so that afterward he was retired from the game because of supposed fatigue. There were three severe blows witnessed in the movies; the specific injury responsible for the tragedy is unknown but it was probably the result of the last play illustrated.

---

* Reprinted from Schneider et al. (43), by permission of the *Journal of the American Medical Association.*

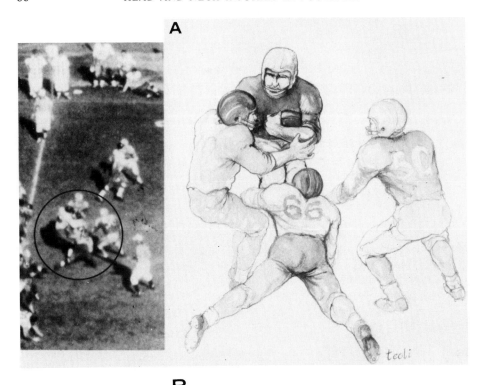

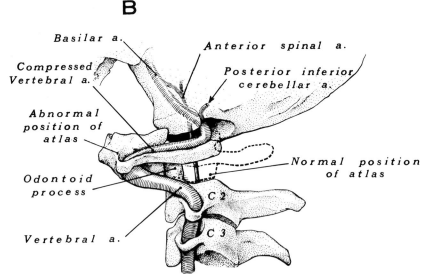

Fig. 31A. Case 22. The tackler, No. 66, dove through the line to make a tackle. His head and neck were thrown back in hyperextension as the ball carrier's right knee struck his chin and faceguard. The left knee hit him another blow hyperextending his neck severely and he lay supine in a dazed state. [Reprinted from Schneider et al. (43), by permission of the *Journal of the American Medical Association*.]

Fig. 31B. Case 22. Lateral view of dislocated atlas on axis showing points of compression of vertebral artery at first cervical intervertebral foramen and point where occipital condyle slides over groove in first cervical lamina. The captive vertebral artery is compressed as C1 dislocates anteriorly. [Reprinted from Schneider and Crosby (41), by permission of *Neurology*.]

The thrust against the face guard, as described before, caused the posterior edge of the helmet to impinge upon the spine at C2-C3 resulting in atlanto-axial dislocation (Fig. 24, C and D) (50) or perhaps a lower cervical fracture-dislocation with spinal cord damage. In atlanto-axial dislocation neurologic symptoms and signs frequently may be delayed, but in this case they were acute. Although this player sustained this injury, he must have had an intact spinal cord which permitted him to walk from the field. As the atlas gradually shifted on the axis he developed tingling in his extremities due to vascular insufficiency in the anterior spinal artery distribution of the cord. Upon looking downward there probably was a further shifting the atlas on the axis causing increased compression of the vertebral arteries and hypoxia to the brain stem (Fig. 31B) (41). As a result the player became belligerent. Coupled with these symptoms there was the final displacement at the dislocation site with subsequent unconsciousness and decerebrate rigidity. It was probably during the last phase of this posturing that the almost total spinal cord transection occurred.

Acute Hyperextension Injury Without Atlanto-Axial Dislocation

A case of this type is presented as a contrast to illustrate how fatality may occur without spinal subluxation.

Case 23.* This college football player was participating in light contact drill without full equipment; he was blocking, using his right shoulder against the midsection of the opponent's body. The play had ended and he was relaxed when two other men struck him from the opposite side, throwing his head into full extension. His respirations ceased but he was fully conscious when he struck the ground. Mouth to mouth resuscitation was immediately instituted, and he was taken to a local hospital where a tracheotomy was performed. At that time he was found to have a complete tetraplegia with a complete sensory loss, a condition which remained unchanged until he died 5 weeks later from an overwhelming pneumonia. In spite of intensive x-ray examinations there was no evidence of bony disruption of the cervical spine.

At autopsy a neurosurgeon performed a complete examination that included the skull, brain and spinal cord; on laminectomy of the cervical spine he found no instability. Although it had been over a month since his injury there was no evidence of any tear of the ligamentous structures or evidence of any resolving hematoma. The odontoid process was in normal relationship to the foramen magnum. The vertebral arteries were dissected at the C1 and C2 vertebral levels and both appeared grossly and histologically normal. A well-defined loculated cystic cavity was demonstrated at the C2 level of the spinal cord (Fig. 32) where it was associated with a complete interruption of the cord.

Comment. This patient was one of the two football players who sustained a serious cervical spinal injury at the same college during one season. The second player lived but was totally tetraplegic. "Stick-blocking" was taught by the coach.

---

* Reprinted from Schneider et al. (46), by permission of the *Journal of Neurosurgery*.

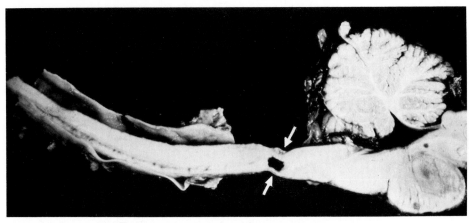

Fig. 32. Case 23. The autopsy specimen of the cerebellum, midbrain, and cervical spinal cord shows the cavitating lesion at the C2 spinal cord segment (arrows). There was no other grossly visible lesion. [Reprinted from Schneider et al. (46), by permission of the *Journal of Neurosurgery*.]

Acute Hyperextension Injury without Cervical Fracture Dislocation: the Acute Central Cervical Cord Injury Syndrome

The following case report is of great importance for the neurosurgeon endeavoring to understand some of the neuroanatomical and clinical relationships affecting the cervical spinal cord. The study of this case history has led to the explanation of the possible etiology central for the acute spinal cord injury syndrome and has perhaps helped in spurring anatomists and neurosurgeons on to new studies of the vascular supply to the cord.

On a Vascular Insufficiency Basis

Case 24.* (42). In November of 1959 at 1:30 P.M. a sturdy 19 year old college football player raced down the field on the opening kick-off and charged into the opposing ball carrier striking him with great force, causing his opponent to lose the ball. The mechanism of injury is shown in a print from the documentary motion pictures of the game (Fig. 33, A–C). The patient was not rendered unconscious. He recalled he struck the other player hard and felt his head and shoulders were thrown backward forcibly as he fell to the ground "numb all over and paralyzed in all four extremities." He remembered he could first move the toes of his left foot and a few minutes later, those of the right foot. The game was interrupted for 10 minutes while he was being examined on the field. He was then carried to the locker room where the team physician noted at 1:50 P.M. that the man was able to move his lower extremities well, but he had some weakness in the arms and profound weakness in the grip of both hands. The patient recalled he had no numbness over the body, but rather a severe burning pain on the outer aspect of both shoulders and along the inner border of his left upper arm.

At the hospital x-rays of the skull and cervical spine revealed no fracture or dislocation. At 4:30 P.M. the author examined the patient and found no

* Reprinted from Schneider and Schemm (42), by permission of the *Journal of Neurosurgery*.

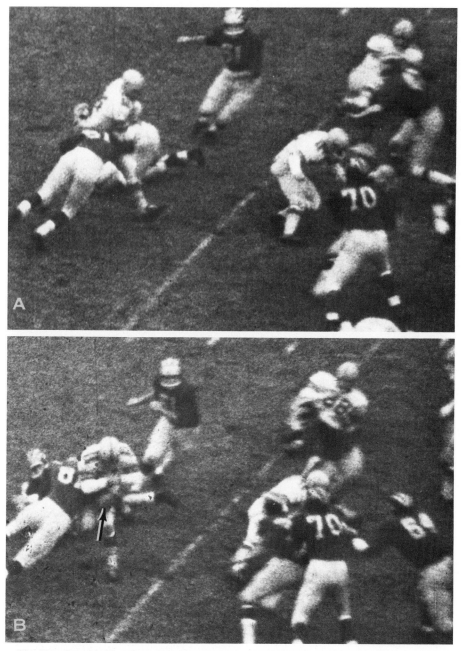

Fig. 33A. Case 24. The white shirted ball carrier is being tackled solidly by the dark shirted player. Simultaneously another dark shirted player is striking the ball carrier on his left side serving as a non-yielding force. The loud crash of the impact suggested that during this tackle the patient sustained his injury.

Fig. 33B. Case 24. The ball carrier has diverged toward his right side with his tackler still clinging firmly to him. The ball has been fumbled (arrow).

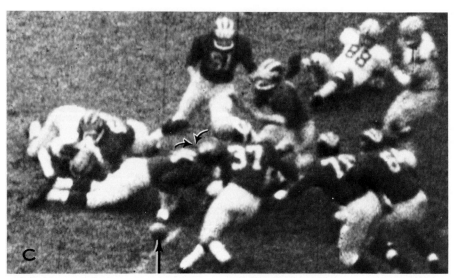

Fig. 33C. Case 24. The tackler has spun around, his head thrown into hyperextension by the face guard caught against one of the opposing players. His arms are dropped at his sides and his legs are extended limply. Note the approximation of the white stripes on the helmet to the white numerals on the tackler's back indicating the degree of cervical hyperextension (small arrows). The ball (large arrow) lies free after the fumble. [Reprinted from Schneider and Schemm (42), by permission of the *Journal of Neurosurgery*.]

abnormality of the cranial nerves, but *hyperalgesia* over the C5 dermatome and the T1 dermatome bilaterally. *Otherwise, sensation was normal in all modalities.* The grip was definitely weak bilaterally. The biceps reflexes were depressed symmetrically, but the remainder of the deep reflexes were equal and active. He had no pathological reflexes. There was little or no tenderness over the cervical spine. By 8 A.M. on the following morning the strength of the grip in both hands had returned almost completely and, with the exception of the hyperalgesia described above, his neurological status was normal. He began to have increasing pain and stiffness in his neck. Lumbar puncture showed normal pressure, cell count, and protein determinations. He was discharged from the hospital on the 5th day after injury with some slight residual stiffness of the neck. His recovery was complete within 7 days of injury.

Comment. This patient has continued to remain in good health years after his injury.

Neurosurgical Data. X-rays of the patient's cervical spine did not show osteoarthritis or a fracture or dislocation. He exhibited *the syndrome of an acute central cervical spinal cord injury without any signs of long tract sensory impairment probably on the basis of vascular insufficiency* (42). This could have been caused by direct trauma with spasm or, as was more likely, by primary compression of the vertebral arteries by the occipital condyles at the point where each vertebral artery passes over the groove in the lamina of the first cervical vertebra (Fig. 34, A and B). Indirectly this would result in a relative insufficiency of blood flow through

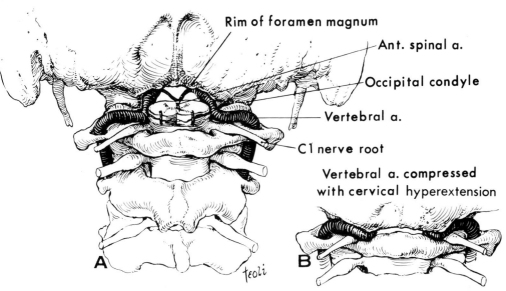

Rim of foramen magnum

Ant. spinal a.

Occipital condyle

Vertebral a.

C1 nerve root

Vertebral a. compressed
with cervical hyperextension

A

B

teoli

Fig. 34A. The vertebral arteries thread through the foramina transversaria, passing over the flattened laminae of the atlas beneath the occipital condyles, and cephalad into the foramen magnum to form the basilar artery. Prebasilarly branches are given off which unite to form the anterior spinal artery. [Reprinted from Schneider et al. (46) by permission by the *Journal of Neurosurgery*.]

Fig. 34B. With hyperextension of the cervical spine and without fracture or dislocation, there is compression of the vertebral arteries between the occipital condyles and the flattened first cervical vertebral laminae. [Reprinted from Schneider et al. (46), by permission of the *Journal of Neurosurgery*.]

the anterior spinal artery (Fig. 34C). The segmental circumferential arterial vessels are derived from the branches of the subclavian and the deep cervical arteries. It will be noted in Fig. 34C that the direction of blood flow from the prebasilar branches and the anterior spinal artery is downward toward the T4 segment of the cord where there may be a zone of poor collateral circulation (Fig. 34C). Such a zone of infarction is well illustrated in the case of an accident victim (Fig. 34, E and F). [This pathologic specimen is another one of four in the entire book which was not found in a football player but which is sufficiently important pathologically to be included (41).] This was nicely demonstrated by Zülch in 1954 (61). Blood flow for the midportion and caudal part of the thoracic cord is through a large radicular vessel, commonly described as the great radicular artery of Adamkiewicz, which may arise from the aorta at a point from T9 through T12 segments. Blood flow is then upward toward the zone of poor collateral circulation at T4 and downward to another such zone at L1, as is shown in (Fig. 34C). The remainder of the lumbar cord and sacral region is supplied by another radicular vessel. If one now makes a section across the cervical cord (Fig. 34G), it may be noted that the anterior spinal artery gives off an anterior sulcal artery which in turn supplies the center of the cord (22), in particular the arm, hand, and trunk portions of the lateral corticospinal tract (41). About the periphery of the spinal cord there are

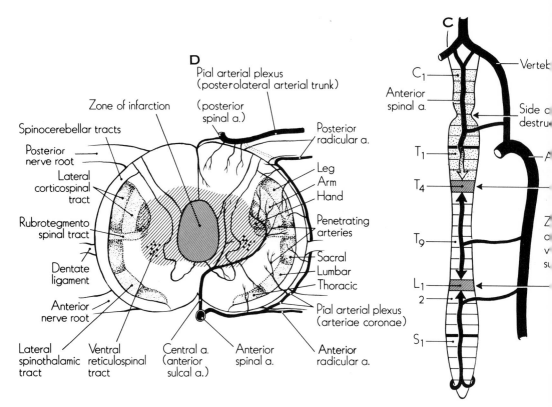

Fig. 34, C and D. (Reprinted from Schneider, R. C.: Concomitant Craniocerebral and Spinal Trauma with Special Reference to the Cervicomedullary Region. *Clin. Neurosurg.*, *18:* 266, 1970, by permission of the Congress of Neurological Surgeons.)

Fig. 34C. The blood supply to the cervical spinal cord is derived primarily from the vertebral arteries, with their prebasilar branches forming the anterior spinal artery. The segmental vessels at C7, C8, and T1 arise from the branches of the subclavian or other arteries of the neck. The remainder of the thoracic cord is supplied by the segmental vessels, one of which is the largest, the greater radicular artery, entering the cord between the T9 and T12 segments. The flow is both cephalad and caudalward, with a zone of poor collateral circulation occurring at the T4 level.

Fig. 34D. The more important anatomical pathways of the cervical spinal cord are portrayed in relationship to their vascular supply. The central (anterior sulcal) arteries supply the center of the cervical cord including the medially placed hand and arm fibers of the lateral corticospinal tract. The pial arterial plexus (the arteriae coronae) is a network of arteries derived from the anterior and posterior radicular vessels which communicate with the anterior and posterior arteries around the periphery of the spinal cord. Perforating branches from this plexus project inward to supply the laterally lying leg area of the lateral corticospinal tract, the lateral spinothalamic tract, and the posterior columns. The darker central cross-hatched zone of infarction or hematomyelia is surrounded by a lighter cross-hatched area of edematomyelia. As the edema subsides the upper extremity symptoms would vanish.

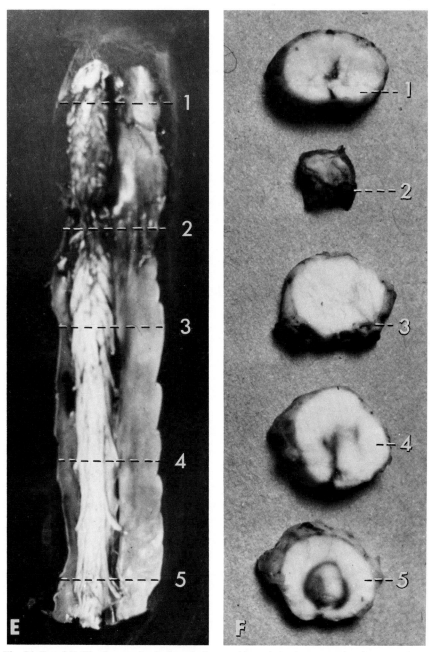

Fig. 34, E and F. The damaged spinal cord of an accident victim is presented to illustrate the pathologic changes occurring secondary to the zone of poor collateral circulation at the T4 level. [Reprinted from Schneider and Crosby (41), by permission of *Neurology*.]

Fig. 34E. The autopsy specimen shows the zone of acute compression and destruction of the cord. The more caudal portions of the cord appeared grossly normal. Sections of numbered levels are shown in the following figure.

Fig. 34F. Cross sections of the above specimen exhibit the zone of almost complete destruction. A segment cephalad and two segments caudally show a relatively less destroyed segment, but further distally, six segments below the site of injury, is a zone of central infarction and necrosis.

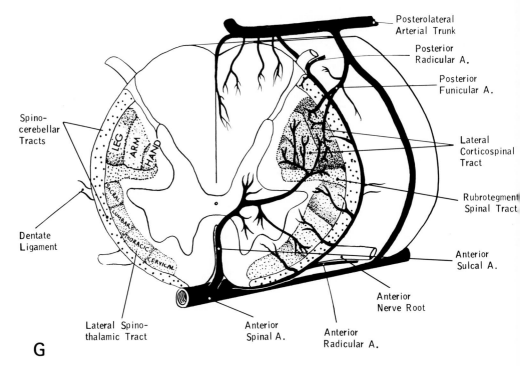

Fig. 34G. A cross section of the cervical spinal cord demonstrates the general pattern of the vascular supply and its relationship to the important motor and sensory pathways.

arterial branches derived from subclavian artery and the radicular vessels lying along both the anterior and posterior roots (57, 58). These are joined about the periphery by a pial arterial mesh (the arteriae coronae of the older literature) which connects the two posterior spinal arteries, the radicular vessels, and the anterior spinal artery about the periphery of the cord. Projections of branches of these vessels inward around the margin of the cord supply the leg component of the lateral corticospinal tract, the lateral spinothalamic tract, and the posterior columns.

Thus the mechanism in Case 24 was one of acute severe hyperextension of the cervical spine as shown in Figure 33C. The patient's headgear was held firmly in place by the chin strap and his solid plastic face guard was caught on the buttocks of one of the opposing players so that the patient's head was thrown backward forcibly (42).

The minimal sensory findings consisting of hyperalgesia exhibited by this patient were caused by compression or "squeezing" of the nerve roots at the C5-C6 and C7-T1 interspaces. These roots were at either end of the arc formed by the cervical spine when forced into hyperextension. There were no sensory signs indicative of direct contusion to any of the long sensory tracts of the cervical spinal cord. The patient made a complete neurologic recovery.

For the sake of completeness it should be noted that there may be several other etiologic factors responsible for the acute central cervical spinal cord injury which may or may not be factors in football injuries. These have been reviewed recently and the concepts brought up to date (48).

On a Cervical Spinal Cord Anterior-Posterior Compression Basis with Acute Cervical Hyperextension

Originally this author and his associates (37) described the acute central cervical cord injury syndrome, believing it was due to acute hyperextension of the cervical spine with inward buckling of the ligamentum flavum [as demonstrated by Taylor (56)] or perhaps the laminae indenting the posterior surface of the cord with simultaneous anterior impingement of an anteriorly placed bony spur, ridge, or body resulting in compression of the cord. In these instances the patients had a pattern of marked weakness or paralysis of the upper extremities with proportionately less motor impairment in the lower extremities and impairment of bladder and bowel functions. It was observed that there was a complete sensory loss in some of these patients and in others, there was no sensory defect. This was extremely difficult to explain. However, from the above study it is apparent that there might be at least two etiologic factors responsible for the acute central cervical cord injury syndrome. With anterior-posterior compression there probably was complete sensory loss whereas with vascular insufficiency a preservation of all types of sensation was more likely.

One thing was certain: in both instances immediate operation seemed contraindicated, for the patients might recover complete function without any operative interference depending upon the extent of central cord destruction, hematomyelia, versus the degree of swelling, edematomyelia (40). In both situations with subsidence of the edema, the lower extremities would regain movement first, the trunk moved next, and motor power reappeared in the arms next with the finger motion returning last of all. In some cases a delayed operation might be necessary for stabilization of the bony spine.

On a Cervicomedullary Pyramidal Decussation Compression Basis. The Cruciate Paralysis Syndrome

In 1970 Bell (5) in an important paper called attention to a syndrome described by Wallenberg (59) and others of paralysis of the ipsilateral arm and contralateral leg due to unilateral involvement of the pyramidal decussation at the lower medulla and upper C1 segment. Bell also related that Nielsen (34) had described two patients with basilar impression who had bilateral paralysis of the arms without involvement of the legs caused by midline lesions. In his report Bell cites three patients, two with associated trauma and one with a suboccipital craniotomy and high cervical laminectomy, for excision of a meningioma, which had presented with this syndrome which he has designated as "cruciate paralysis." Bell called attention to

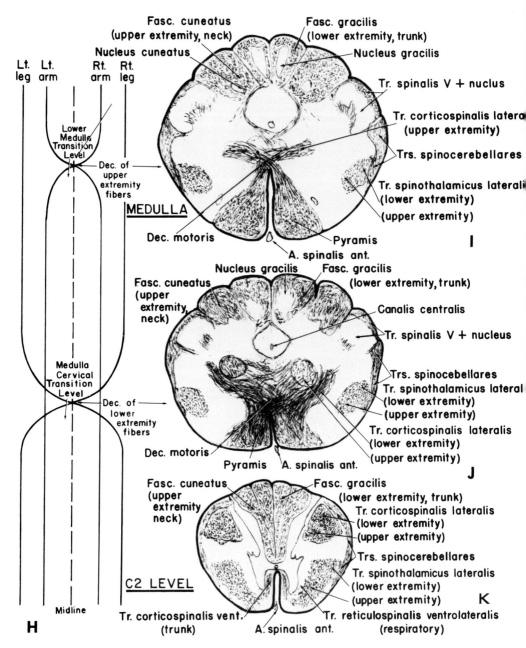

Fig. 34H. This cross section at the cervicomedullary junction shows the pyramidal decussation and its relation to other tracts. At the point of the pyramidal decussation the arm fibers cross at a more cephalad level than the leg fibers. It is therefore possible to get a paralysis in an upper extremity and in the contralateral lower one or bilateral paralysis of the upper extremities—"cruciate paralysis."

Fig. 34I. The level of the cervicomedullary junction is shown.

Fig. 34J. At level of C1 decussation of the arm fibers proceeding to a medial position in the lateral corticospinal tract.

Fig. 34K. At the C2 level the decussation of the lower extremity fibers, as well as the upper ones, is complete with the hands and arms centrally placed and the legs in a lateral position.

the clinical findings and to the neuroanatomical relationships indicating that segmentation occurs in the pyramidal tract at its decussation at the cervicomedullary junction (Fig. 34H) with the upper extremity fibers crossing from a medial position at a higher level than the leg areas (Fig. 34, H–K). The arms then achieve a more medial location than the legs and compression of the cord by the odontoid at this site may cause paralysis of the arms and little or no weakness in the legs. Bell indicated the similarity of his cases to the lesions this author had described in several publications on the acute central cervical cord injury syndrome (37, 42).

On the Basis of Bilateral Avulsion of the Brachial Plexus

This author has emphasized the partial similarity of a case of bilateral brachial plexus avulsion (48) to the acute central cervical cord injury syndrome. In such instances multiple cervical roots have been damaged and there may be paralysis of the upper extremities and yet the patient's lower extremities move readily. Careful neurologic examination and a myelographic study will readily differentiate the two conditions. The former shows combined segmental sensory loss; the latter demonstrates root sleeve avulsion bilaterally.

Tackling by the Face Guard

There is danger of serious injury when a fast moving opponent rushes in and grasps the face mask to make a tackle. If the ball carrier has his feet well placed in the turf with long cleats there is the peril of sustaining either a fracture of the cervical spine or associated cervical spinal cord injury. This is well illustrated by the following case in which the ball carrier was tackled by the face guard.

Case 25. Views from the movie sequence of this play indicate that the tackler in this college football game has completely left his feet and is describing an arc of almost 180 degrees clinging to the ball carrier's face mask so the latter's head and neck is twisted (Fig. 35, A–C). Fortunately the ball carrier remained uninjured on this play, but the 15 yard penalty which should have been called against the opposing team was never evoked.

Comments. This type of play is more frequent than is realized. In Figure 35D a double example of such an infraction of the rules is illustrated in one play. Fortunately attention has been called to the importance of this mechanism in causing serious cervical injury (43), and the popularity of this type of tackling has diminished with the ever greater alertness of officials and their willingness to enforce the rules by applying the appropriate penalties.

"Clotheslining" Technique

"Clotheslining" is an effective method of stopping an offensive player. The defense man on rushing into the ball carrier may merely hold his outstretched arm well extended so the ball carrier's neck is firmly struck, ofttimes directly over the carotid artery (Fig. 20). Such a maneuver may result in transient spasm and unconsciousness to the ball carrier, perhaps eliminating him from the game and even causing permanent neurologic damage. Equally important, but less well known, is

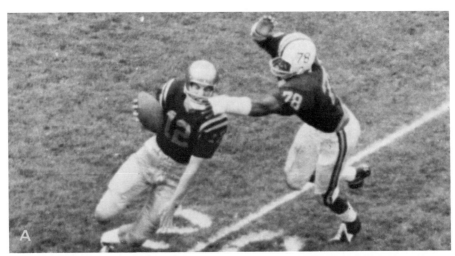

Fig. 35A. Case 25. This series depicts the vicious face guard tackle which might well have resulted in a severe torsion injury to the cervical spine or the major extracranial vessels. The tackler grasps the face guard at the 20 yard line marker.

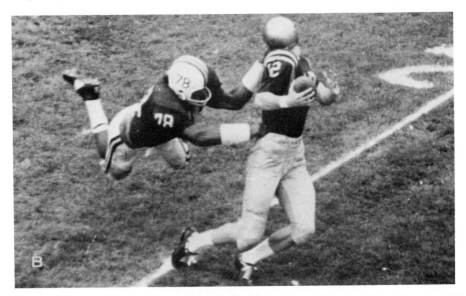

Fig. 35B. Case 25. The tackler has left his feet so that he is approximately midway through a 180 degree arc, twisting the ball carrier's cervical spine acutely.

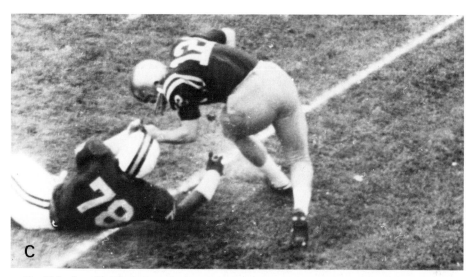

Fig. 35C. Case 25. The ball carrier is now free. Fortunately he was wearing short cleats which enabled him to rotate readily thus preventing a severe neck injury.

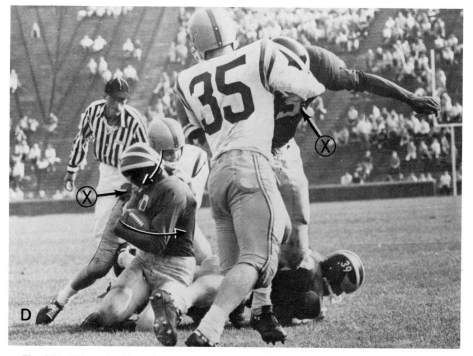

Fig. 35D. This action picture taken from a college game shows two instances of infraction of the rules ("X") where the face guards are being grasped by the opposing defensive players. Presumably the hovering official did not see these, for no penalty was called.

the fact that the tackler may receive a forcible abduction of the arm resulting either in a contusion to or stretching of the brachial plexus (see further discussion, Chapter 13).

Case 26. In a college football game the defensive backfield man rushed forward with his right arm extended and abducted to stop the ball carrier (Fig. 36A). Note there is little attempt to bring the arm about the ball carrier's neck as in a typical tackle (Fig. 36, B and C). Fortunately neither man was injured on this play. More flagrant variations of this technique may be found.

Comment. This is an unnecessarily rough tactic which may cause lasting disability to either player and a technique which could be eliminated by proper coaching and could be outlawed by proper rules of play.

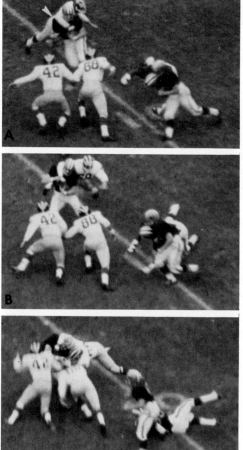

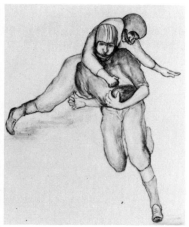

Fig. 36 (A–C). Case 26.

Fig. 36A. Note the ball carrier is being struck a[t] the neck by the tackler whose arm is slightly ben[t as] though he were about to tackle about the neck (arr[ow]), a practice known as "clotheslining."

Fig. 36, B and C. Further serial pictures from [the] movie show there is no attempt by the tackler to b[ring] his left arm upward to encircle the ball carrier.

The "Karate" Blow Technique

With the great enthusiasm engendered by the introduction of judo and karate into our western culture, there has been a tendency to apply surreptitiously some of its principles on the football field. An illustration is presented.

> **Case 27.** In the opening moments of the third period of a college game, the end caught a forward pass and ran it out of bounds (Fig. 37A). A hard charging opponent struck him across the neck with the side of his left hand (Fig. 37B) causing the ball carrier to drop to the turf and roll over and over to a point 4 yards outside of the sidelines (Fig. 37, C and D). His opponent lost his balance and fell to the ground. The ball carrier lay unconscious and did not move (Fig. 37E). People who witnessed the incident thought the man's neck had been broken. The unconscious player did not respond for 4 or 5 minutes but after regaining his senses was able to get to his feet and walk around the end of the field to his own bench while play was resumed. After being examined, he sat there for almost all of the next two periods which were punctuated by numerous time outs. Finally in the last two minutes of the game he was rechecked, found to be in good condition, and returned to the game. He executed several plays very effectively and caught several more passes running them out of bounds to "stop the clock." After the game he suffered no sequelae but was exhausted.
>
> On the following day it was thought advisable for him to have a routine skull and cervical spine x-ray examination. Both were negative. Neurosurgical examination showed no abnormality. However, when the injury was discussed with the man, it was discovered that he had no recollection of the injury, his walk around the end of the field, nor the time spent sitting on the bench. His first recollection was suddenly finding himself on the field again playing football. He has remained neurologically negative and in good health.

Comment. This player obviously sustained an injury to his neck by a karate-like blow with probable vertebral artery insufficiency. The spasm of the vessel must have been sufficiently great to impair not only his state of consciousness for a brief interval but also his awareness of his surroundings for a prolonged period. Even though examined on the field, this state of amnesia could not be detected (35a). The injury might have been worse, for the man might have sustained a permanent arterial thrombosis similar to that described in Case 12.

This was a deliberate injury inflicted on this player outside the field of play and in this writer's opinion should automatically have removed the offender from the game for a personal foul.

Neurosurgical Data. *Internal Carotid Artery Injury.* In the last two mechanisms of injury cited above there was the probability or the actual development of internal carotid artery insufficiency. This problem has already been discussed comprehensively in Case 12. In 1956 Boldrey *et al.* (8) called attention to the fact that with contralateral rotation of the head and neck the internal carotid artery might be compressed against the C1 tubercle causing vasospasm or thrombosis. The grabbing of the face guard with the extreme torsional force exerted on the cervical region, as visualized in Case 25, could readily have resulted in such a vascular injury to this player. If the man had been wearing long cleats on his shoes causing

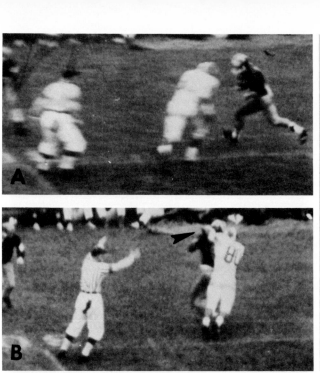

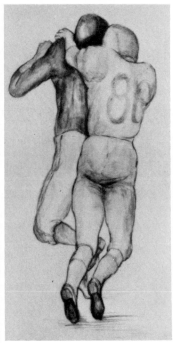

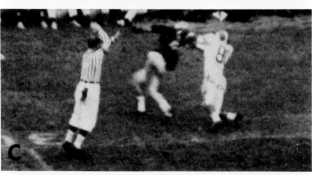

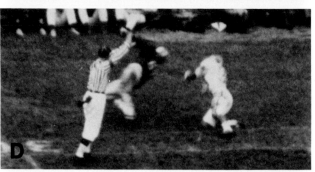

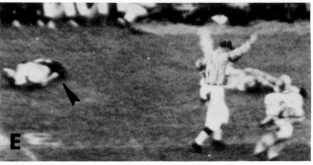

Fig. 37 (A–E). Case 27.

Fig. 37A. The black shirted receiver has caught the ball and is already outside the field boundary stripe.

Fig. 37B. The ball carrier is struck across the neck by the hand and wrist of his white shirted defensive opponent when both are out of the field of play (see insert).

Fig. 37, C and D. The force of the blow whirls the ball carrier downward to his right side as the defensive man loses his balance from the impact.

Fig. 37E. The ball carrier lies limp and unconscious 4 yards off the field of play and his opponent is shown 4 or 5 yards away.

his feet to be firmly planted he could also have easily suffered a fracture or dislocation of the cervical spine. Although this injury is graphically demonstrated the tragedy of internal carotid artery thrombosis (Case 12) due to direct cervical contusion by "clotheslining" is much more difficult to witness and assess. Not only the tackled opponent may be injured but also the tackler exposes himself to a possible serious brachial plexus palsy. The responsibility for diminishing such lesions depends upon coaches teaching clean techniques, indicating the dangers of foul tactics and avoiding them.

Vertebral Artery Injury. Upon reviewing the motion picture films of the player reported in Case 27, the late Dr. Maitland Baldwin (3), both a neurosurgeon and a karate expert, commented on the similarity of the mechanism of injury of a karate blow and that delivered by the side of the extended left hand to the cervical spine of the player just below the mastoid tip causing transient vascular insufficiency with unconsciousness. The site of contusion to the vertebral artery occurs at the atlas or atlanto-occipital membrane (3).

A further comment about the vertebral artery should be made here, for the layman and physician have paid too little attention to this extremely important vessel (12, 24). In two anatomical papers Stopford (52, 53) described the arteries of the pons and the medulla, indicating the number of cases in which there might be hypoplastic (underdeveloped) or absent vertebral vessels. In 1927 DeKleyn and Nieuwenhuyse (14) demonstrated in cadavers that circulation in one vertebral artery could be impaired secondarily if the head were stretched, overextended, and tilted to the opposite side (23). Thirty years later Tatlow and Bammer (55) presented arteriographic evidence of narrowing of the vertebral artery at the atlanto-axial joint during extension and rotation of the head. With these facts in mind it is therefore understandable that much of our knowledge about vertebral insufficiency to the brain stem and spinal cord is derived from the literature on complications related to chiropractic manipulations or mechanotherapy to the cervical spine. Since there is a far-reaching belief in the athletic field that such manipulations can cure almost all headaches and neck pains in football players, it seems appropriate to expand upon the dangers of such practices while discussing the vertebral arteries.

Blaine (7) in 1925 described a case of chiropractic manipulative dislocation of the atlas but no comment was made regarding associated compression of the vertebral artery. In 1947 Pratt-Thomas and Berger (35) presented two cases of patients in their thirties who had sustained chiropractic manipulation and who lost consciousness displaying signs of vertebral or basilar insufficiency and died within 9 and 24 hours, respectively. At autopsy the first patient had thrombosis of the basilar artery, anterior inferior cerebellar and posterior inferior cerebellar arteries with infarction and hemorrhage in the right cerebellar hemisphere. The postmortem examination in the second patient demonstrated basilar artery, right vertebral artery and posterior inferior cerebellar artery thromboses with a left cerebellar hemisphere softening. A 37 year old patient was reported by Ford (15) and Ford and Clark (16) who sustained dizziness, tinnitus, and right homonymous hemianopsia following "non-professional" mechanotherapy by his wife. She had stretched and twisted his neck resulting in the above symptoms which became progressively severe until the patient succumbed 60 hours later. At postmortem examination he had thrombosed his basilar artery as well as his left posterior cerebral and left posterior inferior cerebellar arteries (6). There was associated left cerebellar hemisphere edema. The authors described another patient who was fortunate in that he survived the manipulation by the chiropractor but was unconscious for 24 hours and subsequently developed hemiparesis, ataxia of the right arm and leg, dysphasia, slurred speech, and deafness in the right ear. His symptoms and signs persisted even 10 years later. This paper suggested that the immediate onset of symptoms was due to vertebral artery spasm and thrombosis of the vessel presumably occurred somewhat later.

As was indicated by the second case of Ford and Clark (16) not all of these patients lose their lives but may have severe residual neurologic deficit following manipulation with vertebral artery trauma. Schwarz et al. (49) reported a 28 year old woman who after manipulation developed a posterior inferior cerebellar artery syndrome from which she almost completely recovered. Green and Joynt (19) described two patients, one of whom had multiple sclerosis and the other who was free of associated disease, who were manipulated and showed partial symptoms and signs of a lateral medullary or Wallenberg's syndrome. In neither of the last two reports was there any bony abnormality in the cervical spine. These authors stress the factors involved in cases with such lesions which are reported in the literature: 1) usually the manipulation therapy has been of a violent nature; and 2) they believed bony structures were abnormal by virtue of congenital or degenerative change (although neither of their cases showed any such abnormality).

Grinker and Guy (20) described a case of thrombosis of the anterior spinal artery in a 17 year old boy who sustained a simple sprain of the cervical spine. Yates (60) in reviewing 60 stillborn fetuses chosen at random discovered 24 cases in which there were hemorrhages in the adventitial coat of one or both vertebral arteries. There were some mural hematomas of the vertebral artery due to the tearing of the vertebral artery branches. In only two cases was there any spinal cord damage and both of these instances were in breech deliveries.

There is also a series of cases in which vertebral-basilar problems have arisen with distortion of the cervical spine. Kunkle et al. (27) describe a 35 year old patient who had six adjustments by a chiropractor. The sixth adjustment was unusually vigorous with "stretching, rotatory neck movements, and firm pressure on the right side of the neck" with subsequent symptoms of a lateral medullary syndrome. X-rays showed bony proliferation and vertebral bridging in the lower cervical area. It was believed the patient had infarction of the lateral medullary plate due to thrombosis of the ipsilateral vertebral artery or of its branches. Currier et al. (13) have shown the variability of lesions causing symptoms in studies of seven patients who had spontaneously developed this pattern.

It is indeed clear that the injudicious use of either professional or nonprofessional mechanotherapy (manipulation of the neck), so often resorted to in the treatment of athletes by various cults or trainers, chiropractors or osteopaths, can result in permanent neurologic deficit or death to the football player.

Further discussions of blood vessel injury with head and neck trauma may be procured from the references (4, 10, 11, 15, 21, 31, 47, 51, 54).

"Head Butting" in Lieu of Proper Tackling

The head and neck never can be protected completely to withstand a direct impact force, no matter how good the protective equipment may be. The teaching of the "head butting" technique is one of the most serious errors being perpetuated throughout the country. Two tragic examples are provided.

> **Case 28.** A 17 year old high school defensive football player charged down the field attempting to bring down the opposing ball carrier. He lowered his head and struck the oncoming player with the left temporal region of his head and fell to the ground (Fig. 38, A–C). The boy was able to get to his feet but then suddenly vomited twice and fell to the ground unconscious. He was taken to a local hospital where he was semicomatose. His pupils were equal but reacted sluggishly to light, and his response to questioning was very slow and hesitant. His only other neurologic finding was bilateral pyramidal tract signs. There were no external signs of injury on his head. As he gradually roused it was apparent that he had bilateral blindness, mental confusion, and some bladder incontinence. His lumbar puncture pressure was normal, the cerebrospinal fluid protein was 103 mg. %. His skull and spine x-rays were normal and a left internal carotid arteriogram showed no lesion. An EEG on the day after injury showed a grossly and diffusely abnormal record without evidence of a focal lesion. A subsequent study exhibited some improvement in the pattern with more tendency toward a right temporal localization.
>
> Two months after injury, the patient was admitted to University of Michigan Hospital. The neurologists at first believed him to have cortical blindness, but subsequent evaluation suggested a visual agnosia, marked memory deficit, masking of the facies, poverty of movement and lack of blinking. Evoked visual response were minimal to absent. These findings will be discussed elsewhere.
>
> The above symptoms suggested bilateral diffuse basal ganglia and cortical involvement. The striking contrast in the appearance of the boy prior to injury and a photograph taken 5 months after his trauma suggests the severity of his lesion (Fig. 38, D and E).

Comment. This lad had an extremely severe contusion of the brain probably with multiple, diffuse petechial hemorrhages throughout the frontal and occipital lobes and the basal ganglia. The prognosis for further recovery was hopeless, for 3 years after his injury he still walked with a poverty of movement and had masked facies, loss of associated movements, some partial visual agnosia, and marked retardation although some improvement had occurred within the 7 months of his post-injury period.

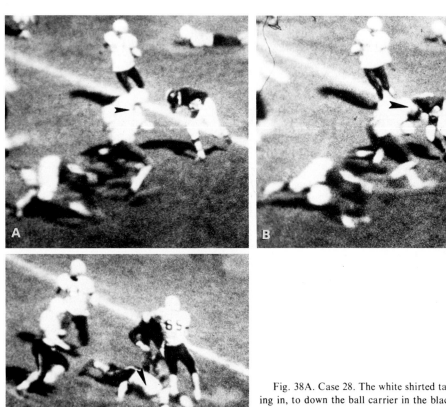

Fig. 38A. Case 28. The white shirted tackler is charg
ing in, to down the ball carrier in the black shirt.

Fig. 38B. Case 28. Instead of trying to tackle the de
fensive player, he forcefully butts the ball carrier in th
head making no attempt to tackle with his arms.

Fig. 38C. Case 28. This frame shows the tackler drop
ping to the ground unconscious (arrow).

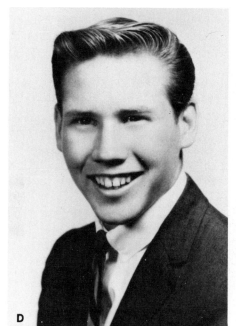 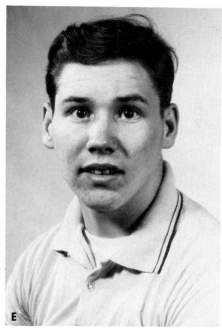

Fig. 38D. Case 28. The injured player's class picture portrays an intelligent appearing, handsome youth before injury.

Fig. 38E. Case 28. The photograph taken 5 months after injury reveals more of a vacant stare, an obvious loss of his mental alertness, and a lack of facial expression.

A second type of injury, similar to that in Case 28 except that it ended in a fatality, is recorded.

Case 29. An 18 year old high school football player charged forward with his head down to tackle the opposing ball carrier. The tackler made no attempt to throw his arms about his opponent but merely lowered his head and drove the right temporal region of his head into the ball carrier's left temporal area (Fig. 39, A–C). He then fell unconscious to the ground. Upon being transported to the hospital he had fixed dilated pupils and, although an acute subdural hemorrhage was drained, he died within 8 hours after his injury.

Comment. This was a completely avoidable injury. Proper coaching techniques might well have saved this boy's life. The intracranial bleeding was so rapid that by the time he arrived at the hospital he was moribund.

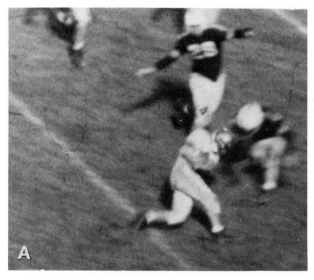

Fig. 39 (A–C). Case 29: "head butting.
Fig. 39A. The black shirted tackler's he
is about to make contact with the ball carrie
helmet. No attempt is being made to thre
the arms forward around the opponent.

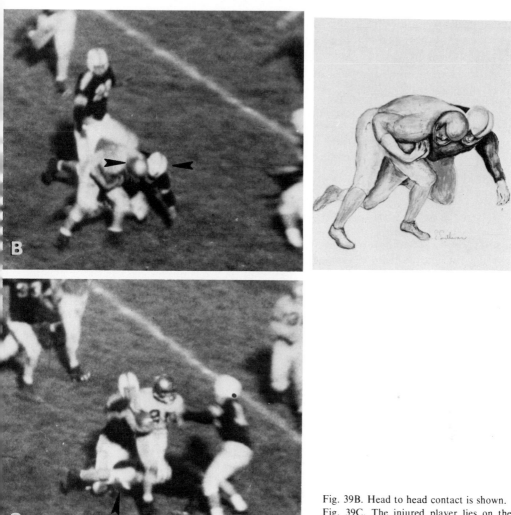

Fig. 39B. Head to head contact is shown.
Fig. 39C. The injured player lies on the
turf (arrow).

Forced Cervical Flexion Injuries

The worst injuries to the cervical spine occur when the football player tends to lower his head and makes acute contact with his opponent with his neck in flexion, a position in which he can withstand a blow less well than if the head and cervical spine are in some degree of hyperextension. The muscles involved in maintaining the latter stance are by far the stronger and better able to withstand the impact.

Case 30. While carrying the ball a right-handed high school football half-back received a neck injury when two tacklers held his arms at his side as he fell with his neck flexed and his head bent downward (Fig. 40A). A third opponent struck the group so that the ball carrier fell forward with the neck so completely flexed that both shoulders rested directly on the ground (Fig. 40, B and C). The halfback had an immediate complete paralysis of all four extremities with a total loss of sensation for a few minutes after injury, but then he began to move his lower extremities. Between the time of injury and admission to his community hospital, the patient gradually recovered all motor power and only noted pain and tingling radiating along the inner aspect of his forearms. After cervical spine x-rays were taken, he was placed in halter traction at a local hospital for 5 days and then was discharged wearing a plastic collar.

Five weeks later, a neurosurgical examination at the University of Michigan Medical Center revealed some right triceps paresis and weakness of his interosseus muscles. X-rays of the cervical spine demonstrated dislocation of C6 on C7 vertebral body with marked subluxation of the facet bilaterally and marked separation between the C6 and C7 spinous processes (Fig. 40D). A fracture of the lateral mass of C7 and possible C6 vertebrae was demonstrated on the stereoscopic views. Vinke tongs were inserted and traction was applied. Two days later a subtotal laminectomy with partial facetectomy was performed at C6-C7 on the right side. The nerve root at this interspace was exposed bilaterally and found to be compressed on the right side. A foramenotomy was made decompressing the involved nerve root. A wire was inserted through the C5 and C7 spinous processes, the latter were drawn together, and bony fusion of the C5, C6 and C7 laminae was performed.

An x-ray examination of the cervical spine taken 12 days postoperatively showed good alignment (Fig. 40E). He is pictured in skeletal traction with another football player who sustained a chronic subdural hematoma (Fig. 13B).

Comment. This injury occurred in the position of forced cervical flexion and the football player was extremely fortunate not to have totally transected his cervical spinal cord. Initially he sustained an acute central cervical cord injury and recovered complete function except for a residual C7 nerve root impairment.

This type of insidious progressive lesion has been seen by this author on several occasions. Serial postinjury x-ray examinations are the only method of excluding such gradual progressive subluxation with symptoms, with or without neurologic deficit. In this instance cautious decompression of the nerve root and realignment of the spine with stabilization by posterior cervical spinal fusion was the treatment of choice.

Flexion injuries of the cervical spine are more frequent than is usually recognized. In Canadian football Melvin (33) has described a mechanism of cervical

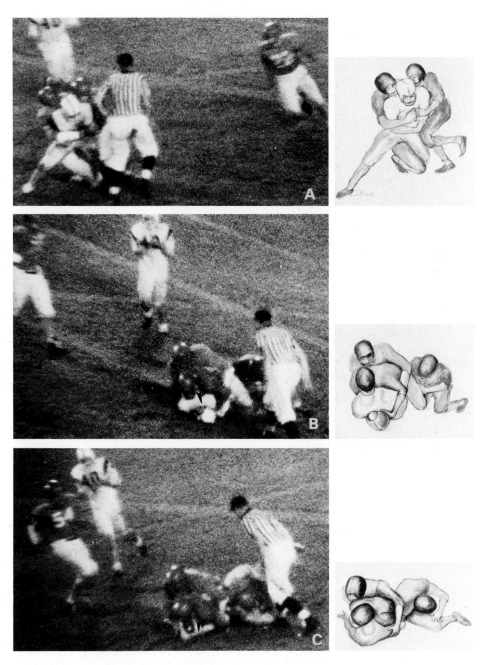

Fig. 40 (A–C). Case 30.

Fig. 40A. The ball carrier in the white shirt is having his arms pinned to his sides.

Fig. 40B. As the referee steps back the third tackler strikes helping to drive the ball carrier's neck into the ground in flexion (arrow).

Fig. 40C. The ball carrier's head seems to have disappeared into the ground. The shoulders are resting directly on the turf (arrow).

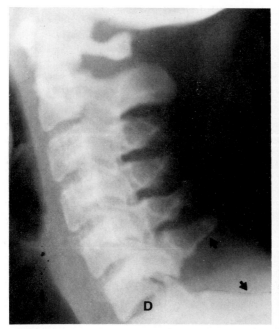
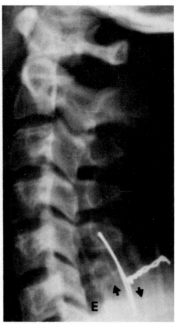

Fig. 40, D and E. Case 30. (Reprinted from Schneider, R. C.: Cervical Spine and Spinal Cord Injuries. *Mich. Med.*, *63:* 773, 1964.)

Fig. 40D. The lateral x-ray shows a fracture-dislocation of C6 on C7 vertebral body with bilateral facet subluxation and a separation between the C6 and C7 spinous processes suggesting an interspinous ligamentous tear (arrows).

Fig. 40E. This x-ray demonstrates realignment of the cervical spine with stability achieved by wire support and posterior cervical bony fusion.

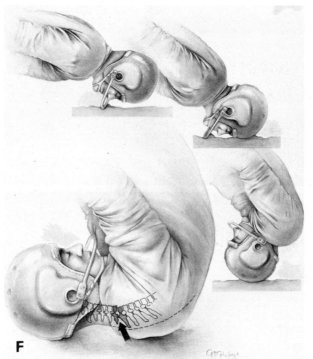

Fig. 40F. Melvin's mechanism of forced flexion of the cervical spine due to impingement of the face guard in mud is shown. The football player with the single face guard may catch the guard in the mud. In spite of desperate attempts to hold the head up and neck in hyperextension there is forced flexion culminating in interspinous ligamentous tear and a fracture-dislocation of the cervical spine usually at the C6-C7 intervertebral space.

hyperflexion due to the single bar face guard catching on the muddy ground. Although his players had been instructed to fall with their heads and necks in hyperextension, their single bar face guards were caught in the ground preventing any attempt at cervical hyperextension. With "forced flexion" they sustained fracture-dislocation injuries (Fig. 40F). This mechanism was responsible for cervical injuries in three of his players resulting in similar fracture-dislocations without neurologic deficits within one year.

Not all cases of cervical flexion injuries terminate so fortunately. One of the more tragic ones is presented here.

Case 31. A 24 year old college football player endeavored to block an onrushing fast halfback (Fig. 41A) by charging forward, thrusting his head downward between the halfback's knees (Fig. 41B). This maneuver transiently rocked the ball carrier backward on his heels only to have him regain momentum and fall down on the blocker who sustained an immediate complete areflexic tetraplegia with a sensory level at the C4 dermatome.

The injured player was placed in traction and carefully transported to the hospital where x-rays disclosed a compression fracture-dislocation at the C4 on C5 vertebra (Fig. 41C). Several hours later a complete cervical laminectomy of C3 through C6 vertebrae was performed and upon opening the dura the spinal cord was noted to be incompletely severed by the posterior margin of the displaced C5 vertebral body. Postoperatively there was no improvement in his neurologic status. A tracheostomy was performed and his respirations were supported with a Bird respirator. Three weeks postoperatively he developed tarry stools, and because of a continually falling hematocrit, he required 60 units of blood during the next 12 days. Seven weeks after his injury, he had a suture ligation of a bleeding gastroduodenal ulcer accompanied by

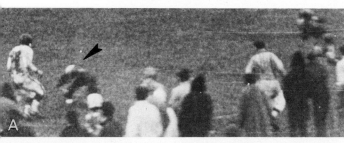

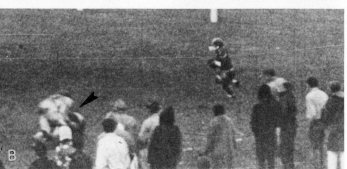

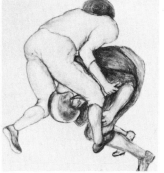

Fig. 41, A and B. Case 31.

Fig. 41A. This shows the low crouch of the black shirted blocker (arrow).

Fig. 41B. The neck is bowed in flexion as the head is driven between the ball carrier's legs (arrow).

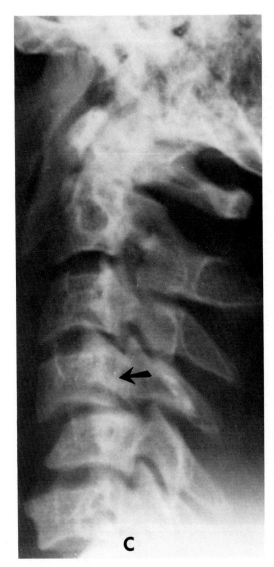

Fig. 41C. Case 31. The cervical spine x-ray
demonstrates a marked fracture-dislocation
of C4 on C5 vertebral body.

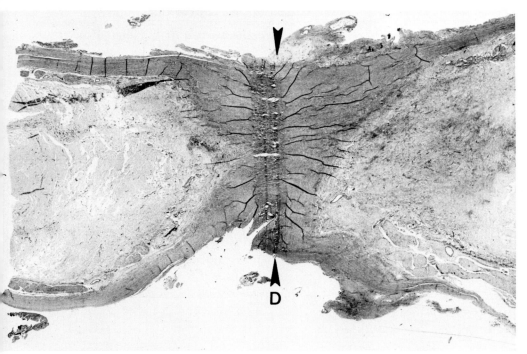

Fig. 41D. Case 31. The microphotograph of a healed transected spinal cord of the high school football player, who died 5 weeks after sustaining an immediate complete paralysis, is shown to demonstrate the thick scar (arrows) which is not traversed by any functional fibers. *With transection there is no regeneration of the spinal cord and no recovery.*

vagotomy, pyloroplasty, and gastrostomy for control of the gastrointestinal bleeding. He subsequently developed air hunger, jaundice, hypotension, and cyanosis and died 2 months after his injury.

At postmortem examination the cervical spinal cord was found to be grossly damaged. Microscopically at the C5 vertebra there was destruction of the neural tissue with gliosis and granulation tissue formation involving the entire width of the cord (Fig. 41D). His immediate cause of death was the hemorrhagic and confluent pneumonitis. Vagotomy appeared complete and the pyloroplasty and gastrostomy were intact. There was no residual duodenal ulcer.

Comment. This case demonstrates the folly of blocking with the head and neck in cervical flexion. In general such an injury should be avoidable with proper coaching techniques. The case is reported rather completely to demonstrate the valiant efforts made by physicians to save a lad who had irreparable damage to his cervical spinal cord and who was doomed to a life of complete paralysis in all four extremities and trunk if he had survived. Occasionally the emotional pressures of our society force the surgeons onward to futile measures in such a hopeless situation. There is no more graphic display of spinal cord damage than the marked scar formation seen here at the site of injury,explaining why the damaged spinal cord in man does not regenerate.

"Stick-Blocking" or "Spearing"

Probably the most single devastating technique to arise as a result of the protection afforded by the plastic helmet and its face guard has been "stick-blocking." The rigid helmet is used as an offensive weapon. "Stick-blocking" consists of the defense man's face being planted directly on the numerals of the offensive man's midsection. If he is carrying the ball, the target for the head is directly on the ball. The head and neck are thrown upward into hyperextension so that the blow may be absorbed by the defensive man with the least chance of injury to himself. Presumably the offensive player will receive a resounding jolt in his abdomen effectively eliminating him from the play or, if he is the ball carrier, cause him to drop the ball. If the defense man is a potential tackler he makes no attempt to throw his arms around the player in the old fashioned tackle, but having done his job merely drops to the ground as his teammates pile on in a "gang-tackling" maneuver.

The author has discussed this practice with coaches. Their comment is that here is the "finest balanced defensive technique ever devised in football. It is perfect."

The term "spearing" refers to the technique of a defensive man driving his head downward and forward into an offensive opponent who is already grounded. The definition means little for the identical mechanism of injury as described in *"stick-blocking"* exists and the same tragic result may occur.

> **Case 32.** In this college game the black shirted offense man (arrow) was almost at a standstill while his teammate was being tackled off on his right flank when a fast moving defense man charged directly into him head on. As the latter struck him he drove his plastic helmet upward abruptly under his opponent's chin (Fig. 42, A–C). With the upward impact of the head there was a simultaneous upward swing of the arms and trunk. As the dark shirted offense man fell over backward in severe hyperextension, the vicious blocker's arm swung upward making it appear to the referee that he had struck his opponent on the chin with his fist (Fig. 42D, arrow). The blocker was ejected from the game for a personal foul. The injured player had his teeth chipped due to the impact.

Comment. This "stick-block" was a perfect one, for the blocker's body did follow a complete arc as he straightened upward. That it was a most efficient technique is seen in the photographs. One may see how difficult it is for an official to determine whether actual slugging happened because of the rapidity with which this vicious block occurred. Actually the defense man's head was responsible for the damage and not the upward driving arm.

Acute Massive Cerebral Displacement*

When a football player runs head on into an opponent who is charging directly at him, the impact may cause instantaneous respiratory or cardiac arrest. The mechanism for such an injury whether due to "stick-blocking" or "spearing" may involve impairment of the vascular supply to the brain stem. There may be diffi-

---

* The following discussion and Cases 33 and 34 are reprinted from Schneider et al. (46), by permission of the *Journal of Neurosurgery*.

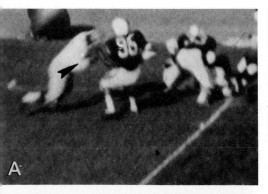

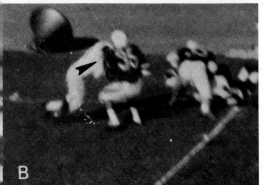

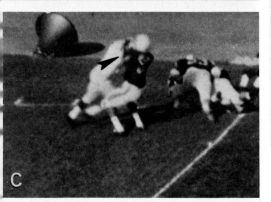

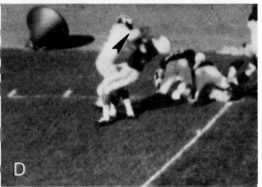

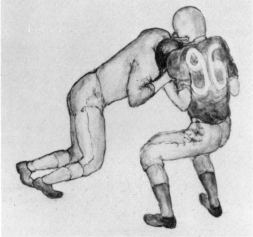

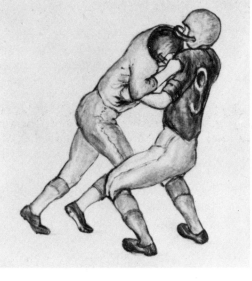

Fig. 42 (A–D). Case 32.

Fig. 42, A and B. The charging white opponent drives his head upward under the face guard of number 96 in a "stick-block."

Fig. 42C. The upward swing or straightening of the blocker's body lends well timed added force as the offensive man is tumbled backward.

Fig. 42D. Number 96 is hurled backward with his head and trunk in hyperextension as the opponent's head and arms fly into the air. The appearance suggests the blocker struck No. 96 with his fist but actually his head has caused the effective blow.

culty in certain cases in differentiating an expanding supratentorial lesion with an uncal herniation from an acute brain stem contusion, infarction, or hemorrhage. Cases 33 and 34 illustrate this problem.

Case 33. This 16 year old high school football player, charging forward with the ball, dove directly into the line, striking the abdomen of an opposing player. He was immediately unconscious and required artifical respiration to initiate breathing. Oxygen was administered as he was rushed to the local hospital where he was found to be semi-comatose, vomiting and with a right hemiplegia. The blood pressure was 110/70, pulse 72, and the labored respirations 24 per minute. The left pupil was 1 to 2 mm. larger than the right. The fundi were normal. The right extremities exhibited spastic extension with hyperreflexia and a right Babinski response. The x-ray films of the skull and cervical spine, including special odontoid views, appeared to be normal. The patient was given mercuhydrin and intramuscular phenergan. A lumbar puncture was performed without difficulty, the spinal fluid was pink and under a pressure of 120 mm. of water.

With a diagnosis made of brain stem contusion and laceration he was placed on a hypothermic regime. Bilateral frontal burr holes were made 36 hours after injury to exclude a supratentorial lesion, and clear colorless fluid under increased pressure was obtained. During the procedure his blood pressure fell, and he progressed to a decerebrate state. Hypotension continued in spite of the administration of vasopressor agents, a careful balancing of his electrolytes and the maintenance of a hypothermic regime with his temperature at 90 degrees. The patient died a week after injury. Autopsy showed a basilar artery thrombosis with infarction of the pons and terminal pneumonia. There was no evidence of any expanding supratentorial lesion other than massive cerebral edema.

Comment. Here the significant factor was the direct transmission of force through the unyielding or non-resilient helmet and the intact skull to the underlying brain causing acute brain stem contusion and basilar artery thrombosis (28, 29).

Case 34. Disparity in Movement of Brain and Cord. A college football linebacker was injured in a scrimmage when he made a head-on tackle leaving the ground and striking a hard-driving ball carrier directly in the abdomen (Fig. 43, A and B). He had an immediate cardiac and respiratory arrest with complete apnea for 20 minutes, but with the aid of cardiopulmonary resuscitation in the form of intracardiac adrenalin and external cardiac massage he regained spontaneous respirations and a cardiac rhythm within an hour at the local hospital. The patient was then transferred to another hospital where an examination revealed an areflexic tetraplegia with no response to painful stimuli. His pupils were equal, and he opened his eyes occasionally. There was frequent irregular twitching of the face and neck muscles, and he had only diaphragmatic respirations. The patient's skull and cervical spine x-ray films revealed no lesion. Although there was an equivocal cardiac enlargement in the chest film, the electrocardiogram was normal. A tracheostomy was performed and a frothy material aspirated from the intratracheal tube. A respirator was used, but he died 17½ hours after injury.

At postmortem examination there was no evidence of any expanding intra-

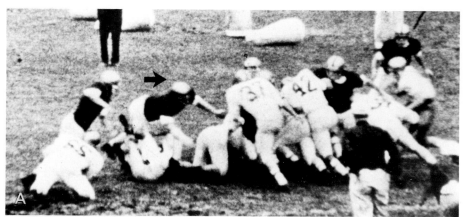

Fig. 43A. Case 34. The defensive tackler (arrow) is beginning to leave his feet to strike the oncoming ball carrier.

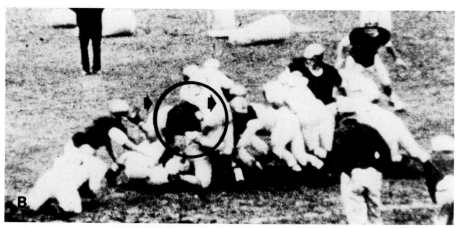

Fig. 43B. Case 34. The tackling player (arrow) has left his feet plunging "head-on" into the ball carrier, striking him so hard that the tackler's head almost appears imbedded in his opponent's abdomen.

cranial hemorrhage. There was bilateral uncal herniation with midbrain compression due to cerebral edema. Pathological sections of the cerebellum showed the type of necrosis in the Purkinje cell layer of the cerebellum characteristic of hypoxia (Fig. 43, C and D). Sections of the cervical spinal cord demonstrated recent traumatic contusion with hemorrhage and necrosis at the C1-C2 level approximately 3 cm. below the medulla (Fig. 43E). These bilateral lesions were in the ventrolateral reticulospinal tract which has a role in normal respiration.

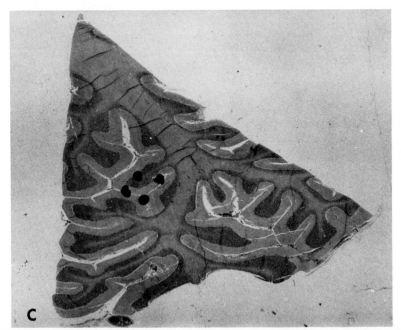

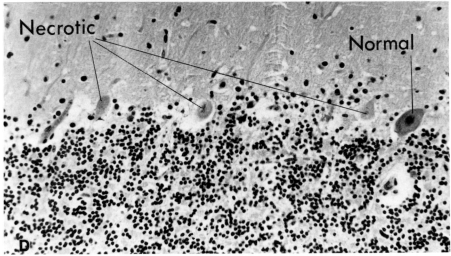

Fig. 43, C and D. Case 34.

Fig. 43C. The study area of the microscopic specimen from the cerebellum is outlined in dots.

Fig. 43D. The pathologic section exhibited the type of necrosis (destruction) in the Purkinje cell layer characteristic of hypoxia (lack of oxygen).

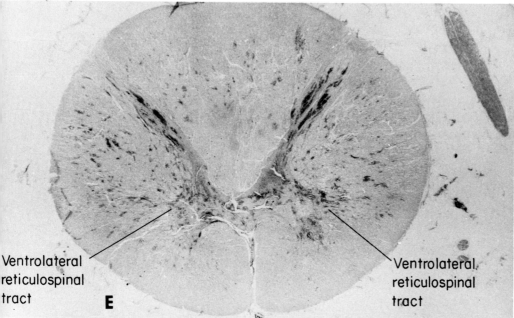

Ventrolateral
reticulospinal
tract

Ventrolateral
reticulospinal
tract

E

Fig. 43E. Case 34. This section of the spinal cord at the second cervical level demonstrates the multiple linear and petechial hemorrhages throughout both the grey and white matter. The bilateral involvement of the region of the ventrolateral reticulospinal tract (the descending respiratory pathway) could be responsible for the patient's death without any other neurologic involvement. [Reprinted from Schneider et al. (46), by permission of the *Journal of Neurosurgery*.]

Comment. The significant kinematic factor in this injury is the tremendous transmission of force on the vertex impact from the hemispheres of the brain to the medulla and upper cervical spinal cord.

At least three isolated or concurrent factors may be present in such cases. Initially the brain moves *en masse* in a cephalad direction but then on impact rebounds (Fig. 43F, see 1) forcing the cerebral hemispheres caudalward so that the uncus is acutely thrust through the tentorial notch (46). This mechanism will cause compression of the posterior cerebral arteries (and possibly even the more caudal superior cerebellar arteries) and result in hypoxia of the cerebral hemispheres and the brain stem (17). The massive caudal shift of the cerebral hemispheres (46) may also transiently occlude the readily compressible subrarachnoid space, straight, and lateral venous sinuses (Fig. 43, see 2) confluens, and thin-walled bridging veins such as the vein of Labbé. The combination of cerebral hypoxia and simultaneous impairment of venous drainage may cause sudden massive cerebral edema and result in the rapid development of a tentorial pressure cone and death.

Superimposed upon this supratentorial problem is a second one, namely, the massive shift of the cerebellum and the lower brain stem during direct vertex impact. The caudal displacement of the cerebellar tonsils through the foramen magnum simultaneously creates a cerebellar pressure cone with direct compression of the cardiac and respiratory centers in the medulla (Fig. 43, see 3) and vascular spasm or compression of the vertebral arteries at the foramen magnum (Fig. 43,

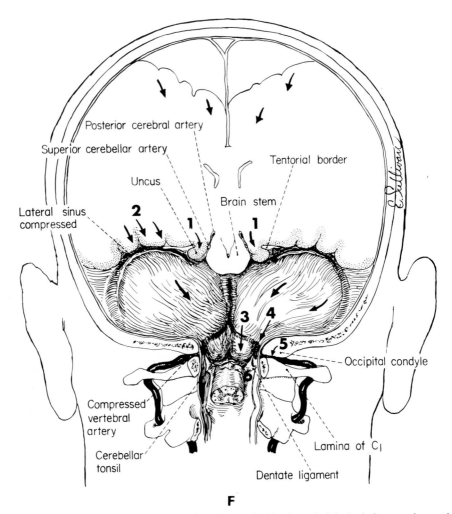

F

Fig. 43F. Case 34. The dynamic mechanisms involved with rebound of the brain in vertex impact injuries are shown: the acute tentorial pressure cone with the uncal herniation (1) compressing the posterior cerebral artery, superior cerebellar artery, and brain stem; (2) the obliteration of the subarachnoid space, bridging veins and lateral sinuses; the acute cerebellar pressure cone (3) with compression of the medullary centers and the vertebral arteries at foramen magnum (4); there may be concomitant occlusion of vertebral arteries between the occipital condyles and C1 laminae (5); the gradient of forces between the thrust of the freely moving brain caudalward and the fixation of the cervical spinal cord by the dentate ligaments (6), resulting in distortion of the cord with petechial hemorrhages. [Reprinted from Schneider et al. (46), by permission of the *Journal of Neurosurgery*.]

see 4). The impact may also cause compression of the vertebral arteries by the occipital condyles against the C1 laminae (Fig. 43, see 5), resulting in further vascular insufficiency as in Case 32. Lindenberg (30) has noted entrapment of the basilar artery in a fracture of the occipital region and Loop et al. (32) have shown a similar ensnaring of the basilar artery in a clival fracture. However, blunt trauma to these vessels on impact may be sufficient to cause damage (Case 27) (21).

A third factor must be specifically considered. With the massive thrust developed on vertex impact, there is a disparity between the marked degree of distortion of the freely movable brain in the intracranial cavity and the relatively fixed upper spinal cord which is rigidly held by the dentate ligaments in the narrow bony canal (Fig. 43, see 6). It was postulated that there was a differential gradient of pressures and the interface of such forces would be at the C1-C2 level directly at the site where the petechial hemorrhages (2) were found in this case (Fig. 43, see 7). Brieg (9) has shown in cadavers that the dentate ligaments anchoring the cervical spinal cord to some degree prevent movement in the cephalad and caudal directions as contrasted to mobility in the anterior and posterior planes of the spinal canal.

Further experimental work by Gosch *et al.* (see Chapter 14) and clinical research will be presented which confirms these concepts and duplicates the lesion seen in Case 34.

The coaches and trainers who have viewed these sequences on the mechanisms of injury have commented that it is impossible to play football without applying these techniques. The enforcement of the rule on clutching the face mask, which was already on the books, has already substantially decreased some cervical injuries. *A similar enforcement of the rule of abolishing "stick-blocking" or "spearing," which has been in the rule books for several years, would avoid many of the fatalities or severe brain cripples due to cervical spinal cord transections and acute subdural hemorrhages, two of the leading causes of tragedy. Lip service has been given to such enforcement, but there has been no decisive action by the coaches and other officials.*

References

1. Bachs, A., Barraquer-Bordas, L., Barrarquer-Ferrers, L., Canadell, J. M. and Modolell, A.: Delayed Myelopathy following Atlanto-Axial Dislocation by Separated Odontoid Process. *Brain*, *78:* 537, 1955.
2. Bailey, P.: Traumatic Hemorrhages into the Spinal Cord. *Med. Rec.*, *57:* 573, 1900.
3. Baldwin, M.: Personal communication.
4. Bell, H. S.: Basilar Artery Insufficiency Due to Atlanto-occipital Instability. *Amer. Surg.*, *35:* 695 1969.
5. Bell, H. S.: Paralysis of Both Arms from Injury of the Pyramidal Decussation: "Cruciate Paralysis." *J. Neurosurg.*, *33:* 376, 1970.
6. Biemond, A.: Thrombosis of Basilar Artery and Vascularization of the Brain Stem. *Brain*, *74:* 300, 1951.
7. Blaine, E. S.: Manipulative (Chiropractic) Dislocations of the Atlas. *J.A.M.A.*, *85:* 1356, 1925.
8. Boldrey, E., Maas, L. and Miller, R. R.: Role of Atlantoid Compression in Etiology of Internal Carotid Artery Thrombosis. *J. Neurosurg.*, *13:* 127, 1956.
9. Brieg, A.: *Biomechanics of the Central Nervous System*. Monograph, Almqvist & Wiksells, Stockholm, 1960.
10. Carpenter, S.: Injury of Neck as Cause of Vertebral Artery Thrombosis. *J. Neurosurg.*, *18:* 849, 1961.
11. Contostavlos, D. L.: Massive Subarachnoid Hemorrhage Due to Laceration of the Vertebral Artery Associated with Fracture of the Transverse Process of the Atlas. *J. Forensic Sci.*, *16:* 40, 1971.
12. Crosby, E. C., Humphrey, T. and Lauer, E. W.: *Correlative Anatomy of the Nervous System*. The Macmillan Company, New York, 1962.

13. Currier, R. D., Schneider, R. C. and Preston, R. E.: Angiographic Findings in Wallenberg's Lateral Medullary Syndrome. *J. Neurosurg., 19:* 1058, 1962.
14. DeKleyn, A. and Nieuwenhuyse, P.: Schwindelanfälle und Nystagmus bei einer bestimmten Stellung des Kopfes. *Acta Otolaryngol., 11:* 155, 1927.
15. Ford, F. R.: Syncope, Vertigo and Disturbances of Vision Resulting from Intermittent Obstruction of the Vertebral Arteries Due to Defect in the Odontoid Process and Excessive Mobility of the Second Cervical Vertebra. *Bull. Johns Hopkins Hospital, 91:* 168, 1952.
16. Ford, F. R. and Clark, D.: Thrombosis of the Basilar Artery with Softenings in the Cerebellum and Brain Stem Due to Manipulation of the Neck. A Report of Two Cases with One Post-mortem Examination. Reasons are Given to Prove that Damage to the Vertebral Arteries Is Responsible. *Bull. Johns Hopkins Hosp., 98:* 37, 1956.
17. Gabrielsen, T. O. and Amundsen, P.: The Pontine Arteries in Vertebral Angiography. *Am. J. Roentgenol., 106:* 296, 1969.
18. Gillilan, L. A.: Veins of the Spinal Cord. Anatomic Details; Suggested Clinical Implications. *Neurology, 20:* 860, 1970.
19. Green, D. and Joynt, R. J.: Vascular Accidents to the Brain Stem Associated with Neck Manipulations. *J.A.M.A., 170:* 522, 1959.
20. Grinker, R. R. and Guy, C. C.: Sprain of the Cervical Spine with Thrombosis of the Anterior Spinal Artery. *J.A.M.A., 88:* 1140, 1927.
21. Gurdjian, E. S., Hardy, W. G., Lindner, D. W. and Thomas, L. M.: Closed Cervical Cranial Trauma Associated with Involvement of Carotid and Vertebral Arteries. *J. Neurosurg., 20:* 418, 1963.
22. Herren, R. and Alexander, L.: Sulcal and Intrinsic Blood Vessels of the Human Spinal Cord. *Arch. Neurol. Psychiatry, 41:* 678, 1939.
23. Holzer, F. J.: Verschluss der Wirbelsaulenschlagader am Kopfgelenk mit nachfolgender Thrombose durch Seitwartsdrehen des Kopfes. Eine Gefahr bei Operationen am Hals mit starker Seitwartsdrehung. *Dtsch. Gesamte Gerichtl. Med., 44:* 422, 1955.
24. Hutchinson, E. C. and Yates, P. O.: The Cervical Portion of the Vertebral Artery. A Clinico-Pathological Study. *Brain, 79:* 319, 1956.
25. Kahn, E. A. and Yglesias, L.: Progressive Atlanto-Axial Dislocation. *J.A.M.A., 105:* 348, 1935.
26. Kahn, E. A.: The Role of the Dentate Ligaments in Spinal Cord Compression and the Syndrome of Lateral Sclerosis. *J. Neurosurg., 4:* 191, 1947.
27. Kunkle, E. C., Muller, J. C. and Odom, G. L.: Traumatic Brain Stem Thrombosis: Report of a Case and Analysis of the Mechanism of Injury. *Ann. Intern. Med., 36:* 1329, 1952.
28. Lindenberg, R.: Compression of Brain Arteries as a Pathogenic Factor for Tissue Necroses and their Areas of Predilection. *J. Neuropathol. Exp. Neurol., 14:* 223, 1955.
29. Lindenberg, R.: Significance of the Tentorium in Head Injuries from Blunt Forces. *Clin. Neurosurg., 12:* 129, 1966.
30. Lindenberg, R.: Incarceration of a Vertebral Artery in the Cleft of a Longitudinal Fracture of the Skull. *J. Neurosurg., 24:* 908, 1966.
31. Liss, L.: Fatal Cervical Cord Injury in a Swimmer. *Neurology, 15:* 675, 1965.
32. Loop, J. W., White, L. E. and Shaw, C. M.: Traumatic Occlusion of the Basilar Artery within a Clivus Fracture. *Radiology, 83:* 36, 1964.
33. Melvin, W. J. S., Dunlop, H. W., Hetherington, R. F. and Kerr, J. W.: The Role of the Faceguard in the Production of Flexion Injuries to the Cervical Spine in Football. *Can. Med. Assoc. J., 93:* 1110, 1965.
34. Nielsen, J. M.: *A Textbook of Clinical Neurology,* 1st ed. Paul B. Hoeber, New York, 1941.
35. Pratt-Thomas, H. R. and Berger, K. E.: Cerebellar and Spinal Injuries After Chiropractic Manipulation. *J.A.M.A., 133:* 600, 1947.
35a. Russell, W. R. and Nathan, P. W.: Traumatic amnesia. *Brain, 69:* 280, 1946.
36. Schneider, R. C.: A Syndrome in Acute Cervical Injuries for Which Early Operation Is Indicated. *J. Neurosurg., 8:* 360, 1951.
37. Schneider, R. C., Cherry, G. and Pantek, H.: The Syndrome of Acute Central Cervical Spinal Cord Injury. *J. Neurosurg., 11:* 546, 1954.
38. Schneider, R. C.: The Syndrome of Acute Anterior Cervical Spinal Cord Injury. *J. Neurosurg., 12:* 95, 1955.

39. Schneider, R. C. and Kahn, E. A.: Chronic Sequelae of Spine and Spinal Cord Trauma. I. The Significance of the Acute "Tear-drop" Fracture. *J. Bone Joint Surg., 38A:* 985, 1956.
40. Schneider, R. C., Thompson, J. M. and Bebin, J.: The Syndrome of Acute Central Cervical Spinal Cord Injury. *J. Neurol. Neurosurg. Psychiatry, 21:* 216, 1958.
41. Schneider, R. C. and Crosby, E. C.: Vascular Insufficiency of the Brain Stem and Spinal Cord in Spinal Trauma. *Neurology, 9:* 643, 1959.
42. Schneider, R. C. and Schemm, G. W.: Vertebral Artery Insufficiency in Acute and Chronic Spinal Trauma. *J. Neurosurg., 18:* 348, 1961.
43. Schneider, R. C., Reifel, E., Crisler, H. O. and Oosterbaan, B. G.: Serious and Fatal Football Injuries Involving the Head and Spinal Cord. *J.A.M.A., 177:* 362, 1961.
44. Schneider, R. C.: Serious and Fatal Neurosurgical Football Injuries. *Clin. Neurosurg., 12:* 226, 1966.
45. Schneider, R. C.: Craniocerebral Trauma and Trauma to the Spine and Spinal Cord. In *Correlative Neurosurgery*, 2nd ed., edited by E. A. Kahn, E. C. Crosby, R. C. Schneider and J. A. Taren, Chap. 25 and 26. Charles C Thomas, Publisher, Springfield, Ill., 1969.
46. Schneider, R. C., Gosch, H. H., Norrell, H., Jerva, M., Combs, L. W. and Smith, R. A.: Vascular Insufficiency and Differential Distortion of Brain and Cord Caused by Cervicomedullary Football Injuries. *J. Neurosurg., 33:* 363, 1970.
47. Schneider, R. C., Gosch, H. H., Taren, J. A., Ferry, D. J. and Jerva, M. J.: Blood Vessel Trauma following Head and Neck Injuries. *Clin. Neurosurg., 19:* 312, 1972.
48. Schneider, R. C., Crosby, E. C., Russo, R. H., and Gosch, H. H.: Traumatic Spinal Cord Syndromes and Their Management. *Clin. Neurosurg., 20:* in press, 1973.
49. Schwarz, G. A., Geiger, J. K. and Spano, A. G.: Posterior Inferior Cerebellar Artery Syndrome of Wallenberg After Chiropractic Manipulation. *Arch. Intern. Med., 97:* 352, 1956.
50. Sherk, H. H. and Nicholson, J. T.: Fractures of the Atlas. *J. Bone Joint Surg., 52-A:* 1017, 1970.
51. Simeone, F. A. and Goldberg, H. I.: Thrombosis of Vertebral Artery from Hyperextension Injury to the Neck. *J. Neurosurg., 29:* 540, 1968.
52. Stopford, J. S. B.: The Arteries of the Pons and Medulla Oblongata. *J. Anat., 50:* 131, 1916.
53. Stopford, J. S. B.: The Arteries of the Pons and Medulla. Part II. *J. Anat., 50:* 255, 1916.
54. Suechting, R. L. and French, L. A.: Posterior Inferior Cerebellar Artery Syndrome following a Fracture of the Cervical Vertebra. *J. Neurosurg., 12:* 187, 1955.
55. Tatlow, W. F. T. and Bammer, H. G.: Syndrome of Vertebral Artery Compression. *Neurology, 7:* 331, 1957.
56. Taylor, A. R.: The Mechanism of Injury to the Spinal Cord in the Neck Without Damage to the Vertebral Column. *J. Bone Joint Surg., 33-B:* 543, 1951.
57. Turnbull, I. M., Brieg, A. and Hassler, O.: Blood Supply of Cervical Spinal Cord in Man. A Microangiographic Cadaver Study. *J. Neurosurg., 24:* 951, 1966.
58. Turnbull, I. M.: Microvasculature of the Human Spinal Cord. *J. Neurosurg., 35:* 141, 1971.
59. Wallenberg, A.: Nerve Fortschritte in der topischen Diagnostik des Pons und der Oblongata. *Dtsch. Z. Nervenheilkd. 41:* 8, 1911.
60. Yates, P. O.: Birth Trauma to the Vertebral Arteries. *Arch. Dis. Child., 34:* 436, 1969.
61. Zülch, K. F.: Mangeldurchblutung an der Grenzzone zweier Getässgebiete als Ursache ungeklärter Rückenmarks schädigen. *Dtsch. Z. Nervenheilkd., 172:* 81, 1954.

chapter seven

Head and Spinal Injuries in Rugby

There has been a growing belief that the armor with which we have clothed the present-day football player may be dangerous. This author has often been asked whether the rugby player is less frequently injured and it seems pertinent to include the meager data which he has gleaned for this response. The rugby player is prohibited by the Laws of the Game from "wearing protective clothing unless the refereee is satisfied that a player requires protection following injury and that the protective pad is not of hard material" (3). For this reason this author contacted the Medical Officer to the Rugby School, J. P. Sparks (9), Mr. Anthony Jefferson, a Sheffield neurosurgeon (5) and Secretaries of the Rugby Football League and/or Unions of England (2, 8), Ireland (3), Scotland (6), and Wales (1) to endeavor to procure statistics of how many rugby players had sustained head and spinal cord injuries during the five year period 1959 to 1964, the interval covered by our statistical football study in the United States. These gentlemen were all most cooperative in presenting their data and this author is greatly indebted to them for this material. Actually the inquiries concerning this topic no doubt startled many of our good friends and colleagues in Great Britain for it was evident that the subject of rugby injuries had not been regarded as being of sufficient interest and importance to warrant special attention. These data have been prepared to stress our own rather unrealistic viewpoint of sports in the United States.

At the outset it should be noted that there are really two different games — rugby football and the game of "rugby league" which is played chiefly in Lancashire and Yorkshire. The latter game differs somewhat in the rules and the composition of the teams; it is played professionally and therefore is different from rugby football. The game is said to be the roughest professional sporting activity in Great Britain. Furthermore, although tackling is performed in rugby, it proceeds in the direction of the player's forward motion. Therefore if the head strikes an opponent it is a glancing or tangential blow to the side of the man carrying the ball rather than by the direct vertex or "head-on" tackling, which is used in the United States and Canada in football.

England

The Medical Officer to the Rugby School, Dr. J. P. Sparks (9), has kindly granted me permission to present an abstract of his injury statistics for the five year interval, 1951 to 1955. During this period he estimated that 630 boarding students between the ages of 13 and 18 years of age played 100,000 boy/game hours with 2046 injuries, most of which were relatively minor ones of all types. From the neurosurgical standpoint there were 99 concussions but these were very mild. There was one player who sustained a spinous process fracture and another player had developed a ruptured lumbar disc. No skull fractures or intracranial hemorrhages were encountered. Mr. Sparks stated: "Injuries to the vertebral column or spinal cord are exceptionally rare at Rugby football. In the last 15 years (prior to 1964) I have only heard of two deaths from injury to the head and neck and spine among thousands of schoolboys in the British Isles." Dr. Sparks then stated that one of these cases was that of a player at Dulwich College who sustained a fracture of the spine with tetraplegia and a delayed death. The second fatal case was that of a 15 year old boy with a congenitally thin skull. It had been reported by Dr. T. A. A. Hunter (4), the Medical Officer for Marlborough College Wiltshire, who was contacted about this case.

Dr. Hunter commented that at the time Marlborough was a residential school with 800 boys ranging from 13 to 19 years of age, each of whom would play two games of rugby a week for the 13 week term. There is a routine arrangement that any boy who sustains a head injury involving any interference with consciousness, a concussion, is admitted to the school sanatorium and kept under observation for at least 24 hours. In two years there were 11 such cases of uncomplicated cerebral concussion admitted without any serious sequelae. In the entire 17 years there, he had never seen a spinal injury and had admitted but one complicated head injury. This was a 16 year old boy. "He tackled an opponent while he was kicking the ball and his temple made contact with the moving knee. An hour after admission to the infirmary he became restless and developed irregular pupils. He died in an ambulance on the way to the hospital half an hour after the onset of the above symptoms. An autopsy revealed a very large extradural hemorrhage from a middle meningeal artery." It should be noted that the nearest neurosurgical unit was 40 miles away.

From Mr. Fallowfield (2), the Secretary of Rugby League Football of England, Mr. Anthony Jefferson (5), one of England's distinguished neurosurgeons, received permission to communicate with the insurance company which is responsible for the injury coverage of the League, Mr. Jefferson procured the lists of injuries from 1953 to 1962 with lists of the diagnoses. There was a total number of 3845 injuries of all types for this interval. The neurosurgical diagnoses could be broken down into "concussions" 49; "head injuries," 73; and "neck injuries," 44. Emphasis should be placed on the fact that during this 10 year interval there were in the second category, "head injuries," only five serious or possibly fatal neurosurgical injuries listed: "hemorrhage of the brain," 3; and "fracture of the skull," 2. Unfortunately there were no man/game hour estimates similar to those available from the Rugby School report. To seek a further breakdown of this data by Mr. Jefferson seemed to this author to be an excessive request, since he had recollections of the two years devoted to collecting his own data on American football statistics.

In 1964 Potter (7) reported that of 1500 head injuries admitted to the Radcliffe Infirmary, Oxford, in the year 1963 to 1964, there were 10 rugby players, none of whom apparently sustained any serious neurosurgical injury.

Ireland

In response to an inquiry word was received from Mr. R. Fitzgerald (3), Secretary of the Irish Rugby Football Union, indicating that the incidence of head and spinal cord injury was low in Ireland. During the five years (1959–1963) with 10,000 players participating per season, there were nine serious head and spinal cord injuries recorded: fracture dislocation of the cervical spine without residual paralysis, 2; fracture dislocation of the cervical spine with quadriplegia, 3, with 2 fatalities; depressed fracture of parietal area, 1; depressed fracture of anterior wall of frontal sinus, 1. Two other injuries were not recorded by diagnosis. Of the total of nine cases, three of these had resulted in fatalities.

Scotland

The Secretary of the Scottish Rugby Union, Mr. John Law (6), reported that in the decade 1955 to 1965, he could only recall one fatal accident. "The player careened, . . . was injured when a scrimmage collapsed . . . the injury which was to his spinal column proved fatal and he died in the Royal Infirmary, Edinburgh within a day or so." As to the incidence of play: "Approximately 11,000 individuals play Rugby in club football in Scotland and it is also played at many of our schools."

Wales

From Mr. W. H. Clement (1), the Secretary of the Welsh Rugby Union: "It was estimated that, from School to Senior level, between 18,000 to 20,000 players play Rugby Union football at least once per week during September to April (inclusive) annually. An Injury Registry was just being developed in connection with insurance matters that year (1964)."

From World War II (1945–1964) there had been four serious neurosurgical rugby injuries in Wales: fractures of cervical spine, 2 (complete permanent paralysis, 1, partial residual paralysis, 1); head injuries, 2. "In both these cases the injured players died, but it was established that one of these players suffered from an inherent head weakness and that consequently, the injury merely accelerated the death and was not the cause." The etiologies remain unknown.

Summary

It is apparent that a true comparison of the incidence of serious and fatal neurosurgical injuries cannot be made between rugby and American football because of the differences in man/game hours and the variations in the methods of defense in halting the opponent in the two sports. However, it does seem abundantly clear that the unprotected head and neck of the rugby player in the British Isles, similarly to the sandlot football player in the United States, fares better than the currently protected American football players with hard shell helmets which lack sufficient resiliency to dissipate the impact of a blow.

References

1. Clement, W. H., Secretary, Welsh Rugby Union: Personal communication, October 28, 1964.
2. Fallowfield, W., Secretary, English Rugby Football League: Personal communication to Mr. Anthony Jefferson, November 1, 1962.
3. Fitzgerald, R., Secretary, Irish Rugby Football Union: Personal communication, December 8, 1964.
4. Hunter, T. A. A., Medical Officer, Marlborough College, Marlborough, Wiltshire: Personal communication October 16, 1964.
5. Jefferson, A., Sheffield, England: Personal communication. January 8, 1965.
6. Law, J., Secretary, Scottish Rugby Union: Personal communication, October 19, 1964.
7. Potter, J., *Head Injuries in Students*, p. 30, British Student Health Association—16th Conference, Oxford, 1964.
8. Prescott, R. E., Secretary, English Rugby Union: Personal communication, October 19, 1964.
9. Sparks, J. P., Medical Officer of the Rugby School: Personal communications, October 8, 1964.

chapter eight

The Psychological Aspects of Football

ROBERT A. MOORE, M.D. AND
RICHARD C. SCHNEIDER, M.D.

In any sport the psychological factors are as important or perhaps even of greater significance than the physical ones; this is particularly true in a team sport such as football (3). All good coaches and trainers are obviously keenly aware of this problem and often resort to varied techniques in an effort to procure the maximum of a team's potential at crucial times. Perhaps there may be the attention to finer details such as a key player's mental attitude before a weekend game, for he may require reassurance and the instillation of a feeling of security or aggressiveness to achieve his finest performance. Or perhaps the coach may have to decide whether the player has a bona fide injury. Frequently the physician must participate in many complex psychological situations and serve as a consultant to the coach or trainer in order to provide an understanding analysis of the player's physical and emotional problems. The failure of these three individuals to cooperate and achieve a harmonious relationship with regard to the athletes' basic difficulties may result not only in a physical but also sometimes an even more significant psychological or psychiatric catastrophe (4, 5).

In 1960 Moore made the following statements (2). "In our increasingly 'civilized,' that is, constricted and repressive culture, we find ourselves having to give up certain personal freedoms for the general good of society as a whole. Basic biologic drives cannot be given free reign of expression without coming into serious conflict with the taboos of our time (1). We are perhaps more familiar with the limitations of sexual freedom, realizing that random gratification of this natural urge leads to serious and dramatic consequences. Today, we find various diversions of the sexual drive a common symptom in the effort of individuals to reach a compromise between drive and prohibition.

"Less dramatic, but equally important is the conflict over expression of aggressive drives. Our distant cave-dwelling ancestors had no problems here—to be aggressive meant to survive a bit longer. In our times, however, uncontrolled aggressive behavior subjects one to incarceration or extinction, or at least to severe censure. The mature and civilized adult is seen as a calm and composed individual who rises above the strife about him—he sublimates his aggressivity into a useful assertiveness in his social and business conduct . . . ."

"Each growing child must learn how to achieve an uneasy compromise between his urges to be actively aggressive, motor-wise, and his wishes to be pleasing to his parents. The distinction between sexes in the expression of aggression used to be more clear, but today this is blurred with women assuming male prerogatives and men sharing the woman's role in the home in the worship of 'togetherness.' It isn't as easy for the child to know that women are like this and men are like that and as a result we seem to be breeding a generation where men assume more feminine behavior and women more masculine behavior. This makes the definition of what is acceptable aggressive behavior in the boy less easy to achieve. His father likes baseball games, plays golf, but also washes dishes and doesn't always seem as powerful as his mother. His father seems to approve his son's interest in sports and even seems a bit pleased, though outwardly critical, when he gives the boy next door a bloody nose. At the same time, in a middle-class community at least, this will result in considerable conflict with the desire that all the children be 'well-adjusted' that is, 'well controlled.'

"The child soon learns that uncontrolled aggressive behavior brings him not gain but pain as he is punished by withdrawal of love by his parents, by stern criticism from his teachers, and loss of comradeship with his peers. The equation becomes clear: that to express aggression means to receive aggression in return— perhaps greater than the child can tolerate or defend against. The child incorporates this disapproval and so develops guilt and anxiety if he is too aggressive and finally feels uneasy even if he contemplates aggression. He is now civilized.

The Problem of Aggression

"There are two areas where modern man can take off his coat and roll up his sleeves: in war time military service and in competitive sports. In these areas, like the caveman, to be unable to be aggressive may mean a short span of survival. Unfortunately, it is not a simple task to switch suddenly from an existence where aggression is bad to an area of endeavor where aggression is good. Some can do it and some cannot.

"We now turn to the other area where aggression is both permitted and rewarded: competitive athletics. Since participation is voluntary, the situation is not quite similar to war time military service. We would then expect that a distinguishing feature in athletes would be their freedom of restriction in the expression of aggression. Certainly team sports put a high premium on aggressiveness, especially such sports as football and hockey. In addition, the good athlete has a certain confidence that his expression of aggression will not be repaid by overwhelming retaliation, translated into a feeling he will win, or at least not be demolished, even when facing long odds. A football halfback who anticipates with each stride a bruising tackle or a hockey wing who on each rush awaits a hard check will not be very successful.

"Since the athlete is a volunteer, in fact an eager one, it might be expected no problems are to be found here. In the world of the psyche, however, everything is relative, and the degree of this conflict is relative too. The very urge that forces the young athlete to suffer the many long hours of practice with its concomitant wear and tear on his body is an amalgam of his underlying competitiveness and his fear. This is manifested by his conscious pretense that he is not afraid.

"To be athletic is to be manly in our culture. To the adolescent, the epitome of what is masculine is the athlete, with hero worship and mimicry a common phenomenon. As pointed out earlier, perhaps a greater problem in our culture than in others is the difficulty a young boy faces in defining himself as male in contradistinction to female. What better solution could there be than to become an athlete?

Thus we see problems in expression of both aggressive and sexual drives as they face a growing youth about to embark on an athletic career."

Moore then goes on to list possible dangerous situations.

Situations of Potential Danger

"It would be very useful to coaches, team trainers, and team physicians if they could anticipate such situations before they occur. Unfortunately this is a difficult process since hindsight is better than foresight. Still, being aware of this problem may be of some use in understanding the accident-prone athlete or the one whose bruises seem slow to heal. A few possible situations and examples can be listed which should alert one to the possibility of injuries:

"**1.** A situation is loaded where the degree of athletic ability is grossly out of proportion with the individual's willingness to be aggressive. A boy who wants to play so badly but hasn't much ability or a boy with loads of ability who doesn't want to play very badly are good candidates for the injury file."

> **Case 35.** A number of years ago a stocky 20 year old, right-handed college junior sustained numerous blows to the head and body while playing at the guard position during the first two quarters of a football game. At half time the player, who had become progressively more dizzy and drowsy, started to crawl out of the stadium on his hands and knees toward the dressing room. He was then assisted by a trainer and some players to the training room where he was permitted to lie down until the last quarter. The team physician stated the player had never been rendered unconscious but had complained of a "pressure in the left side of the head."
> Upon arrival at the emergency room of the hospital, the player was unresponsive to painful stimuli. Fearing that he had an extradural hemorrhage, the team physician had a neurosurgeon summoned. When the latter examined the player, touching of his eyelids caused slight twitching and, as the sole of his foot was stroked to elicit pathologic reflexes, he suddenly became very alert, kicked strongly, looked at his hands, and then was

completely oriented. Although his neurologic examination was normal, he was admitted to the hospital overnight as a precautionary measure at the request of the team physician. On the following morning he was asymptomatic and he flew back to his university with the squad.

Comment. This was a bona fide case of conversion hysteria. The player rebelled at sustaining such a severe beating. It was learned subsequently that he was an art student and although he was playing football he was doing so only to maintain a scholarship and pay his way through school. Other sources of support were procured for him by the administration. He gave up football and returned happily to his art work.

"**2.** One should be alerted by a family where the boy's ability to be aggressive or his athletic ability is way out of line with that of his father. Every coach has been plagued at one time in his career by the athletically successful father who ambitiously pushes his not-too-capable son into sports, forcing the boy into competition for which he is unprepared. As dangerous may be the situation where a boy's ability and aggressivity are much greater than the father's, so that his superiority puts him into the potentially frightening position of defeating his father. Occasionally a parent has the excellent insight into the situation and takes proper action as is noted in this report of a player involved in the former problem."

Case 36. A college football player, the son of an outstanding intercollegiate player, sustained several relatively minor blows to the head during scrimmage at which time he rolled about on the ground holding his head. Since the boy was well-liked by his teammates and the coach they were particularly concerned about him. Fearing a possible chronic subdural hematoma the team physician referred him to a neurosurgeon. Upon taking a careful history, it was clearly evident that the player was fine during the first day or so of the week, but then headaches developed during the latter part of the week when more body contact occurred in scrimmage. It also was quite obvious that the boy's ability was such that he could never hope to achieve the same fame in football as his father had done. His grades had begun to suffer and he was quite unhappy. The neurosurgeon called the father and explained the situation. The latter agreed the boy should give up football "on doctor's orders." The player took the advice of the neurosurgeon and he immediately became symptom-free. For the next two years he excelled in a minor sport earning several letters and was very happy with his accomplishment.

The following case of delayed recovery from injury illustrates the opposite disparity between father and son.

Case 37. This is a case of a much more successful athlete. He was an outstanding high school football player, much sought after by several colleges before he enrolled at a large university. Despite his great success, he never felt he achieved sufficient acclaim from his father. His father was a rather distant, non-demonstrative man who emphasized the gloomy side of life with the central theme being that their family wasn't meant for big things. An overall picture of passivity pervaded the family with only this boy not fitting the pattern. The much less successful and much less aggressive siblings were given considerably more praise by the father. So the message began to get across to this athlete—the more successfully aggressive he was, the more alien and non-understandable he became to his family. He started off his sophomore year in college by running with the first string before the opening game. Unfortunately, he suffered an injury to his leg and missed the opening game. Somehow, the leg didn't respond to treatment and the discouraged athlete limped through drills with the scrubs, no longer noticed by the coaches, until he finally quit the team.

Comment. While the injury itself may or may not have had a purposeful reason behind it, certainly the recovery from the injury was prolonged as a solution to the problem. He was now safe from further straying from his father's demand to remain passive. Later he turned to track as a dash man and long jumper. In the "big meets," he never reached his dual meet times and faulted in the jumps.

"**3.** The too-aggressive athlete who lacks sufficient control of himself may rush blindly into the fray with the result both he and an opponent or two are stretched out on the turf. Watching film strips of football injuries has suggested to some observers that some players develop "tunnel vision" and in their "mad charge" to make a tackle fail to see blockers who are slightly off the direct line of vision. This would amount to an hysterical denial of the dangers inherent in his aggression.

"**4.** A history of previous athletic attempts which is full of repeated injuries should give pause to permit that player to continue in the sport. We must assume he will be injured again and a serious injury may be the next one on the schedule for him."

Case 38. This 18 year old college football player was rendered unconscious during a football practice and was amnesic for 3 days. He was told that after being injured during the scrimmage he became violent requiring restraint by several teammates. The boy was entirely asymptomatic for 6 months when he noted soreness of the neck, fleeting dizziness, and severe generalized headache. After receiving sedation he became confused and talked about a friend whom he had seen drown while he was a lifeguard. The patient described his dizziness as "things going around me counter-clockwise." When he closed his eyes he felt he was turning in that direction. X-rays of his skull and spine and ophthalmologic and otolaryngologic examinations were normal except that his right pupil was minimally larger than the left. Lumbar puncture studies revealed no abnormality. An EEG exhibited some rare spike waves with 3 to 4 per second single waves in the right posterior quadrant, but there was no evidence of an expanding intracranial lesion. Six months later another EEG demonstrated identical findings in both posterior temporal regions.

The psychiatrist stated: "This patient has rather severe emotional conflicts related to his need to be successful in football and has anxiety concerning playing again. His reaction is largely a conversion mechanism. He should be advised against further participation in body contact sports. If this approach to treatment is presented some of his symptoms will be relieved, otherwise he will have to have some psychotherapy." It is rather interesting that prior to his discharge from the hospital he had been advised not to play football in the spring, but he would be able to return to football practice again in the following fall, which he did. While again playing football he was tackled, falling backward striking his occiput on the ground. Upon regaining consciousness a minute later he wildly threw himself about appearing disoriented and shouting "We are going to beat—!" This episode of hyperactivity lasted only a few minutes after which he seemed to sleep, a situation which was repeated six times while en route to the hospital and after his arrival on the hospital ward. Although he threw himself about violently swinging his arms, he did not injure himself. During a "lucid interval" the patient complained of double vision, but a few minutes later removed his ankle tapes with relative ease and precision. Breath-holding was observed with each of his attacks.

After a third hospital admission with almost identical attacks, a psychiatric interview disclosed that the lad's father had been an All-American halfback who had played professional ball. The patient himself had been named All-State back in his native state but had been unable to make the first team at his college. A diagnosis of a severe emotional problem was made and, although psychiatric therapy was advocated, it was refused.

Three months later he dropped unconscious in front of one of the college buildings and was hospitalized for a fourth time. A few days later he fell from a chair in a doctor's office and subsequently, after discharge, had a similar experience in class. Thereafter he displayed a left-sided facial and hand paralysis and an equivocal left extensor plantar reflex. Skull x-rays and an air study (pneumoencephalogram) were normal and after the latter his neurologic symptoms cleared.

He was discharged on an anticonvulsant regime and although psychiatric aid again was recommended the patient and his family refused. His life was fraught with increasing difficulty in his studies and his grades declined. The patient had returned home for his Army induction physical examination. A month later the patient was readmitted to the hospital with pounding headaches of 10 days' duration. On his arrival at the hospital the boy had a paralysis of the *left* arm and his speech was slightly slurred. Horizontal, vertical, and rotatory nystagmus were observed on extreme lateral vertical gaze with simultaneous contractures of the eyelids. When not following an object during conversation, no nystagmoid jerks were present; the pupils were myotic and normal. There was a flaccid paralysis of the left upper extremity. The Romberg was positive, but it was the impression of the examiner that it was simulated. There was complete glove anesthesia of the left upper extremity. The remainder of the physical examination was normal. A repeat EEG revealed an abnormal pattern suggestive of a convulsive disorder.

The neurologist believed there was no doubt the patient had a conversion hysteria but there was also a definite post-traumatic convulsive disorder. A vascular anomaly or slow growing tumor was considered and studies to exclude such a lesion were suggested, but this was refused just as psychiatric counseling had not been accepted. It was requested that the player's studies be forwarded to a distant neurosurgical consultant and this was done. Approximately 6 weeks later this consultant returned all of the data and films reporting that the appointment had been cancelled at the request of the patient's parents.

Comment. In this author's opinion this case was treated poorly from the beginning. The coach, the team physician, the neurologist, the neurosurgeon, and the boy's parents should have had sufficient insight into his problem to have denied him the opportunity to play football. The player should have had earlier psychiatric help and the parents should have been made to understand the seriousness of his problem. The EEG demonstrated that he also had organic convulsive seizure which demanded attention. He probably had a contrecoup injury with temporal lobe damage possibly to the amygdala and hypothalamus. We have improved our approach to these problems in 20 years but much remains to be done in diagnosing the aggressive-assaultive state in football players. This case also illustrates Situation 2—where there is a serious disparity between father's and son's athletic ability.

"5. A frequently voiced complaint is that, contrary to exaggerating their injuries or prolonging their recoveries, many athletes make light of their injuries and want to return to action too soon, even concealing rather serious injuries. Such bravery and devotion are commendable within limits, but one should watch carefully when an athlete carries this to extremes. Is he, by overdoing it, trying to prove he isn't afraid because he is afraid? Is he actually seeking to be seriously injured as a punishment for some deep feeling of guilt, perhaps over his previous conflicted expression of aggression?"

> **Case 39.** An 18 year old sophomore college football player sustained pain in his neck after a "head-on" blow while charging into an opposing lineman. X-rays of his cervical spine revealed very slight or equivocal compression fracture of the C5 vertebra. A surgical consultant noted the player had local stiffness and pain in the neck at the site of the x-ray abnormality. He discussed the problem with the coach and it was suggested the player give up football for that season.
>
> During the next summer the athlete worked exhaustively to improve his physical condition for the coming football season. This program was under the direction of his brother, a masseur, who also provided physical therapy for patients who had diseases of the central nervous system, some with post-traumatic tetraplegia. The football player read his brother's books and learned about the anatomy of the brain, spinal cord, and nerve roots and he witnessed the ravages of damage to these structures.
>
> Early in the fall of his junior year the man returned to his campus in excellent condition, and after a few weeks of practice, the student newspaper ran a large picture of him as "the hero of old—." He played hard, sustaining a head injury with unconsciousness for several minutes with a residual headache. Upon examination he had a sensory loss to the C6 dermatome, bilateral symmetrical hyperreflexia in all four extremities, and bilateral extensor plantar reflexes. X-rays of the cervical spine displayed an equivocal offset of the C5 on the C6 vertebra, *the same site of his injury of the previous year*. The neurosurgeon who saw the boy believed he should give up football since the neurologic signs were consistent with the diagnosis of injury at the site suspected as being abnormal in the x-ray examination. However, a committee of five physicians met, the neurosurgeon was overruled, and the boy returned to the football squad after a 5 day rest.

During his first day's return to practice he dressed, jogged about the field, and passed the ball back and forth with other players. On the following day, a Saturday, he watched two of his teammates collide "head-on" in a scrimmage and both lay transiently unconscious on the field. It left a profound impression on the boy. After eating breakfast the following day he arose from the training table and as he walked down the hallway with his companions his knees began to shake and slowly buckled under him causing him to drop to the floor. He was taken to the hospital where the neurosurgeon re-examined him and a diagnosis was made of conversion hysteria with paralysis of his lower extremities. Another member of the surgical committee, who had returned him to the game, was called to examine the lad, and as he walked out the door of the room he muttered, "He's yellow; he'll never go back to the football field. He's through." The boy overheard this unfortunate comment. After hospital admission and sedation for a few days he was discharged without any neurologic abnormality. The lad was reassured that he would remain well but was advised that he should retire from the football squad.

The neurosurgeon lost track of the boy for a year. Suddenly one day the telephone rang and a professor at his college asked whether the neurosurgeon knew the former player. When told of the young man's football problem during the previous year the professor stated that the boy had been brooding and his grades had dropped consistently lower and lower so that he was afraid the boy would not graduate from college. Fortunately the athlete did manage to pass his examinations and procured his degree.

Six years later the neurosurgeon received a letter from the former football player now residing in another state stating he was still having headaches and wondering whether these could be real and related to the injury he had received or whether they were purely imaginary. The neurosurgeon answered the letter saying he would be glad to see the man and re-examine him, but a return letter from the former player stated the distances were too great for an examination at that time.

Comment. This was a tragedy which could have been averted if either the coach or any of the physicians had taken the time to discuss with the player his summer's work with his brother, the masseur. It was obvious that he had seen a number of patients with severe spinal cord injuries during that interval. Upon his return to college he had tried to suppress his recollections of the patients he had seen with neurologic sequelae from spinal cord injuries. He continued to play football with great motivation and the desire to help his teammates win. His second head and neck injury set the stage for further physical and emotional stress. The result was the hysterical paralysis the day after seeing his two teammates injured. The crowning blow to this young man's psyche was overhearing the surgeon's unfortunate comment as he walked out of the hospital room door. The fact that the man still wondered about his headache and neck pain 6 years after graduation when he wrote to the neurosurgeon demonstrates the profound influence this distressing event had had upon his whole life! This young man might well have profited by judicious psychiatric counseling soon after his injury. Such evaluation should have been mandatory after his hysterical episode.

"**6.** Fear of or exaggeration of injury should be taken seriously. As accident prone is the overly timid athlete who halts almost imperceptibly just before being tackled and, having lost his momentum, is more likely to suffer injury on contact. Then there is the cry-baby whose every little bruise needs immediate attention. He's scared and perhaps would be better out of the game before he has to take himself out with a real injury.

"**7.** Sometimes an athlete with promise seems to slip and finds himself more frequently on the bench. Perhaps his dwindling skill represents his inability to allow himself the success he did and could continue to experience. Maybe when he seems to be trying too hard to regain his position he will solve the conflict through injury. This inability to tolerate success, in fact to seek out failure, is one of the more common symptoms seen in psychiatric practice and is certainly one of the most resistant symptoms to treat (1). It may be manifested in ways other than athletics, as in the case of the young man who needed one hour for his college degree, but twice failed a two hour course that would have obtained it for him; then he quit college completely.

"Another risk is the anxiety the slipping athlete feels. This may impair his sleep, particularly his dreaming sleep. One effect of this may be a slowing of reaction time which makes him vulnerable in a confrontation with a faster reacting athlete who may also be physically quicker and stronger.

"**8.** An athlete who seems to relish danger with eager anticipation and who shows an omnipotent feeling of invulnerability may be demonstrating a counter-phobic reaction which will require his taking unnecessary risks until he is finally injured.

Counterphobia is a defense against extreme fearfulness. The person must deny any danger exists. He becomes "hipped-up" before facing real danger and ex-hilarated by his actual escape, then again uneasy until he can again deny his terror by confronting danger (6). Various daredevil performers and athletes may demonstrate this. Because they cannot acknowledge fear, they must disregard normal safeguards (it was a long time before professional hockey goalies would allow face masks to be introduced and there were still those old pros who disdained the football helmet up to World War II)."

Summary

Excluded here is a discussion of the frankly psychiatrically ill boy where being injured may satisfy some perverse masochistic need or be representative of a bizarre psychotic fantasy. These situations listed may be found among the kind of boys that try out for every high school, college, and professional athletic team or who engage in various individual sports.

Considerable space has been devoted to these few pertinent case reports because of the failure of all concerned to understand that more of these serious problems exist than is realized. The problem is one of having an understanding and informed group of people cooperate in diagnosing and excluding such players from football before they do themselves, their loved ones, and the sport harm.

There must be thoughtful athletic and medical teams behind the football player and his teammates (2, 3).

References

1. Beisser, A. R.: *The Madness in Sports.* Meredith Publishing Company, New York City, 1967.
2. Moore, R. A.: Psychological factors in athletic injuries. *J. Mich. S. Med. Soc. 59:* 1805, 1960.
3. Moore, R. A.: *Sports and Mental Health.* Charles C Thomas, Publisher, Springfield, Ill., 1966.
4. Ogilvie, B. C. and Tutko, T. A.: *Problem Athletes and How to Handle Them.* Pelham Books Ltd., London, 1966.
5. Pierce, C. M., quoted in: Football Injuries Seem High—but Could Have Been Higher. *Med. Tribune,* March 13, 1969.
6. Yablonsky, L.: Where is Science Taking Us? *The Saturday Review, 46:* 54–56, Feb. 2, 1963.

chapter nine

A Physical Basis for Aggressive-Assaultive Behavior in Football Players

**RICHARD C. SCHNEIDER, M.D. AND
ELIZABETH C. CROSBY, Ph.D., Sc.D.**

In the previous pages the psychological factors which may be responsible for a football player's behavior have been discussed. Occasionally there may be a pathologic physical basis for a player's vicious reactions during a game. The primitive responses of rage, fear, and pain are present both in animal and in man. The degree to which these emotions are controlled depends largely on a rather delicate balancing or interaction of various areas of the brain. When control is lost in a rough sport such as football, a rare type of pathologic aggressive-assaultive response, which has been concealed for a time, surfaces and recurs chronically, resulting in particularly violent acts. *Fortunately only a minimal degree of the roughness in football, as witnessed on a television program, "Mayhem on a Sunday Afternoon," may be due to such a factor.* Nevertheless it is particularly pertinent for football coaches and the athletic team physician to recognize the pathologic player who presents a set of symptoms which has been described as forming the "dyscontrol syndrome." Mark and Ervin (13) have set forth this pattern as having the following characteristics, *not all of which are present simultaneously*: 1) a history of physical assault; 2) a pathologic intoxication with alcohol triggering senseless brutality; 3) a history of impulsive sexual behavior, at times including sexual assaults; and 4) a history of many traffic accidents. Obviously not all of these reactions are witnessed in one individual nor can they be seen on the football field. However, what the player does off the field may be even more significant than what he does while in the game. The tragedy is that he cannot control his aggressive and assaultive actions.

    Case 40.* A set of twins were unusually good high school football players who were noted for their toughness and great ability on the field. Upon enter-

---

* Of all the case histories presented in this monograph, *this is the only one* in which documentation had to be partially relied upon by reports of the news media rather than by the player's record.

ing college they continued their same aggressive tactics, but one of them was particularly singled out for his violence. He sustained multiple moderately severe head injuries and it was discovered that he had a chronic subdural hematoma which could not be definitely attributed to any single specific episode of trauma. This blood clot was successfully removed and he returned to football.

In one game this player "piled on" an opponent, who was already downed outside the field of play, striking him with an elbow and fracturing his nose and maxilla. A penalty was not even assessed against the assaulting player or his team. The motion picture films of the play clearly demonstrated that the action was avoidable and actually deliberate. This "most flagrant violation" led to heated discussion about this player's conduct. In 2 years of intercollegiate play he had been ejected from four games because of the same assaultive unsportsman-like tactics. Public apologies were made by the president of his institution and even the governor raised questions relative to dirty football in this particular game.

This writer has only slight information of the player's extracurricular or social activities for the remainder of his life. However, it is a matter of public knowledge that this player subsequently was involved in a serious automobile accident sustaining a severe head injury. At operation an acute subdural hematoma was removed but there was marked underlying brain damage so that the patient lingered for months before he succumbed.

Comment. This player had two of the four criteria for the "dyscontrol syndrome" (13) described above. The unfortunate thing was that in those days there was no recognition of this syndrome or the possible mechanism of triggering off the limbic system of the brain resulting in this aggressive assaultive behavior. *The player, and most important, his distraught family, might have been spared the heartaches of undue publicity and tragedy if the problem had been identified.*

Discussion

Injury to the orbital surface of the frontal lobe and the tip of the temporal lobe, the frontotemporal area, may result not only in damage to these regions but also trigger off their connections with the limbic system (see anatomical details, p. 143). If the patient survives such injury an aberrant behavior problem may result.

In the case cited above there could have been a completely hidden or forgotten physical factor responsible for the player's aggressive-assaultive reaction. The player was one of a set of twins. It is well known that either both (5) or, more frequently, the second of a set of twins may be subject to neurologic or psychiatric disorders such as epileptic seizures (11, 15) (see Case 43), cerebral palsy (17), mental deficiency (1, 16), psychoses (10), mongolism (11), and asocial behavior (16). Lennox and Lennox (11) cite prematurity, abnormal intrauterine conditions, difficulty with parturition, and embryonic structural defects as etiologic factors responsible for these conditions. Earle et al. (7) reported that 64% of 157 cases of temporal lobe epilepsy, that were operated upon, showed that inferior and mesial portions of the temporal lobe were atrophic or sclerosed to varying degrees. Since the posterior cerebral arteries and the anterior and posterior choroidal arteries cross the tentorium to supply part of the temporal lobe, the herniation of the uncus, as passage of the child occurs through the birth canal, may compress those vessels and cause hypoxia to this region of the amygdala and hippocampus. Many of these patients develop focal atrophy and progressive epileptogenic foci appear later in life causing temporal lobe seizures, which are often characterized by various types of hallucinations, dreamy states, automatisms, and, on rare occasions, by rage states (18, 19). Sweet et al. (19) have indicated that clinical seizures may not necessarily be present and yet the limbic system may be fired under such conditions.

In a series of 500 consecutive twin deliveries Macdonald (12) found breech delivery occurred with 142 first twins and 222 second twins. Prolapse of the cord occurred 10 times with first twins causing four deaths and 7 times with second twins causing death each time. Malpresentation, foetal distress, and traumatic delivery are much more common with the second twin. Prematurity may be a major factor in mortality of either twin (11). Although we do not know whether our football player, described above, was a first or second twin, on the law of averages he could have sustained some hypoxia to the amygdala-hippocampal complex at birth resulting in abnormal behavior later in life.

Although aggressive-assaultive behavior may be related to birth trauma in twins, one need not look that far afield to find an answer for this football player's problems. *Multiple severe head injuries could have occurred in damage to the frontotemporal area of the brain resulting in chronic scarring involving the amygdala-hippocampal complex directly or the fiber pathways leading to and from it.*

In a pathologic study of 206 fatal head injuries Courville (4) discovered 84 injuries to the basal region of the frontal lobe and contusions to the tip of the temporal lobe. The mechanism of these lesions was believed to be a contrecoup contusion of the frontotemporal region against the sharp sphenoid ridge. Gosch et al. (Chapter 14) have visualized this movement of the brain in the experimental animal using a Lexan calvarium as shown in Figure 66 on page 219. A specimen from an auto accident victim (one of only four non-football photographs in the book) graphically demonstrates the site of such pathologic lesions (Fig. 44). On the right side of the brain the cut section reveals the amygdala unharmed. The left side has been sectioned slightly more anteriorly showing the hippocampal gyrus with some residual frontotemporal cerebral destruction and clot. McLaurin and Helmer (14) have described a syndrome of temporal lobe contusion which was seen in 12 patients with severe head injury. All of the patients were lethargic and had progressive neurologic deterioration with progressive hemiparesis and expressive aphasia, if the lesion was on the dominant side. This study was significant in the fact that seven of these patients were "restless, combative, and uncooperative." McLaurin and Helmer (14) adhered to Botterell's teachings (2) that pulped brain should be removed from this region by anterior temporal lobectomy. These writers believed that such cerebral excision reversed the neurologic deterioration and minimized the ultimate deficit. The authors (E.C.C. and

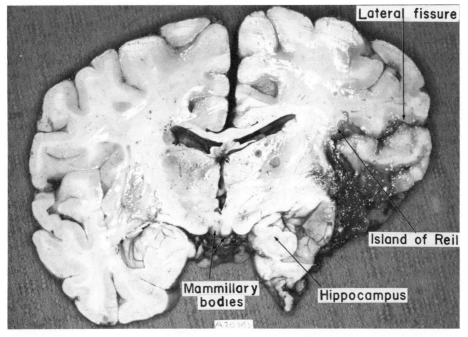

Fig. 44. This sagittal section of the brain is that of an auto accident victim who had a severe head injury with removal of a left temporal intracerebral clot. The temporal lobe is grossly subtotally destroyed but microscopically all the fibers to the amygdalo-hippocampal complex and the temporal operculum of the island of Reil have been badly damaged. If the patient had survived he would have been a fine candidate for the "dyscontrol syndrome" because of the location of the lesion. (This is one of only four specimens in this book not procured from an injured football player, but it shows an important anatomical landmark.)

R.C.S.) agree with Botterell and have found that with such surgical excision there is an improvement from the combative state—with a more docile type of individual in both the acute and chronic states following head injuries (18). Clinical recovery may be due to ablation of an irritative focus, which had stimulated the amygdala. Such a loss of stimulation to the amygdala eliminated its overdischarge to the hypothalamus or released inhibition of it.

   Anatomical and physiologic considerations. This rather complex study has been included so that the medical student and physician may have a better understanding of some of the anatomical pathways involved in behavior, a topic which is currently being discussed by the layman without any background for his conclusions. Also in a day when anatomy is fast disappearing from the curricula of our medical schools, it emphasizes the need for some anatomical background and also a broad general understanding of the field of medicine, not only of the central nervous system but even of obstetrics in cases such as these.
   The amygdala (Fig. 45A) is an almond-shaped mass of neurons situated in the medial part of the anterior one-third of the temporal lobe (as the term is used by clinicians) and largely underneath a protuberance called the uncus. The amygdala in reality belongs to the limbic lobe and is a part of a nuclear circuit, including the septum, the cingulate gyrus, the hippocampus, the hippocampal gyrus, the mamillary body, and the associated fiber paths (Fig. 45, A–C), concerned with building up emotional states and stimulating the rest of the cortex. The amygdala can be subdivided into various secondary parts, with different functional significance. It is not surprising then

that irritation of appropriate portions of it (such as possibly the large celled part of the basal nucleus), but certainly not of all parts of it, should result in a build-up of unprovoked rage.

The amygdala is interconnected with the adjacent parts of the temporal cortex (including the hippocampus through the hippocampal gyrus) and with the base and septal areas of the frontal cortex (Fig. 45 A and B). Space has not permitted illustration of all of these connections, particularly those between the frontal cortex and the amygdala, which include fibers relayed from the olfactory bulb and the lateral part of the anterior perforated space, as well as those indicated in the ventral leaf of the uncinate fasciculus (Fig. 45C), and by way of the association bundle, the cingulum (Fig. 45B). The cingulum [coursing for much of its extent through the cingulate gyrus (Fig. 45B)] interrelates various cortical regions and provides for some interconnections between frontal areas and the hippocampal gyrus (and through the gyrus, to the amygdala and hippocampus).

The efferent paths of the amygdala to the hypothalamus include the stria terminalis. From the amygdala this path circles around the floor of the lateral ventricle, in company with the tail of the caudate nucleus, until the plane of the anterior commissure is reached (Fig. 45A). Then some fibers cross in the commissure to distribute to the amygdala of the other side. Other fibers of the stria terminalis, with or without decussating, pass down in small amounts in front of the anterior commissure to the septal, to the preoptic, and probably to the anterior hypothalamic area and, behind the commissure, to terminate chiefly in the anterior hypothalamic area and the ventromedial hypothalamic nucleus (Fig. 45A).

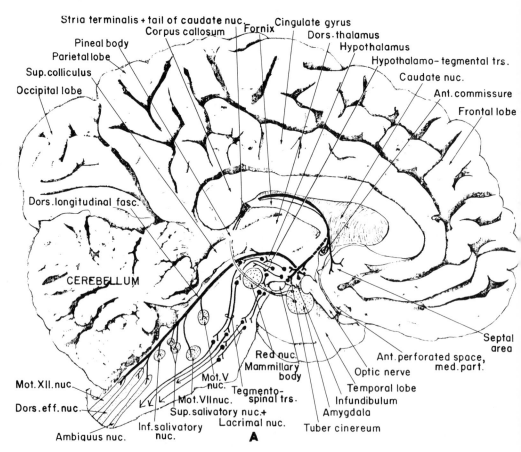

Fig. 45A. This diagram shows certain discharge paths from the amygdala through the hypothalamus to motor and preganglionic areas of the brain stem and spinal cord.

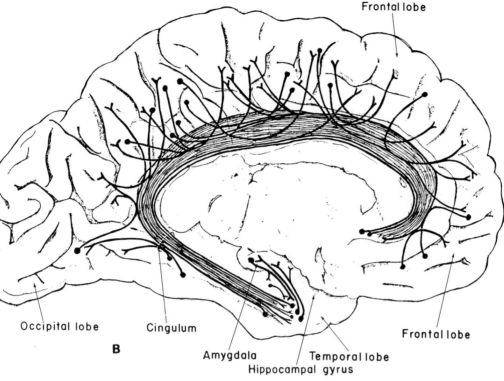

Fig. 45B. This diagram of the cingulum indicates the richness of its fiber constituents.

From these hypothalamic areas, there are two main avenues of discharge to brain stem and spinal cord levels. 1) One of the major discharge paths is formed by fascicles in the dorsal longitudinal fasciculus (Fig. 45A). Certain of such fascicles end in the motor nuclei of cranial nerves (V, VII, IX, X, XI, and probably XII) to provide for emotional smiling, frowning, convulsive swallowing, and other like emotional responses. Other hypothalamic discharge fascicles coursing in the dorsal longitudinal fasciculus terminate on the preganglionic parasympathetic nuclei (such as the Edinger-Westphal, superior and inferior salivatory, and lacrimal and dorsal efferent nuclei). Stimulation of such parasympathetic nuclei results in pupillary changes, tearing, flow of saliva, slowing of the heart rate, increased peristalsis and the like. 2) The second major system of discharge from the hypothalamus is represented by a series of multisynaptic paths (hypothalamotegmental and tegmentospinal tracts) with several synapses in course (Fig. 45A). These latter tracts end on motor and preganglionic sympathetic centers of the spinal cord. The paths to motor centers permit the expression of emotional states by body movements, such as clenching of the fists, rapid walking, kicking, and the like (3). The discharge to and through the preganglionic sympathetic centers provides for increased heart rate, pallor (through the innervation of the smooth muscles of the blood vessels), and similar responses. The amygdalae of the two sides are interconnected through the anterior commissure.

One knows what another man thinks only by the overt behavior of the person being watched, by what he does, what he says, and how he looks (9). The emotional state is built up (Fig. 45 A and B) by the interplay of various limbic areas, such as the cingulate gyrus, the septum, the hippocampal gyrus, the hippocampus, and the amygdala, and by the anterior nuclear group of the dorsal thalamus and the mammillary body of the hypothalamus. The hypothalamic areas receiving impulses from these various regions are concerned in emotional expression and in relaying the impulses reaching them to motor and autonomic centers to provide the complex responses constituting behavior.

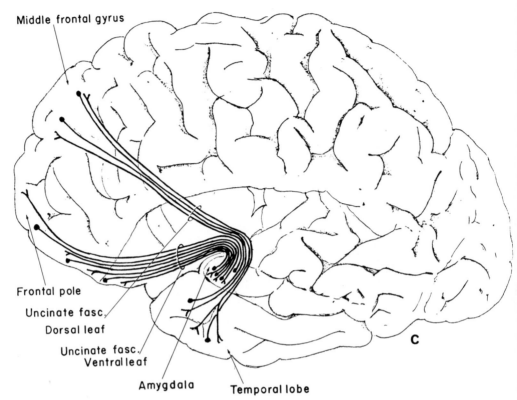

Fig. 45C. This diagram shows the two major parts of the uncinate fasciculus.

It is not surprising then that irritation of the appropriate part of the amygdala directly or by more than normal discharges to it from other areas, such as the temporal lobe or portions of the septum, may produce unwarranted rage. Also lesions at the base of the frontal lobe (including the anterior perforated space or the olfactory tubercle and/or the posterior orbital gyrus) release from inhibitory discharges the magnocellular part of the basal amygdaloid nuclei and uninhibited rage may result.

The lateral part of the frontal cortex is concerned more with intellectual than with emotional responses. It regulates the emotional responses relayed through the hypothalamus by discharging to it by direct corticohypothalamic paths and by multisynaptic paths to the hypothalamus by way of the dorsal thalamus. It also monitors amygdaloid discharges 1) by relay through the dorsal leaf of the uncinate fasciculus to the temporal cortex (Fig. 45C) and from temporal areas to amygdala and 2) by way of the cingulum (Fig. 45B). The lateral surface of the frontal lobe is also connected with its basal areas and these, with the amygdala. In the normal individual rage is controlled by an intelligent appreciation of the results of its indulgence in certain cases.

[Documentary literature for the fiber connections is available in the anatomical descriptions in *Correlative Anatomy of the Nervous System* by Crosby et al. (6) and in the anatomical discussions in *Correlative Neurosurgery* edited by Kahn et al. (8, 18).]

Although the author has never performed temporal lobectomies with amygdalectomy for aggressive-assaultive states *alone*, in a series of 67 such operations on carefully selected patients with severe intractable temporal convulsive seizures, there were six patients who had marked aggressive-assaultive behavior. In the latter half dozen cases the temporal lobectomy, including amygdalectomy, resulted in marked amelioration of their abberant behavior or a complete return to normal (18). It suggests that the amygdala and its connections to the hypothalamus plays an important role in such cases.

References

1. Berg, J. M. and Kerman, B. H.: The mentally defective twin. *Br. Med. J.*, *1:* 1911, 1960.
2. Botterell, E. H.: Brain-Injuries and Complications. *Br. Surg. Proc. 2:* 349, 1948.
3. Cannon, W. B.: *Bodily Changes in Pain, Hunger, Fear and Rage.* Appleton-Century-Crofts, New York, 1920.
4. Courville, C. B.: Coup-Contrecoup Mechanism of Craniocerebral Injuries. *Arch. Surg. 45:* 19, 1942.
5. Critchley, M. and Willimas, D.: Identical Twins, One Suffering from Petit Mal, Both with Abnormal Electro-Encephalograms. *Proc. R. Soc. Med., 32:* 1417, 1939.
6. Crosby, E. C., Humphrey, T. and Lauer, E. W.: *Correlative Anatomy of the Nervous System.* The Macmillan Company, New York, 1962.
7. Earle, K. M., Baldwin, M. and Penfield, W.: Incisural Sclerosis and Temporal Lobe Seizures Produced by Hippocampal Herniation at Birth. *Arch. Neurol. Psychiatry, 64:* 27, 1953.
8. Kahn, E. A., Crosby, E. C., Schneider, R. C. and Taren, J. A., Editors: *Correlative Neurosurgery,* Charles C Thomas, Springfield, Ill., 1969.
9. Kahn, E. A. and Crosby, E. C.: Korsakoff's Syndrome Associated with Surgical Lesions Involving the Mammillary Bodies. *Neurology, 22:* 117, 1972.
10. Kallmann, F. J.: The Genetic Theory of Schizophrenia: An Analysis of 691 Schizophrenic Twin Index Families. *Am. J. Psychiatry, 103:* 309, 1946.
11. Lennox, W. G. and Lennox, M. A.: *Epilepsy and Related Disorders,* Little, Brown & Company, Boston, 1960.
12. Macdonald, R. R.: Management of the Second Twin. *Br. Med. J., 1:* 518, 1962.
13. Mark, V. H. and Ervin, F. R.: *Violence and the Brain,* Harper and Row, Publishers, New York, 1970.
14. McLaurin, R. L. and Helmer, F.: The Syndrome of Temporal Lobe Contusion. *J. Neurosurg., 23:* 296, 1965.
15. Rosanoff, A. J., Handy, L. M. and Rosanoff, J. A.: Etiology of Epilepsy with Special Reference to Its Occurrence in Twins. *Arch. Neurol. Psychiatry, 31:* 1165, 1934.
16. Rosanoff, A. J., Handy, L. M. and Plesset, I. R.: *The Etiology of Child Behavior Difficulties, Juvenile Deliquency and Adult Criminality with Special Reference to Their Occurrence in Twins, Psychiatric Monograph No. 7,* California State Printing Office, Sacramento, 1941.
17. Russell, E. M.: Cerebral Palsied Twins. *Arch. Dis. Child., 36:* 328, 1961.
18. Schneider, R. C., Crosby, E. C. and Calhoun, H. D.: Surgery of Convulsive Seizures and Allied Disorders. In *Correlative Neurosurgery,* 2nd ed, ed. by E. A. Kahn, E. C. Crosby, R. C. Schneider, and J. A. Taren, Chap. 16. Charles C Thomas, Publisher, Springield, Ill., 1969.
19. Sweet, W. H., Ervin, F. R. and Mark, V. H.: The Relationship of Violent Behavior to Focal Cerebral Disease. In *Aggressive Behavior,* ed. by W. Garattini and B. Siggie, pp. 336-352. Excerpta Medica Foundation, Amsterdam, 1969.

chapter ten

The Role of Electroencephalography (EEG) in Sports

KENNETH M. KOOI, M.D., HAZEL D. CALHOUN, B.A., M.A. AND RICHARD C. SCHNEIDER, M.D.

For the uninitiated, electroencephalography (EEG) is the recording of brain wave potentials similar to the electrocardiogram (EKG) which registers the comparatively higher potentials from the heart. These recordings of the electrical activity of the brain (the EEG) provide valuable information about its functional state. Following head trauma, in the presence of brain tumors, vascular diseases, infectious and metabolic disorders, or degenerative diseases of the brain, this electroencephalogram (EEG) has the advantage of being an objective test. However, certain limitations of the procedure must be borne in mind. The data which are gained are of a physiologic (electrical) nature so that any conclusions made about the type of abnormality in the brain are based upon a variety of abnormal brain wave patterns. Secondly, it is known that the EEG is most sensitive to disturbances which involve the upper convexity (the superficial surfaces of the paired cerebral hemispheres) of the brain. The abnormalities which lie deep within these hemispheres may be either inevident or shown by the secondary effects on cortical functioning (within the more superficial and more definitive layers of these hemispheres).

The brain wave potentials are picked up from the scalp and amplified by the electroencephalograph. When these tiniest of potentials are amplified with enough strength they can be measured in microvolts (μV) and in frequency of occurrence, that is, cycles per second (cps), and can be obtained as a permanent written chart. The small electrodes attached to the scalp are placed in a pattern to cover the important lobes of the brain.

The Normal and Abnormal EEG

The general features of the normal electrical patterns have been outlined in detail elsewhere (9). In brief summary, the various areas have characteristic wave forms, the most distinctive of which is the dominant rhythm of the occipital lobes. It is called the alpha rhythm. In the normal, awake, adult brain, its amplitude ranges from 10 to 100 μV and its frequency ranges from 9 to 12 cps (Fig. 46A). The other areas have their own amplitude and frequency parameters. Fast, low voltage rhythms of 20 to 30 cps (beta rhythms) may predominate over the frontal areas of the brain. Slow waves below 8 cps are usually not prominent. A highly important normal characteristic of the EEG is in the similarity of wave patterns at corresponding points over the two paired hemispheres.

Any condition which disturbs the environment of these potentials will change their characteristics. Many of these changes when correlated with clinical signs and symptoms can be significant guideposts although none is, by itself, diagnostic of any given entity. The more dramatic and abrupt the changes in the brain are, the greater are the EEG changes. For this reason it is easy to understand why an epileptic discharge may cause a marked response in the EEG (Fig. 46B).

Every organism, including man's central nervous system, has its threshold for response to stimulation. Any harmful agent, be it injury, drug insult, or disease, when potent enough, can lower this threshold and cause a seizure. In order to accentuate the lowered threshold in some patients, mild forms of stimulation may be used during the EEG recording. It is important to have the subject breathe deeply and rapidly for a period of time in order to ascertain whether hyperventilation will trigger the abnormal activity that may lead to the attack. A sensitivity to the changes in blood carbon dioxide levels associated with rapid breathing may be the mechanism by which a seizure may be initiated (Case 41). Photic stimulation (flashing a light) is another form of stimulation which is used. And finally, the pattern obtained during drowsiness or light sleep may reveal additional information.

Occasionally a patient has an inherited tendency toward convulsive episodes and, when head trauma occurs or there is hyperventilation during participation in a sport, the seizure threshold may be exceeded. This is illustrated in the following case report.

Case 41. An 18 year old, right-handed, high school youth had had convulsive seizures since the age of 6 years. During the past 4 years, he had averaged 12 to 45 seizures per year in spite of all types of anticonvulsant medication. Both his father and maternal grandmother had seizures. His typical seizure pattern was one of halting whatever he was doing, turning to one side, becoming unconscious and falling down with occasional incontinence of bladder and the sustaining of bruises. The seizure, lasting 3 to 5 minutes, was followed by prolonged postictal stupor. Upon recovery, the patient was weak and short winded. In spite of phenobarbital, 30 mgm. q.i.d., Dilantin sodium, 100 mgm. q.i.d., and Mysoline, 125 mgm. q.i.d., the patient continued to have seizures especially following exertion when playing touch football, basketball, and baseball. His EEG revealed an abnormal pattern characterized by numerous bursts of diffuse and bilaterally synchronous spike-wave discharges. Hyperventilation greatly increased their incidence (Fig. 47A; please note Fig. 46 for head diagram and electrode placement).

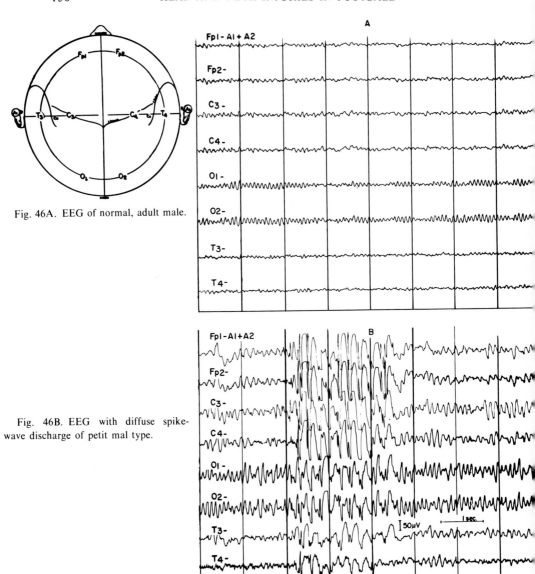

Fig. 46A. EEG of normal, adult male.

Fig. 46B. EEG with diffuse spike-wave discharge of petit mal type.

Comment. This patient with a family history of epilepsy had convulsive seizures which were not precipitated initially by football injury. This case is one of those which belies the statement that exercise is actually good for the seizure patient and that it tends to prevent convulsive episodes (6, 14, 15). In this instance the youngster apparently exerted himself in athletic activity, altering the acid-base balance of the blood, and thereby causing the seizure.

The EEG in Head Trauma

When a football player has a blow to his head which causes him to become momentarily dazed, one would not expect to find dramatic EEG changes. If

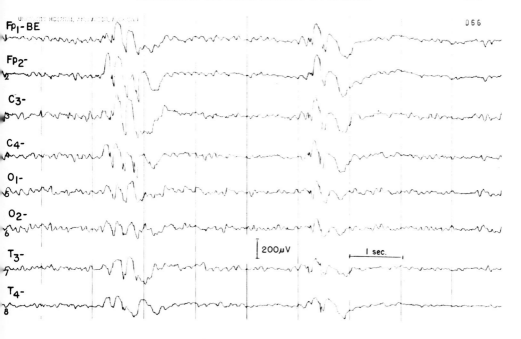

Fig. 47A. Case 41. Bursts of diffuse and bilaterally synchronous spike-wave discharges during hyperventilation (see head diagram for electrode placements on Fig. 46A).

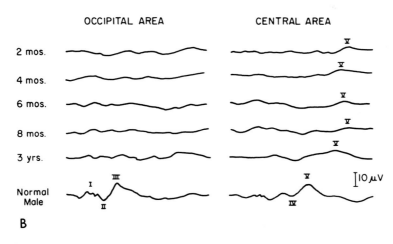

B

Fig. 47B. Case 28. These are the visual evoked responses from a high school football player who had sustained a severe head injury from a "head butting manuever" (Case 28). The interval between head trauma and examination is given in the left hand column. In the next column the occipital visual evoked responses are poorly formed and variable. The vertex wave (V) has latencies ranging from 200 msec. initially to 180 msec. at the time of the last study, normal values being 120 to 170 msec. The typical normal responses are represented below those of this patient showing components I through V. Stimulus (flash) is given at onset of trace. The analysis period is 250 msec. Each trace is an average of 50 individual responses.

his injury is severe—with a loss of consciousness and even with seizures—one would be justified in expecting marked EEG changes (2). On occasion, a severe injury which renders the player unconscious may be in an area of the brain (midbrain) which may not cause major EEG changes.

If an EEG after trauma can be compared to a baseline (initial) record the electroencephalographer is in a much better position to evaluate the findings. The next best method of correlation is serial recording following the injury. Sometimes the EEG signs are very subtle and are manifested by a slight amplitude discrepancy in one or more areas or by a difference in frequency of wave forms in one or more areas.

Because head injuries tend to occur in adolescents and young adults, it is necessary to draw attention to certain EEG features in this age group. The alpha rhythm may be expected to fall within the usual frequency range but may be rather labile in terms of moment to moment variability and show transient left-right asymmetries of amplitude and pattern. The faster beta patterns are apt to show their usual amplitude and distribution. On occasion, intermediate range activity of 14 to 16 ps may occur with a spindle-like form in the central areas in adolescents. The theta range activity (4 to 7 ps) with its bilateral anterior distribution may be somewhat more prominent than in older individuals. Even some delta activity (1–3 ps) may be acceptable, especially if it is in the form of single delta waves in the posterior regions. These delta waves may be preceded by an exceptionally large alpha wave and have been termed alpha-delta complexes. Some apparently normal teenagers and even young adults may have rhythmic delta activity underlying the alpha rhythm.

In evaluating the EEG tracing for evidence of a paroxysmal cerebral disorder, there are three patterns which must be distinguished from true paroxysmal activity. At this age, the hypersynchronous slow waves of drowsiness tend to occur in very short runs and may be mistaken for abnormal discharges if careful attention is not paid to the subject's level of consciousness. In conjunction with this type of drowsiness pattern, or occurring quite separately, one may encounter runs of rhythmic and sometimes sharp theta components in the temporal areas. It remains uncertain whether these wave patterns are entirely normal or not, but they clearly bear no direct relationship to head trauma. A spikey pattern which must be differentiated from true spikes is the 14 and 6 ps discharge. This can be recognized by its frequency characteristics and its location over the parietotemporal regions. Its tendency to shift between the two hemispheres with an overall preponderance on the right side is also notable. Again, this is a pattern that quite commonly occurs in the records of individuals in this age group and no special significance can be attributed to it.

In considering the EEG effects of hyperventilation, the slow-wave build-up may be quite prompt and marked in individuals of this age, making the response abnormal only when it has rather definite focal characteristics or when it shows specific paroxysmal patterns (spikes or spike-waves).

It is also worth mentioning that central sharp activity seems to be a prominent finding in this particular age group. Careful evaluation of this activity is necessary since it may represent normal vertex responses to various events occurring in the recording situation.

Acute EEG Effects of Trauma. The severity of a head injury is usually reflected quite closely by changes in the electrical activity of the brain. Minor effects are evidenced by a slight increase in generalized slow activity or by intermittent sharp discharges or spikes. Little or no change of intrinsic patterns is to be expected. With a more severe cerebral insult, the incidence of slow activity becomes greater and the proportion of delta components to theta components is relatively larger. The slow activity again may be either diffuse or focal. Background patterns may be slow and disorganized. Asymmetries of intrinsic rhythms are produced by local voltage depression and disorganization. Very severe cerebral trauma ordinarily results in marked disorganization of pre-existing activity with replacement either by high voltage very slow activity or by low amplitude ill defined undulations. Cerebral activity over one or both hemispheres may be essentially flat.

The mild focal changes may occur in close relationship to the site of the trauma or appear at a directly opposite location (contrecoup effect). The site of the focal changes should be carefully noted since it may provide a clue as to the basis of certain of the patient's symptoms. For example, difficulty with finding the right word (aphasia or dysphasia) may be associated with slow-wave activity in the low left frontal area, the usual area of the motor center for speech. EEG changes in the occipital region may be observed in individuals who report that their vision is blurred or indistinct (not to be confused with double vision). With actual cortical blindness, there is usually a profound disruption of occipital activity (Fig. 47B; see Case 28). As already mentioned, an unusual situation may exist where there is an apparent dissociation between the character of the EEG and the level of consciousness, the EEG showing relatively normal characteristics in the face of a deeply comatose state clinically (2). In this situation, the EEG may exhibit what appears to be a waking pattern with a dominant alpha rhythm or the pattern may be one of sleep with episodic spindling, vertex waves; and serial slow patterns. In either case, it is believed that the discrepancy is explained by the principal location of the brain injury, the effect being predominantly on the brain stem. In some instances of severe head trauma, the EEG patterns may vaguely resemble those of normal sleep, the usual activity being distorted and poorly formed. One may encounter REM (rapid eye movement) activity during types of EEG sleep patterns not ordinarily associated with the REM stage of sleep. This indicates a loss of the normal integration between forebrain and brain stem aspects of sleep mechanisms.

Resolution of the EEG changes requires from a few days to a week in the case of minor slowing to several months when marked changes have occurred. It has sometimes been held that once the EEG has returned to normal and slow activity has subsided further clinical improvement is not to be expected. While this may be accepted as a rough generalization, certain exceptions are encountered. It may be noted that the EEG can return to "normal" on the basis of empirical criterion but that subsequent tracings may reveal further changes in the direction of better organization and increased frequency of intrinsic rhythms. The disturbing situation may occur where serial EEGs have shown a return to an entirely normal pattern only to have a subsequent tracing reveal sporadic paroxysmal activity.

In the immediate period following the head injury, the EEG is not useful in determining the presence or absence of a subdural hematoma or other space occupying lesion (17) although it may provide localizing information. Following the immediate post-traumatic period—two weeks or more is a rule of thumb—careful attention should be paid to EEG changes that 1) are out or proportion to the severity of the head injury or 2) consist of a combination of focal signs and diffuse slow waves since these findings greatly enhance the possibility of a subdural hematoma. This situation is illustrated by Case 5 (Fig. 47C).

Although one might wish to vary the schedule depending upon the patient's clinical course, it is ordinarily desirable to obtain an EEG tracing within the first week after the injury with follow-up tracings at one month and six months in the event of significant findings on the initial study.

Chronic EEG Changes Following Trauma. Although it is usual for the EEG to return to normal at a variable interval—from hours to weeks—following head injury, there may be residual focal or diffuse abnormalities. If these are of a true paroxysmal character, i.e., spike or spike-wave formations, the patient will need periodic follow-ups because of their potentially epileptogenic nature. Even in the absence of clinical seizures, sharp-wave foci also deserve careful observation since they may evolve into more frank paroxysmal discharges. The athlete presents a somewhat unique situation in respect to multiplicity of head injuries so that the EEG changes after any given injury may represent a combination of acute and chronic effects. In a patient suspected of having post-traumatic

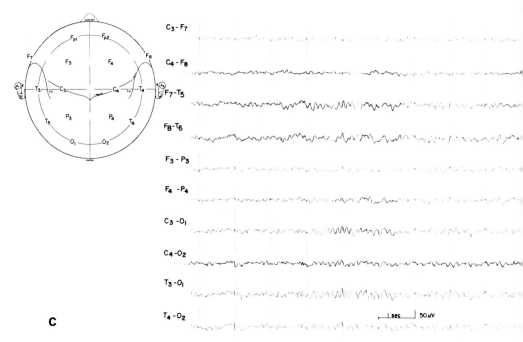

C

Fig. 47C. Case 5 The EEG showed rather subtle changes of suppression of the right-sided voltage with a brain wave pattern suggesting a diffuse right-sided abnormality. To the uninitiated this would not suggest the presence of a large subdural hemorrhage.

epilepsy, a single normal tracing should not be taken to exclude the possibility of convulsive disorder or any expanding intracranial lesion such as a blood clot (see Case 4).

Epilepsy and Participation in Football

In the furor of discussing epilepsy in athletics one must calmly consider and assess several significant factors. First, the correct definition of epilepsy is important. In 1870 J. Hughlings Jackson (7) stated, "A convulsion is but a symptom and implies only that there is an occasional, an excessive, and a disorderly discharge of nerve tissue on muscles. . . . " The sporadic occurrence of convulsive seizures as a symptom complex related to a bout of elevated temperature in an infantile infection must be differentiated from the patient who has had a severe episode of trauma, cerebritis, or some other precipitating cause followed by scarification of the brain and chronic recurrent convulsive episodes. For example, Jennett (8) believed that a child's brain is more liable to react to a variety of noxious stimuli with convulsions without this indicating brain damage or future epilepsy. Thus the liability of young children to have early fits was not thought to be the precipitation of "idiopathic epilepsy" by cerebral injury. In general, the chronic recurrent convulsive episodes may be designated as true epilepsy but couched in less ominous terms for the layman as "convulsive disorder" which seems to cause less of a stigma. In addition to idiopathic epilepsy (a term meaning "for which there is no known cause"), there are other etiologies for such seizures, some of them previously mentioned, congenital deformities of the brain, birth trauma, subdural hematomas, brain tumors, abscesses, cysts, arteriovenous anomalies, and degenerative cerebral diseases.

Throughout the years there have been many well oriented paramedical, as well as medical, groups that have valiantly and admirably endeavored to rid patients with neurologic handicaps from the stigmata of the diagnosis associated with their disease with the hope of enabling the patient to achieve a satisfactory place in society (1, 11, 14). This situation has been true particularly in fields of cerebral palsy and epilepsy. In order to provide some reasonable guidelines for the physician who has encountered the athlete with convulsive seizures, the author contacted three neurosurgical colleagues who are world renowned for their work in the surgery of convulsive disorders, posing the question whether the athlete who had chronic recurrent convulsive seizures should be permitted to engage in contact sports. This resulted in this statement in the *Journal of the American Medical Association*"... young people with convulsive disorders, once the seizures are under reasonable control, should be encouraged to lead as normal and active a life as possible." The summary included the comment: "Participation should include any sports of interest with the exception of boxing, tackle football, ice hockey, diving, soccer, rugby, and lacrosse and other activities where chronic recurrent head trauma may occur."

Livingston (14, 15) takes issue with the statement for he has declared that he had had hundreds of patients who have participated in boxing, lacrosse, wrestling, and tackle football with the participant exposed to blows on the head and in not one single instance has there been evidence of recurrence of epileptic seizures related to a head injury in any athlete. He cites a case in which a football player was denied the opportunity to play and developed anxiety and depression. This state was presumably relieved by permitting him to re-enter college and to play the sport. The reader is referred to Case 38 for just the reverse situation in which the football player trying to excel was so emotionally distraught with frustration that he continued to play football with the subsequent development of conversion hysteria. He finally had true post-traumatic seizures.

The EEG plays an important role in the evaluation of an athlete with a possible or established convulsive disorder. When the diagnosis of epilepsy is in doubt, the EEG may provide confirmatory evidence by showing abnormal wave patterns suggestive of a cerebral paroxysmal instability. Even when there is little doubt that a seizure has occurred, an EEG should be obtained to give information as to the degree of the cerebral disturbance and its location in respect to the various brain areas. Location of the abnormal discharges over the temporal regions of the brain suggests that the seizures may take a more subtle form, so-called temporal lobe or psychomotor seizures, and therefore may be less readily recognized whereas diffuse discharges are likely to be associated with generalized motor seizures or, less commonly, brief lapses of consciousness termed petit mal.

The role of the EEG in providing a prognosis following a head injury is less definitive since even a rather severe disturbance of the electrical functioning of the brain is not incompatible with complete recovery. Further, minor atypical electrical patterns may have actually predated the injury. Nonetheless, it is probably ill-advised to permit a full return to athletic activities when a significant disturbance of the EEG is still present. Careful follow-up is required when the abnormalities are of a paroxysmal and potentially epileptogenic type and when they are out of proportion to the severity of the head injury. In the latter case, subdural or intracerebral hemorrhage is always to be considered.

In a further discussion of this topic a few case histories may be cited as a basis for further review of the topic.

Case 42. An 18 year old, right-handed, college freshman football player was participating in sandlot ball when he had a tonic seizure with both arms and legs extended during which he became apneic and cyanotic and struck his left temporal region. He was unconscious for 3 to 4 minutes during this episode. On arrival at the hospital small abrasions of the left temporal and right forehead were noted and except for a postconvulsive stupor he was found to have no neurologic abnormality. He was admitted to the hospital merely for overnight observation and was then released.

Two weeks later a neurosurgeon examined him and noticed a ptosis of the left eyelid and flattening of his left maxillary and mandibular areas, a condition said by his mother to have been present for years. Careful birth history disclosed that he had had a greatly misshapen head at birth and that he had been cyanotic and subsequently was very slow in talking compared to the remainder of the children in the family. His EEG was abnormal, paroxysmal, and indicative of a convulsive tendency because of rare diffuse spike-wave discharges with a right-sided gradient and paroxysmal response to photic stimulation (Fig. 48, A–C). He was placed on the anticonvulsant, Dilantin sodium, three times daily and he remained seizure-free for 2 years. After discussing the problems of the hemiatrophy of the face suggestive of birth trauma, and the abnormal EEG with relation to his career this intelligent youngster and his parents decided he should give up contact sports. He was perfectly fine until 2 years later when he sustained a brief convulsive episode while running on the track. He recovered and his EEG again was suggestive of a convulsive tendency.

Comment. This boy was an excellent high school football player who probably could have done well in college. However, with the history of birth trauma, demonstrable neurologic deficit, and an abnormal EEG in adulthood, he was judged to be a poor candidate for repeated head contact blows. For the advocates of exercise having a beneficial effect on the seizures it should be pointed out that he sustained his next seizure while running on the track (14, 15). This occurrence may have some relationship to his atypical EEG response to hyperventilation (Fig. 48C). There is no doubt that non-contact exercise may be of some value to these patients with convulsive seizures.

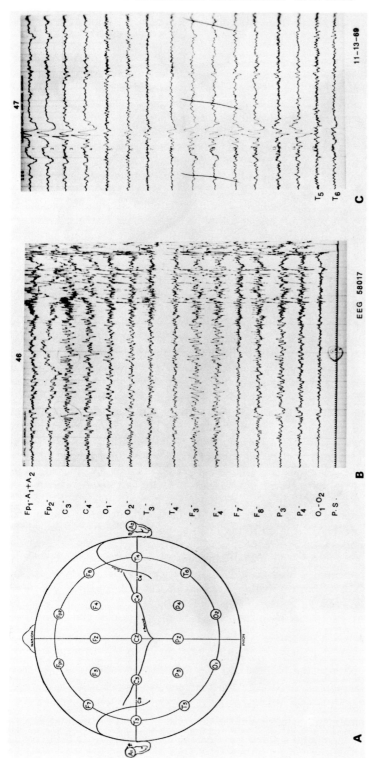

Fig. 48 (A–C). Case 42.

Fig. 48A. The diagram at the left shows the sites of electrode placement.

Fig. 48B. This was abnormal and paroxysmal suggestive of a convulsive tendency because of rare diffuse spike-wave discharges with a right-sided gradient and paroxysmal responses to photic stimulation.

Fig. 48C. The above pattern was the response noted to hyperventilation (deep breathing); although this one was not as abnormal as the photic stimulation, it too produces spike waves.

It is always interesting to provide contrasts in order to fairly present a problem. Consequently another case history is presented.

Case 43. A 23 year old, right-handed professional football player tackled an oncoming opponent in the fourth play of a game causing him to be thrown into the air and then to strike the ground hard. Upon arising he was dazed, dizzy, and quite unstable in his gait and was ordered to the bench. However, he recovered rapidly and re-entered the game. Within 3 minutes of the end of the game and with no time outs left for his team, he dove for the football on an "on-side" kick. He was rendered unconscious and was picked up rapidly, dragged off the field, and taken to the locker room. After this episode he had a bitemporal headache but managed to shower and take the bus to his motel. While en route he vomited. Upon arrival at the motel he went to the bathroom to vomit again but lost consciousness and after falling in the bathtub had a full-blown grand mal convulsive seizure biting his tongue bilaterally. He was rushed to a hospital where he spent 24 hours in the intensive care unit. He was neurologically normal except for the right-sided hyperreflexia as noted by his neurosurgeon. Skull x-rays were reported as normal and he was placed on anticonvulsant therapy. An EEG revealed some bitemporal spikes, but three days later he was believed to be sufficiently recovered to travel to his home.

Upon arriving in the neurosurgeon's office at home on the 4th day after the injury the player seemed to be dazed. The doctor had known the player and when he arrived in the office the doctor apologized to the young man for being late. The player commented, "Yes, it is really awfully late" and looked at his watch. He was asked how late he thought the neurosurgeon was. After glancing in a rather puzzled fashion at his watch he replied slowly, "About an hour and a half." Actually he had waited 10 minutes. In addition to the distortion of time he stated that he felt "unreal" as though he "was present in the world but somehow standing off in the background looking in." Two years before he recalled he had sustained a head to knee injury in a college game, had been rendered dizzy, and had played automatically for 1¼ quarters but did not feel that he had a full sensation of awareness of what was going on around him. He volunteered that as he played the game he had a feeling that he had been in this position and played there before. It was a strange dreamy feeling. He had no previous convulsive seizures but *a twin had had convulsions as a little child* which were outgrown without the use of anticonvulsant medication. His only neurologic abnormality was a right hyperreflexia without any extensor plantar reflex. The patient had a brain scan and EEG which appeared normal and a week later he was neurologically negative. A diagnosis of frontotemporal contusion with associated transient grand mal convulsive seizure was made.

Comment. There was a question whether this player after his injury vomited, slipped, and fell into the bathtub striking his head and then had a seizure or whether the seizure preceded the fall in the tub and secondarily the patient struck his head. Regardless of the sequence of events there is little doubt that he sustained a frontotemporal contusion as demonstrated by his feelings of unreality (12, 13). An incidental finding was that of an inability to tell time or a disorientation in time (4). Spiegel et al. (19) have termed this condition "chronotaraxis." In performing 30 cases of dorsomedial thalamotomy they discovered that 19 of the patients had transient disturbances in temporal orientation. In most instances it lasted only a few days or weeks. This young professional athlete and his wife were told that he had had several severe head blows with a bruise to the brain but was recovering. They were advised that he might be subject to permanent brain damage if he had further injuries. However, he elected to take that chance and he has played 3 more years of professional football without any apparent incident.

Discussion

The individual evaluation of football players with head injuries which may be complicated by convulsive seizure problems is important. In Case 42 the player already had a sufficiently compromised brain from birth so that he demonstrated chronic neurologic deficit. It is believed that such a brain could not withstand chronic recurrent blows to the head without further sequelae. Fortunately the lad and his parents accepted the physician's suggestion and he gave up the game. Despite admonition to the young professional, Case 43, that he might sustain permanent seizures or other neurologic disability, he persisted in playing stating that this was his whole livelihood and he would take these chances. It was a risk that he chose to take in spite of medical advice.

Case 44. A 19 year old, right-handed college football player was about to enter his junior year transferring from one college to another because of the possibility of entering a pre-professional program and being tendered a football scholarship at the second school. His father, a physician, was concerned about the young man's welfare due to his history of multiple severe head injuries and sought neurosurgical consultation.

During his freshman year he had been scrimmaging when he was struck on the head and was rendered unconscious for an indefinite but apparently brief interval. Following the blow he had bifrontal headache and dizziness without nausea or vomiting. After examination at the health service he was discharged and told to stay in bed and out of classes for one day; he then returned to football and played at center the rest of the year. He received another head injury in a game sustaining bleeding from the left side of his nose and mouth. Although not unconscious he again sustained dizziness and a 30 minute anterograde amnesia (loss of memory for events for a 30 minute interval following the injury). During this time he was laughing and had no recollection of it. Again he stayed out of practice for a week; upon his return he reported dizziness after vigorous exercise, but completed his freshman season.

During spring practice he charged into someone on the first play and received another head injury without unconsciousness or a period of amnesia but remained glassy-eyed. He was sent to a nearby medical center where an EEG was made which was reported as revealing minor asymmetry but no focal lesion. He was kept out of football during the remainder of spring practice to avoid head contact.

After the history of these three concussions the neurosurgeon found the player to have no neurologic signs but ordered and EEG. The record was abnormal and paroxysmal with emphasis in the right temporal area. During hyperventilation in the small triangle epochs 3–4 burst of 4–5/sec spike-waves with right temporal emphasis were noted. (Unfortunately his EEG was stored on microfilm and it was impossible to reproduce it satisfactorily.) On the basis of the history of repeated dizziness, amnesia, headaches, and the EEG study a diagnosis of right frontotemporal contusion was made and he was advised to discontinue football. A 10 year follow-up disclosed that he took this advice and has had no seizures. He is a very successful businessman who is married and has one child.

Comment. This football player presented with an excellent history of multiple head injuries with dizziness, most probably due to a contusion of the vestibular centers in the superior temporal gyrus of the temporal operculum, a symptom which has been noted and reported from this clinic (18). Ten years ago a neurosurgeon specifically inquired about other symptoms of temporal lobe phenomena, such as: feelings of unreality, *deja vu* phenomena, olfactory, auditory, and visual hallucinations, macropsia, or micropsia. These symptoms are ofttimes not volunteered but must be actively sought by the examiner. It is only recently that a central source of dizziness has been localized to the temporal operculum, as one of the cortical vestibular association centers and active sources of this symptom (18).

Contrary to Livingston's belief (15), this player would have seemed to be a fine candidate for permanent temporal lobe scarring with a permanent seizure involvement, if he had sustained further head contact with injury.

The mechanisms of the formation of cerebral contusions and their morphology have been described by Martland and Beling (16) and Lindenberg and Freytag (12) with the frequent occurrence of such lesions in the frontal or temporal lobes or directly at the frontotemporal junction. The professional player presented in Case 43 had a very severe convulsive episode following a blow on the head. Presumably he had a marked contusion to the frontotemporal area for he still had feelings of unreality and could not tell time four days later. On his initial EEG 3 days after injury he had a very few minor spikes and he had a normal EEG study 7 days after trauma. This finding supports the statement made by Gibbs et al. (5) made over a quarter of a century ago that subjective complaints after head injury certainly do not correlate significantly with EEG abnormalities.

The high school player reported in Case 5 had a chronic subdural hematoma without convulsive seizures. His EEG showed a subtle but definite depression of voltage over the side of the lesion. It has been the author's experience (KMK) that approximately 90% of the patients with subdural hematomas have abnormal EEGs and correct lateralization of a single hematoma is possible in better than three-fourths of the patients with abnormal tracings. Diffuse abnormalities occur with unilateral hematomas, and unilateral emphasis may occur even though bilateral hematomas are present. Chusid and de Guitierrez-Mahoney (3) have indicated that part of the difficulty with the diagnosis of subdural hematoma by electroencephalographic methods may be due to association with other brain alterations due to cerebral lacerations, intracerebral hematomas, etc.

Gotze et al. (6) have studied adolescent epileptics with EEG telemetry and note that with hyperventilation during physical exercise there is a shift of the nerve cell environment toward acidosis with a decrease in voltage, an increase in frequency, and a diminished evidence of seizure discharge. Pediatricians and neurologists have accepted this work and on the basis of it have recommended participation in sports, even the contact ones (10, 14, 15). In the light of these concepts the patients reported in Cases 41 and 42 are of particular interest. In both instances the patients had latent seizures and were precipitated into clinical ones while exercising. The player in Case 41 had seizures which "were caused by overexertion while playing football, basketball and baseball," this despite a heavy anticonvulsant regime.

Bower (1) has emphasized the importance of consultation between the boy, his parents, and the physician; however, the parents must know the truth about recurrent seizures in athletes as described above. It is one thing to encourage physical activity in an epileptic athlete in non-contact sports but quite another thing to subject him to multiple episodes of chronic recurrent blows to a brain, which is already damaged, in football, hockey, lacrosse, boxing, etc. The need for serial EEGs (20) after head injuries is nicely demonstrated by the player in Case 44. After three concussions he had two EEG studies; the first one was normal but the second showed spike-wave bursts in the right temporal region. The study plus the clinical history caused this boy to give up football. Ten years later he is well and seizure-free, probably reprieved from a life of post-traumatic temporal lobe epilepsy which he might have developed with further recurrent trauma.

Finally there is the dreadful problem of differentiating between the possibility of hysteria or brain damage from multiple head injuries. In Case 38 the patient obviously had both functional and physical problems; the latter were confirmed by serial EEG examinations. The behavior might have been judged abnormal on a physical basis, such as assaultive-aggressive behavior as described with limbic lobe stimulation, but there were also true hysterical components. In Case 28 the player's brain was badly damaged as demonstrated by clinical findings and serial EEGs, but the question arose as to whether he had hysterical blindness. In the interval early after his injury his evoked visual potentials were shown to be definitely abnormal which strongly suggested the blindness was not on an hysterical basis. As he gradually recovered his sight there was also some degree of visual agnosia.

References

1. Bower, B. D.: Epilepsy and School Athletics. *Dev. Med. Child. Neurol., 11:* 244, 1969.
2. Chatrian, G. E., White, L. E. Jr. and Daly, D.: Electroencephalographic Patterns Resembling Those of Sleep in Certain Comatose States after Injuries to the Head. *Electroenceph. Clin. Neurophysiol., 15:* 272, 1963.
3. Chusid, J. G. and de Guitierrez-Mahoney, C. C.: The Electroencephalogram in Head Injuries with Subdural Hematoma. *Neurology 6:* 11, 1956.
4. Crosby, E. C., Humphrey, T. and Lauer, E. W.: *Correlative Anatomy of the Nervous System.* The Macmillan Company, New York, 1962.
5. Gibbs, F. A., Wegner, W. R. and Gibbs, E. L.: The Electroencephalogram in Posttraumatic Epilepsy. *Am. J. Psychiatry, 100:* 738, 1944.
6. Gotze, W., Kubicki, M., Munter, M. and Teichman, J.: Effect of Physical Exercise on Seizure Threshold Investigated byy Electroencephalographic Telimetry. *Dis. Nerv. Syst., 28:* 664, 1967.
7. Jackson, J. H.: *Selected Writings of Hughlings Jackson*, Vol. 1, ed. by J. Taylor. Hoadder and Stoughton, London, 1931.
8. Jennett, W. B.: *Epilepsy After Blunt Head Injury.* William Heinneman Medical Books, Limited, London, 1962.
9. Kooi, K.: *Fundamentals of Electroencephalography.* Harper & Row, Publishers, New York, 1971.
10. Kugel, R. B., et al. (Committee): The Epileptic Child and Competitive School Athletics. *Pediatrics 42:* 700, 1968.
11. Lennox, W. G. and Lennox, M. A.: *Epilepsy and Related Disorders.* Little, Brown & Company, Boston, 1960.
12. Lindenberg, R. and Freytag, E.: Morphology of Cortical Contusions. *Arch. Pathol., 63:* 23, 1957.
13. Lindenberg, R. and Freytag, E.: The Mechanisms of Cerebral Contusions. A Pathologic-Anatomic Study. *Arch. Pathol., 69:* 440, 1960.
14. Livingston, S.: Convulsive Disorders and Participation in Sports. *J.A.M.A., 207:* 1917, 1969.
15. Livingston, S.: Should Physical Activity of the Epileptic Child Be Restricted. *Clin. Ped., 10:* 694, 1971.
16. Martland, H. S. and Beling, C.: Traumatic Cerebral Hemorrhage. *Arch. Neurol. Psychiatry., 22:* 1001, 1929.
17. Rodin, E. A.: Contribution of the EEG to Prognosis after Head Injury. *Dis. Nerv. Syst., 28:* 595, 1967.
18. Schneider, R. C., Crosby, E. C. and Calhoun, H. D.: Surgery of Convulsive Seizures and Allied Disorders. In *Correlative Neurosurgery*, 2nd ed., ed. by E. A. Kahn, E. C. Crosby, R. C. Schneider and J. A. Taren, Chap. 16. Charles C Thomas, Springfield, Ill., 1969.
19. Spiegel, E. A., Wycis, H. T., Orchnik, C. W. and Freed, H.: The Thalamus and Temporal Orientation. *Science, 121:* 771, 1955.
20. Whelan, J. L., Webster, J. E. and Gurdjian, E. S.: Serial Electroencephalography in Recent Head Injuries with Attention to Photic Stimulation. *Electroencephalogr. Clin. Neurophysiol., 7:* 495, 1935.

chapter eleven

First Aid and Diagnosis — —
The Treatment of Head Injuries

RICHARD C. SCHNEIDER, M.D. AND
FREDERICK C. KRISS, M.D.

Football is a rough sport and regardless of how thoroughly trained, well protected, and experienced the personnel may be, there will always be a certain number of players who will sustain serious and fatal injuries which cannot be avoided. However, it is surprising how little has been recorded in the way of basic medical instruction for the officials, coaches, trainers, and team physicians who are associated with the game. The early preparation for and recognition of a possible impending tragedy may prevent serious disability and death. Several fundamental concepts are presented which may serve this group as guidelines in such situations.

First Aid

The term in this instance means the immediate diagnosis, treatment, and transportation of the injured player from the field. In order to assess properly the patient's condition, a few important definitions must be clarified so that all physicians, coaches, and trainers have some common terminology which may be effectively used.

In Head Injuries

One of the most crucial and vital decisions that has to be made in head injuries is the differentiation between "cerebral concussion," a non-operable condition, and the occurrence of a "rapidly expanding intracranial blood clot," an emergency surgical situation.

Cerebral Concussion*

For many years the term cerebral concussion in the patient with a head injury implied to most neurosurgeons the impairment of the state of consciousness which might vary in its duration from a few transient seconds to a number of minutes.

---

* Material on cerebral concussion reprinted from Schneider and Kriss (24) by permission of *Medicine and Science in Sports*.

163

Ofttimes the length of this interval was regarded as an index of the severity of the head injury and the use of the term itself implied complete recovery. Such a definition seems improper, however, since the head injury patient may show other symptoms which prove equally significant and he may *not* lose consciousness. In fact the use of the term concussion is so confusing that it has been reported that the British neurosurgeons (30) have recommended abandoning it. However, it would be difficult to expurgate a word which is so firmly entrenched in the medical literature.

In 1964 the Congress of Neurological Surgeons designated a Committee on Head Injury Nomenclature to clarify and classify types of head trauma and thus to standardize terms wherever possible. The definition of cerebral concussion which this group decided upon was: "Concussion, brain: a clinical syndrome characterized by immediate and transient impairment of neural function, such as alteration of consciousness, disturbance of vision, equilibrium, etc., due to mechanical forces" (6). While this nomenclature committee was discussing the problem, the Subcommittee on Classification of Sports Injuries, of the Committee on the Medical Aspects of Sports of the AMA was in session attempting to clarify the terminology which is used in athletics. In order to promote the use of identical definitions, permission was sought of the Nomenclature Committee of the Congress of Neurological Surgeons to use their description of "cerebral concussion." This request was kindly granted. *The term concussion no longer requires the patient to have had a complete loss of consciousness and presents a much more realistic approach to the problem* (1).

The significant point is that with uncomplicated cerebral concussion there is a transient or reversible physiologic condition (6). It is due to a very temporary interruption of transmission of impulses within the brain with brief neurologic dysfunction.

For practical use in athletic injuries the authors found it expedient to subdivide this newly defined term further into first, second, and third degrees of concussion based upon the duration and severity of the symptoms. Those definitions have been published by the AMA in the Standard Nomenclature of Athletic Injuries but have been re-evaluated recently and more realistically outlined with stress placed upon the rate of recovery (1).

It should be emphasized that these criteria are highly artificial. Any one of several of them may be lacking in any given degree of concussion in athletes who have sustained injury. Time no doubt will alter these standards, but this classification hopefully will provide a starting point (1).

The player who has sustained a first degree or mild cerebral concussion usually may be returned to the game after a play or two but should be carefully watched for undue fatigue, signs of disorientation, or any peculiar behavior. Such vague symptoms may first be observed by an alert teammate and it may be wise to take one of the stable players aside and advise him to watch his friend for any unusual signs.

TABLE I

Cerebral Concussion

	1st Degree, Mild	2nd Degree, Moderate	3rd Degree Severe
Consciousness	No loss	Transitory loss (up to 3–4 minutes)	Prolonged loss (over 5 minutes)
Mental confusion	Slight	Momentary	For 5 or more minutes
Memory loss	None or very transient	Definite mild retrograde amnesia*	Prolonged retrograde amnesia*
Tinnitus	Mild	Moderate	Severe
Dizziness	Mild	Moderate	Severe
Unsteadiness	Usually none	Moderate	Marked
General recovery rate	Very rapid	Complete in 5 minutes	Slow (longer than a period of 5 minutes)

* Please note subsequent definition.

The second degree or moderate concussion victim probably should be removed from the game for a period and observed. Retrograde amnesia is defined as a loss of memory for events immediately preceding the injury. It has been presumed that the longer this interval persists, the more severe is the injury. In this instance it may be a matter of up to 5 minutes (1). If the player recovers completely within 5 minutes he may be returned to action after a suitable rest.

The player with a third degree or severe concussion should be sent directly to the hospital for observation. In such cases unconsciousness may be more prolonged, lasting for 5 or more minutes. If there is marked confusion, which lasts more than 10 or 15 minutes, a severe loss of memory for an interval prior to that injury (12, 17, 22, 32), and marked dizziness and unsteadiness (4, 18, 23), the player must no longer be regarded as having just a severe concussion but possibly a contusion or an intracranial hemorrhage (15). Immediate hospitalization is then indicated.

The thoughtful neurosurgeon cannot help but think of the dichotomy in standards set for the average citizen and football player. In many hospitals the traffic accident victim is unequivocally hospitalized for 24 hours if there has been a blow to the head with unconsciousness. However, with football players it is obviously offtimes "necessary" to return them to the game if they have only sustained a first or second degree concussion.

As much as one would like simply to compartmentalize head injuries, no hard and fast rules can be made (6). The general condition of the player is vital and this may be judged only by experience. For example, Quigley (19) stated that three severe concussions sustained in football automatically should remove the player permanently from the sport. This author agrees, but often circumstances are such that the player may have only one severe concussion and yet good judgment will rule that he should be excluded from playing any more football.

The above criteria are merely empirical ones and do not have current medical proof. *They are not to be construed as being established unequivocally for each and every situation* but may serve as guidelines.

The Presence of an Expanding Intracranial Hemorrhage

During this early interval of evaluation the coach, trainer, or team physician should check on the equality of the patient's pupils. *If they are unequal at any time, regardless of whether the patient is mentally alert or disoriented, he should be seen by a physician and under no circumstances should he be returned to the game.* It has been particularly gratifying to this author currently to observe the team physician or trainer on the field cupping his hands on either side of the injured player's face to shield the player's eyes from extraneous light and check for pupillary equality on the field shortly after an equivocal or transient interlude of unconsciousness.

A simple check of the blood pressure, pulse, and respiratory rate taken over a minute's span every 5 or 10 minutes is a wise precaution.

Signs demanding EMERGENCY ACTION:

1. Increasing headache, nausea, vomiting
2. Inequality of the pupils
3. Disorientation
4. Progressive impairment of consciousness
5. Gradual rise in the blood pressure
6. Diminution of the pulse rate

Such a player is no longer suffering from a simple concussion or contusion of the brain but rather from an expanding blood clot within the skull (24, 25).

Fortunately convulsive seizures occur very rarely but the physician and trainer should be prepared for such an emergency. The more frequent use of the midline bar coupled with the two or more horizontal ones of the face guard make insertion of a mouth gag almost an impossibility. Either an instrument, such as a size "0" bolt cutter, should be available to cut off the face guard or the helmet while the head is supported (Fig. 49, A and B) or, if the player is wearing a pneumatic type of helmet, it may be readily deflated by inserting a knife and puncturing its inner pneumatic support (Fig. 85, A and B). This ease of removal of the headgear is important, for the patient may have a spinal as well as a head injury requiring careful extraction techniques. Even with the helmet removed it is at times difficult to insert a mouth gag or perhaps several tongue depressors wrapped together at the tip with gauze sponges in order to prevent the patient from biting his tongue and perhaps to ensure a better airway.

Pulmonary and Cardiac Resuscitation

A good airway is essential in all head and neck injuries and a plastic one should be available for such insertion. There may be the rare instance for the need of the two way resuscitube (Fig. 49C) if there has been cardiac and pulmonary arrest. This former type of tube is more readily applicable to this situation and certainly is more hygienic than the mouth to mouth technique depicted

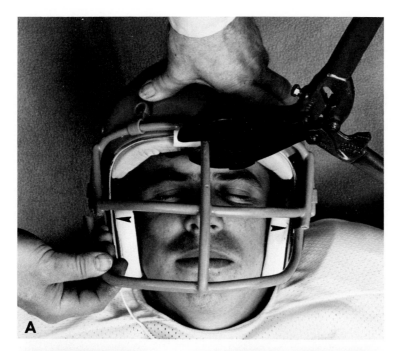

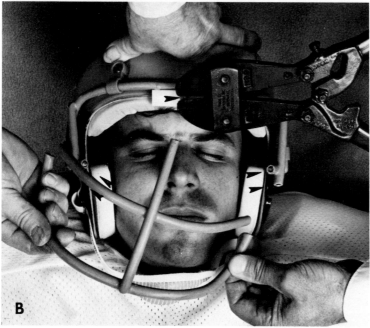

Fig. 49. *An important item of equipment* should be available for rapidly removing the face guard if an emergency cardiac or pulmonary arrest occurs.

Fig. 49A. A size "0" bolt cutter is used to cut directly across the bars of the steel face guard. No attempt should be made to save time by cutting across a joint for the cutter must be *perpendicular* to the bar to be transected. A protective towel should be placed across the face under the guard (not shown here). The head should be firmly steadied.

Fig 49B. The last of the five cuts has been made and the face guard is free. If done properly it can be accomplished in less than a minute.

167

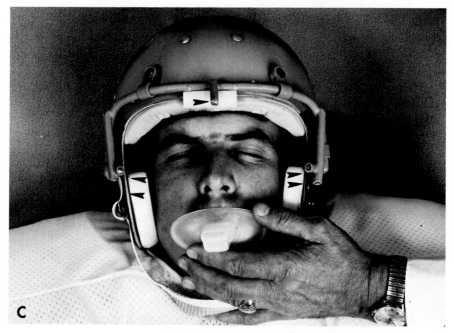

Fig. 49C. This airway has been inserted, being sure the tongue was pulled well forward while lipping it into place. The victim is now prepared for mouth to mouth resuscitation.

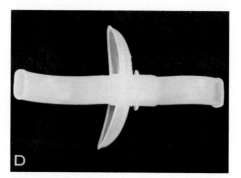

Fig. 49D. A plastic two-way resuscitube is shown.

on the usual resuscitative charts (Fig. 49D) (11). (In very rare instances in which the player has a severe seizure and the jaws cannot be opened successfully for the insertion of a plastic pharyngeal airway, an emergency "needle tracheotomy" is valuable if properly inserted just below the thyroid cartilage at the thyrocricoid junction in the exact midline by experienced and trained personnel. However, the frequent occurrence of penetration of the lung, esophagus, or a large blood vessel has led to other hazardous complications and has resulted in the abandonment of the procedure.) For cardiac arrest cardiopulmonary resuscitative measures must be instituted (Fig. 50) (2, 16).

Occasionally the heart will not start again with external massage alone (3). There are a few isolated large universities and other facilities in the country where a defibrillator (an electric device to give the heart a quick jolt when external cardiac massage is unsatisfactory) and an electrocardiogram (EKG, for

EMERGENCY MEASURES IN CARDIOPULMONARY RESUSCITATION

Place Victim Flat On His Back On A Hard Surface

IF UNCONSCIOUS, OPEN AIRWAY

LIFT UP NECK
PUSH FOREHEAD BACK
CLEAR OUT MOUTH IF NECESSARY

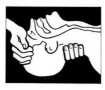

Fig. 50. These emergency measures in cardiopulmonary resuscitation may be followed with only the *vital reminder* that if the patient has sustained head trauma and a concomitant cervical spine injury is suspected, the neck *may not be lifted* as noted in the first step. It must be maintained in the plane of the body and the angle of the mandible must be elevated. A hand operated resuscitation bag or respirator may be necessary to continue artificial ventilation. [Courtesy of the American Heart Association (2).]

IF NOT BREATHING, BEGIN ARTIFICIAL BREATHING

CONTINUE AT A RATE OF
12 INFLATIONS PER MINUTE

**CHECK
CAROTID PULSE**

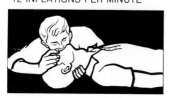 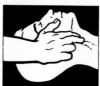

IF PULSE ABSENT, BEGIN ARTIFICIAL CIRCULATION

LOCATE
PRESSURE
POINT

DEPRESS STERNUM 1½" TO 2"
60 TO 80 TIMES PER MINUTE

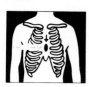

ONE RESCUER
15 compressions
2 quick inflations

TWO RESCUERS
5 compressions
1 inflation

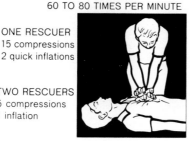

 American Heart Association • 44 East 23 Street • New York, N.Y. 10010

scanning the wave form rhythm) are available in the stadium emergency unit (Fig. 51) (5, 10, 13). Cooper (7) has presented an extremely unusual personal experience within one afternoon of two such patients with cardiac arrest, one an official and the other a football player. He has been kind enough to permit the author to recount the story here.*

In the first instance a head linesman collapsed and lay motionless. He was unconscious, somewhat rigid, quivering, apneic, and pale with no palpable pulse. An airway was maintained and external cardiac massage was instituted. Mouth to mouth resuscitation was carried out until a respirator arrived, and the patient was transferred to a student health center where a cardiac monitor revealed the presence of a ventricular fibrillation. After defibrillation and the continuous administration of oxygen, the patient was placed under the care of the internist who had been called.

The team physician returned to the football field and within approximately one minute was involved in the following situation.

Case 45. A defensive football player intercepted a pass and started running for the goal line when, after moving with extreme exertion for 60 to 70 yards, he was tackled from the rear by an opponent, causing him to fall to the ground. He immediately arose with assistance from his teammates, walked 5 to 10 feet, and then collapsed, becoming unconscious. He quivered in a semi-convulsive manner with his mouth clenched tightly, there were no respirations, and a mouth guard was lodged in his pharynx. A screw-top mouth gag was used to pry open the mouth and the removal of the mouth-

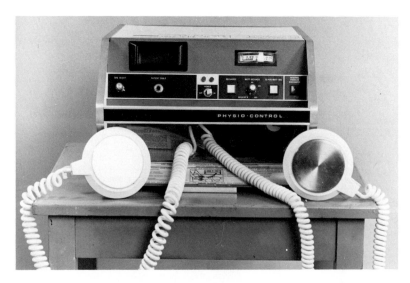

Fig. 51. Portable defibrillator shows the two electrodes for the chest. The EKG sweep is noted in the upper left-hand corner. The patient's electrode ground cord (not shown here) is inserted in the jack in the left lower corner of the machine.

---

* Part of the following material was abstracted and reprinted from Cooper (7) by permission of the *Journal of The American College Health Association.*

guard was accomplished. Although an adequate airway was developed, the player did not breathe and there was no pulse. His uniform was stripped off and external cardiac massage instituted. Mouth to mouth resuscitation was continued until respirator control was instituted and he was transported to the health center emergency room. Here the player was cyanotic, comatose, apneic, and without a pulse. When a cardiac monitor was applied, no heart contractions were noted. After the defibrillator was applied and electrical shock was administered, independent cardiac activity was re-established. Oxygen was administered through the airway and 15 cc. of sodium bicarbonate solution was injected intravenously. About 2 to 4 minutes after defibrillation his blood pressure increased, his color improved, and his pupils returned to normal. After a few minutes he began to answer questions but was confused and had difficulty with his vision and his speech was slurred. By the following morning his cardiovascular status was normal.

The student finished his academic quarter, although he had to reduce his course load. His vision apparently cleared completely, but there was difficulty with phonation when he was fatigued.

Comment. This report is a remarkable saga concerning the importance of a well educated physician and a carefully trained team, who ably met the challenge of possible fatality on two occasions and achieved a 100% salvation for these potential victims. This is a vital report for all personnel since the brain is unable to function without oxygen and must rely heavily on the re-establishment of both pulmonary and cardiac function. Equipment such as the defibrillator must be used by a trained medical team. In addition to the circumstances described above, the defibrillator has been successfully applied by Carveth (5), Cooper (7), Fors (13), and Rose and Dunn (21) to save officials, spectators, and players.

It would seem presumptuous to mention that all persons involved should be knowledgeable about the importance of these measures and that in our society such equipment is readily available. Yet not too long ago, a professional football player lay on the field afflicted with a cardiac arrest before thousands of spectators in a large city and it was evident that total confusion reigned without a definite plan to meet the emergency. *However, it should be re-emphasized that the needle tracheotomy and the defibrillator are of value only in the hands of personnel who have been taught to use them properly. If not, the complications of improper use far outweigh the benefits and merely compound an extremely serious situation.*

A mere glance at the statistical tables with reference to the time intervals (Chapter 3) between injury and operation or injury and death should provide evidence for the urgency of some of these situations. After rapid assessment of the seriousness of the player's condition and transferal of the patient to the readily available ambulance, the emergency room of the hospital to which he is being sent should be notified and the condition of the patient described. Currently this communication has been easily achieved by a two-way radio from the ambulance to the hospital center. At the University of Michigan Medical Center such an alert now sets in motion an emergency plan, which is outlined in the following case history.

Case 46. A 14 year old high school football player sustained a head injury while scrimmaging at 5:30 P.M. in Saline, Michigan. His chief complaint was dizziness. Three minutes later he fell over unconscious with a dilated right pupil. There were two coaches on the scene who remained unshaken and performed magnificently. One of them ran to a telephone and called the local physician to meet the injured player at the local hospital emergency room. The second coach loaded the boy onto a stretcher and into a station wagon, dispatching him rapidly to that community hospital about half a mile away; he arrived at 5:50 P.M. The local physician made a rapid survey of the situation, noted the dilated pupil, inserted a plastic airway, and started the boy on his way to the Medical Center in Ann Arbor 10 miles away.

Then the physician called ahead to the Center and told the neurosurgeon of the incident and related the fact that the right pupil was dilated. The neurosurgeon called the emergency room instructing that a stretcher be at the door. The hair clippers and razor were laid out. Cross-match and typing material was procured and the blood bank technician was sent to the emergency room to stand by. Two intravenous sets were hung with No. 18 needles readily available. Two 50 cc. syringes were filled with 50 cc. of 50% glucose and two No. 18 needles were applied to them. The neurosurgery resident and other house staff personnel were notified to proceed to the emergency room. The Anesthesia Department was alerted and the operating room team was ordered to open a pre-sterilized trephine set with its rapid action electric trephine drill available.

The unconscious boy arrived at 6:05 P.M. At the emergency room door a quick glance showed the right pupil was dilated and fixed to light; the left was normal. He was placed upon the waiting stretcher and, by the time he was wheeled to the emergency room 25 yards away where the team was waiting, the left pupil had dilated also and was fixed to light. The 100 cc. of 50% glucose were administered rapidly intravenously and both pupils constricted to normal size and reacted to light within 3 minutes.

The head was shaved, an intracheal tube was inserted, the specimen of blood for the cross-match and type was procured, the two intravenous sets were started, and the patient was rushed by a waiting elevator to the operating room. The head was prepared hastily and draped and four burr holes were made by 6:30 P.M. releasing a 125 cc. acute subdural blood clot, 1 hour after the injury had occurred 10 miles away. Drains were inserted and a tracheotomy was performed. The boy is shown 3 weeks postoperatively (Fig. 52). He was neurologically intact and made a complete recovery. The neurosurgeon attended the player's high school graduation 4 years later and was delighted to find that the boy ranked high in his class.

Comment. Although the use of 100 cc. of 50% glucose intravenously to reduce the increased intracranial pressure has been regarded as antiquated by some neurosurgeons "because of a secondary overswing with pressure eventually becoming elevated above the level at the time of its administration" the drug has its place in acute intracranial emergencies such as these. The much discussed "overswing" occurs a few hours later after the intracerebral clot has been removed. Then there is adequate space for the expanded edematous brain. The critical difference in the use of the hypertonic glucose in preference to urea, man-

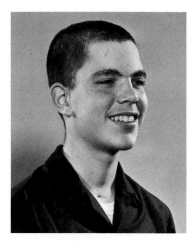

Fig. 52. Case 46. This fortunate young man's life was saved by the teamwork of rapid transportation *from the site of the game to the hospital 10 miles away* where early diagnosis and drainage of an acute subdural hemorrhage were accomplished within 1 hour after injury. He was neurologically negative, graduating high in his class 3 years later. Note the tracheotomy scar.

nitol, and other agents lies in its availability without added preparation, the speed of administration, and the truly remarkable response within 3 to 5 minutes. There is no wasted time in transferring fluid from one bottle to another, shaking the container to dissolve powder, as in the case of other agents, and then permiting the drug to be infused intravenously by drip. Speed is a vital factor.

The successful outcome in this case is not a tribute to the neurosurgeon but rather one to a well informed team of athletic, nursing, paramedical, and surgical personnel that could, and did, function extremely efficiently. For this reason it is vital that all the individuals involved in the sport be educated to the problems related to such injuries. *It is only through a sense of urgency, maintained at all levels, that the mortality rate in acute subdural hemorrhages will diminish.* It used to be as high as 90% in some of the best clinics in our country (25). There are probably two reasons for this. 1) There was a failure to recognize that here is one of the few instances in which *time in minutes and even seconds* may be a factor in the patient's survival. To pause for cerebral angiography in many cases is to court disaster. 2) The football player with acute subdural hemorrhage is much more salvageable than most high speed vehicular traffic victims. In the case of the player the forces at impact frequently are not as great and ofttimes only a single large bridging vein is disrupted, whereas the traffic victim may have not only this source of hemorrhage but also a considerable amount of underlying brain damage. Fortunately with an emergency plan such as that used above, the mortality rate should be lowered to 8 to 10% for acute subdural hemorrhage in football players.

The above case report is not an isolated incident. Another player fell over unconscious within seconds after a head injury in Ypsilanti, Michigan. He was rushed to the Medical Center in Ann Arbor seven miles away. In the interim the neurosurgeon was notified immediately by telephone that the boy was unconscious and had a dilated right pupil. His condition was so tenuous that cerebral arteriography could not be performed. A similar routine to that described in

Case 46 was followed and a large acute subdural hematoma was evacuated with recovery. The player is shown 10 days postoperatively (Fig. 53).

Emergency Operative Treatment. After careful consideration the following discussion of the operative sites and technique is described. Often after a personal presentation of much of the material in this book in over half of the states in this country this author invariably was asked, "I am a trained general surgeon, act as a team physician, am 200 miles from the nearest neurosurgeon and I have a player who falls over unconscious with a dilated pupil and upgoing toe signs as you have described. Air transportation is not available and, if time is such an important factor as suggested, what will I do?" This author is convinced that the following reply, or one similar to it, is essential.

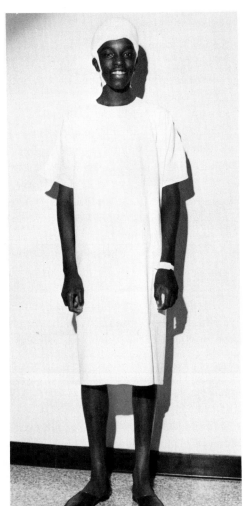

Fig. 53. This high school player fell over unconscious after a tackle. He was rushed seven miles to the medical center and an acute subdural hematoma was removed within 1½ hours.

"*If* the general surgeon is skilled, *if* blood and proper operating room facilities are instantly at hand, and *if* there is no way in which to transport the player to a neurosurgeon, it may be necessary for the local *general surgeon* to proceed in such desperate cases."

For operation the patient should be intubated promptly for control of the respiration, and the head should be shaved completely and prepared. Two large bore needle intravenous infusions are inserted. The midline of the head is identified by a superficial scalp marking and the sites for burr hole incisions sketched out bilaterally as shown on the diagram (Fig. 54). With the use of local anesthesia the scalp is infiltrated at the site and the incision is carried down to the skull, the scalp layers are separated, and a mastoid retractor is inserted. In less than usually experienced hands the burr hole is most safely made under such circumstances by the hand perforator and burr rather than by the mechanically powered instruments, with special care being taken not to plunge into the underlying brain. If the hemorrhage is on the dura (extradural), a bleeding vessel may be identified on the surface which may be cauterized or packed with a hemostatic agent. Occasionally this is not the case and it is necessary to pursue the point of the middle meningeal artery's entrance into the base of the skull through the foramen spinosum, which must be plugged with bone wax or a tiny cotton pledget. If the hemorrhage underlies the dura, the latter should be

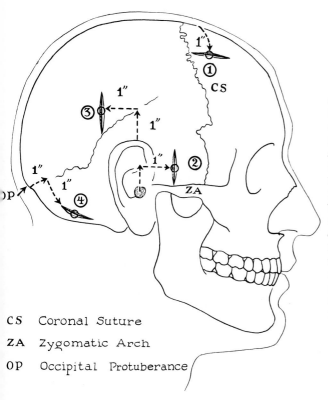

Fig. 54. Diagram of the skull shows sites of exploratory burr holes. 1) Incision 1 in. lateral to the midline and just anterior to the coronal suture. 2) Incision 1 in. above the external auditory meatus and 1 in. anterior to it. The lowermost point of the incision lies on the zygomatic arch. 3) Incision 1 in. above and 1 in. behind the ear, The lowermost point of the incision should be at the level of the top of the ear. 4) The suboccipital incision should lie 1 in. lateral to the external occipital protuberance and begin at a point one inch below the lateral sinus. [Reprinted from Schneider (26) by permission of Charles C Thomas, Publishers.]

CS   Coronal Suture

ZA   Zygomatic Arch

OP   Occipital Protuberance

cauterized slightly and then opened cautiously with a scalpel so that the underlying brain will not be damaged. Subdural hemorrhage will pour forth through the hole and a rubber Penrose drain is usually inserted to permit the blood to continue to drain out. Burr holes may be made in this manner at the sites 1, 2, and 3. The number 4 site lies over the source of the fewest surgical hemorrhages and should not be trephined by the occasional surgeon for fear of causing more harm than good. After the head dressing is applied the patient should be promptly transported to a neurosurgeon for further observation and treatment. Recurrent hemorrhage is much more difficult to handle.

Resumé

In first aid for the successful emergency care of the football player three cardinal points must be stressed:

1. Communication. A telephone with a direct outside line must be available at the field to call an ambulance.

2. Transportation. An ambulance or some other suitable vehicle, such as a station wagon or pick-up truck, must be available immediately to move the player to the hospital.

3. Notification. The hospital to which the patient is directed *must be informed of the player's status* even while the patient's immediate needs are being administered to, so that proper facilities and personnel will be available on his arrival.

Often there is an acute state of confusion with such emergencies and one of these important measures is forgotten. The first letters of this triad, "*CTN*," might well call attention to these important steps, which are to be immediately initiated, by the phrase "*Coaches Take Note*." Appropriately placed placards in the locker rooms may call attention to the routine and serve as a constant reminder when the excitement of an emergency causes confusion. (The word "citizens" might be substituted for "coaches" for situations in which vehicular accidents and other emergency conditions are present.)

It is perhaps pertinent to point out here that for many years the members of the medical profession have devoted much time and interest to the care of athletes, usually with little or no remuneration and too frequently without any recognition of them "until something goes wrong." There are few people who have been more dedicated to the care of football players or other athletes. Yet they have been completely forgotten by the populace. In many smaller communities there are insufficient physicians to have one attend each football game, but in many such instances the doctor will leave word where he may be contacted. If present at the field, or if his presence is required there, then he should be recompensed for his professional services just like any other official connected with the game. For some reason such medical service has been rather routinely accepted as a charitable gift, too often without the slightest expression of gratitude.

One of the most difficult problems is that of differentiating an acute expanding intracranial lesion, as in Case 47, from cerebral concussion which has been defined as an immediate and transient impairment of neural function, such as alteration of consciousness, disturbance of vision, equilibrium, etc., due to mechanical forces.

Case 47. A 19 year old All-American sophomore quarterback played an unusually fine game of football. In the third quarter he was struck on the head but was not rendered unconscious. He continued to play throughout the entire game and had incomplete recall of all events. After the game as he was about to board the bus he felt dizzy, fainted, and, upon being taken to the hospital, complained of left fronto-orbital headache. During this 3 hour interval he vomited only once. The only positive neurologic finding was an equivocal right Babinski sign (an upgoing toe on stroking the side of the right foot). He was roused hourly to check his state of consciousness, his blood pressure, pulse, respirations, and equality of pupils. The neurosurgeon stayed in an adjacent room all night checking the nurse's evaluation of the patient at intervals. On the following morning the player roused to eat a huge breakfast with great relish and appeared much better than the weary nurse and the neurosurgeon who had checked him all night. He was discharged 24 hours after his injury.

Comment. Only relatively recently have association and projection areas for vestibular function (dizziness) become recognized as being located in the brain at the frontotemporal junction in the superior operculum of the temporal lobe (Fig. 55) (4, 9, 18, 23). These symptoms occur when the player falls on the back of the head and the brain rebounds and smashes this frontotemporal area against the sharp sphenoid ridge leading to concussion, contusion, or, in more severe cases, intracerebral hematomas [blood clots in the brain (8, 20, 25, 29, 31)]. The result is dizziness or an unstable gait. Many football players have continued the game and have even played well after a head injury, although they subsequently remember nothing of that part of the game which followed the concussion (17, 32).

This patient (Case 47) made a good recovery from his mild contusion. He continued to play 2 more years of college football and 6 years as a professional without difficulty.

Occasionally the guidelines for the responsibility of the football players' welfare are not well defined among the team physician, the coach, and the trainer. Regrettably there is the team physician who because of timidity and insecurity withholds any injured player from the game even though the injury has been slight. On the other hand there is the coach or the trainer who overrules the doctor and urges the injured man to return at any cost. Fortunately as more and more first aid programs have been conducted, there are fewer such problems; the athletic-physician group work as a team. An example of a failure of understanding and assignment of responsibility may be found in the next case.

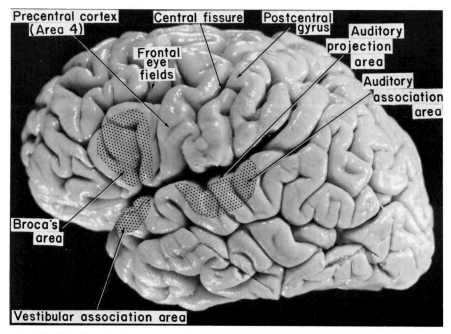

Fig. 55. This diagram demonstrates the vestibular association area along the superior temporal gyrus, which is frequently contused with contrecoup injuries resulting in dizziness and, in some cases, with rotational movements (4, 9, 18, 23). Broca's motor speech area, the motor strip (precentral area, area 4), the sensory cortex (postcentral gyrus), and the auditory projection and association areas are shown.

In a large city on the day following a full day's symposium on football injuries for physicians, coaches, and trainers in which the emphasis was placed on the mechanism of injury, the importance of prompt diagnosis, and early treatment of the injured player, the following situation occurred.

Case 48. A halfback sustained a rather severe head injury when kicked in the head by an opponent. He was markedly confused and extremely unstable on his feet, but nevertheless he was led from the field weaving from one side toward the other (Fig. 56A). In spite of his disorientation he received the classical treatment of neck massage (Fig. 56B), an ice bag to the head (Fig. 56C), and the final touch of a whiff of smelling salts (Fig. 56D). These touches of superficial therapy probably did no harm in this case for they were not too vigorous, but rather they indicated desire on the part of the trainers to "do something" for the poor fellow. Furthermore, instead of the player being retired to the locker room where he could lie down and be watched, he was permitted to sit on the bench in a semi-stuporous condition. At the close of the first half-time period he arose with his teammates heading for the locker room. He still staggered as he walked and lurched into the iron railing on the way to the locker room. It was not until that evening after the football game that he was admitted to the hospital and only then neurosurgical consultation was sought (although it was known to the officials and coaches that several neurosurgeons were available in the stands during the game). Fortunately the player recovered

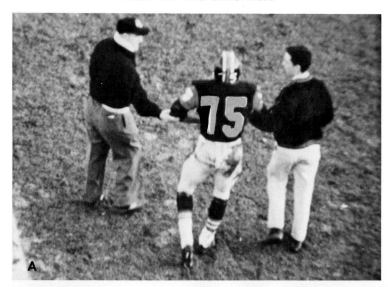

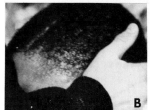
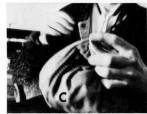
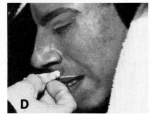

Fig. 56. Case 48. The usual or customary routine for cerebral concussion is shown.

Fig. 56A. The staggering and unsteady player is assisted from the field.

Fig. 56B. Massage to the head and neck gives the trainer a sense of aiding the injured. (The neck may be fractured.)

Fig. 56C. An ice bag possibly reduces the swelling.

Fig. 56D. The final touch is the ampule of spirits of ammonia which clears up any mental confusion.

completely from his severe concussion or contusion to the brain and was released from the hospital 24 hours later.

Comment. Currently the proper course of action would be to remove the patient from the field promptly. In this instance it would have been preferable to carry him off the field to prevent his falling and injuring himself further, but this course of action seems to be unpopular, perhaps being regarded as unmanly. The patient should have been examined in the locker room by the team physician and the neurosurgeon and then transferred to the hospital for observation.

In Cervicomedullary and Spinal Injuries

Hopefully the classically artificial division of craniospinal trauma into head and spinal injuries is vanishing. Currently there is increasing recognition that either one of these areas may be injured or very often their junction, the cervicomedullary region, may be damaged (27, 28). As has been demonstrated in these pages most of such injuries result in a fatal outcome.

Spinal Injuries

Although speed of transportation to adequate facilities for the proper treatment of all injuries to the central nervous system is important, it must be emphasized that the spinal cord is a captive within the confines of the relatively rigid bony canal. With injury there is no region of the body in which even a slightly untoward movement may be so devastating due to partial or complete transection of the cord, the latter resulting in complete permanent paralysis of the trunk, extremities, and all bodily functions below the site of injury (Fig. 57, A and B). To some extent haste should be sacrificed for extreme care in proper immobilization and movement of the patient. *The current trend of speed in transportation is being emphasized to enhance early operation and proper splinting may be overlooked.*

Diagnosis. The presence and the level of a spinal cord injury may be determined on the football field provided the examiner knows a few fundamental facts. If the patient has a fracture or dislocation of the cervical spine without any spinal cord injury there may be local tenderness and muscle spasm. No deformity is usually palpated on gently feeling the neck. If there has been spinal cord damage the player complains of little or no pain but may merely have complete paralysis and a loss of sensation. With a relatively few movement tests and a brief sensory examination with a safety pin (see dermatomes Fig. 22F) by a knowledgeable physician or a trainer, the level of the injury may be ascertained (10a). Such an examination should include the face and head (27).

1. C3-C4 level. Usually the player has a complete paralysis of the trunk and extremities with a complete loss of all normal unassisted respirations due to a paralysis of the diaphragmatic and thoracic musculature, and a loss of pain to pinprick to a point just below the clavicle including the upper extremities (10a).

2. C4-C5 level. He can only shrug his shoulders while the arms, the lower extremities, and trunk will lie without movement with the toes pointed outward; he will have only abdominal breathing. The progression of spinal cord swelling or hemorrhage of only one more segment toward the head may mean the cessation of spontaneous respiration. The absence of pain sensation is present to the level of the outer border of the upper extremity between the shoulder and elbow.

3. C5-C6 level. At this level the player will be able to bend the arms at the elbows, and they will tend to remain flexed in that position unless they fall downward with gravity. Attempted movement of the hands results in hyperextension at the wrists with inability to voluntarily close the fingers. Extension of the arms is markedly impaired. There may be a loss of pain on pinprick over the region of the thumb and index fingers of the hands.

4. C6-C7 level. With injury at this site the patient will be able to very weakly

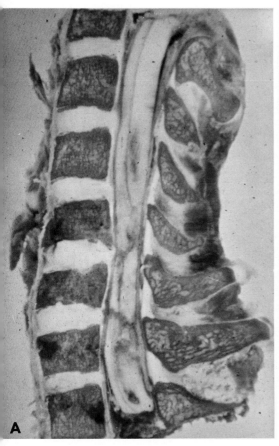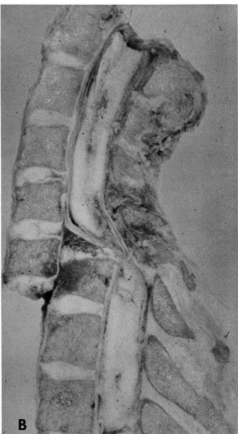

Fig. 57. These are two of only four figures in this book which are not related to football, but which are so graphically illustrative of such injuries that they are included. (Courtesy of the Museum of the Royal College of Surgeons, London.)

Fig. 57A. A compression fracture of C5 vertebral body demonstrating the extent of linear hemorrhages cephalad and caudad despite minimal encroachment on the spinal cord by the posterior margin of the vertebral body.

Fig. 57B. Marked fracture-dislocation of C5 on C6 vertebral body displaying severe spinal cord damage.

close the hands and grasp with the fingers. The arms can be flexed and extended weakly at the elbows. He is unable to spread the fingers apart strongly. Pinprick sensation will be intact over the thumb and index fingers but usually is lost over the middle and the radial half of the ring fingers.

Rarely do fracture-dislocations of the thoracic or lumbar spine or spinal cord injuries occur in football players. In the "Statistical Survey;" (Chapter 3) there were no fracture-dislocations or spinal cord injuries to the thoracic region. The support of the thoracic rib cage, the strong paraspinous muscles in this region, and the protective shoulder padding almost reaching the hip padding are probably preventive factors. Only a single fracture-dislocation of the lumbar spine was reported in the survey.

5. L1-L2 level. Good movement is found in the upper extremities. There is paralysis of the thighs, inability to extend and flex the legs on the thighs, and paralysis of any movement of the legs and feet. Pinprick sensation is impaired from the middle or inner part of the thighs downward to include the inner part of the legs, the feet, and the outer portion of the thighs and perhaps the saddle area (over both buttocks).

These rather simple tests, which are far from a complete neurologic examination, are meant only as a quick field test. If there is any doubt as to whether such neurologic findings are real or due to hysteria, the player should be treated as having a true physical lesion.

Movement and Immobilization. If a broken neck is suspected, the helmet may be left in place with the chin strap firmly attached, that is, provided the removal of the headgear is not essential for special attention to respiratory function. The in situ examination having been completed, the patient must be moved cautiously to a long board specially used for immobilization in emergency vehicles. Such movement is thus accomplished by one person applying steady traction on either side of the head with the fingers along the mandible providing a pull in the plane of the body while three other people standing on the same side may insert their hands and forearms under the player raising him rigidly so there is no sagging of the body (Fig. 58). The patient is then applied to a special long board and immobilized.

Careful attention is directed toward immobilization of the head and neck. Certain models of helmets may be removed readily by the excision of the face guard as previously described (see Fig. 49, A–C). Simple deflation may be achieved by puncturing with a knife any pneumatic inflated inner supports (Fig. 85 A and B).

A method, which may be used satisfactorily if carefully supervised by knowledgeable personnel, is the use of chin strap sling traction. This may be achieved by the firm bolting of a temporary metal frame with a small wheel to the head of one of the long emergency boards. A chin strap sling is then applied to the patient and the rope from the sling hung over the grooved wheel of the frame with the application of sufficient weight to maintain a constant pull of the head and neck in the plane of the body. The board is then fastened firmly on the stretcher and the weights hang freely. Gooding (14a) has designed a new calibrated spring traction attachment to the usual long board for emergencies. This device has the desirable features of increased stability by avoiding swinging traction weights and requires less space (Fig. 59, A and B) (14a). The conveyor, whether ambulance or helicopter, must provide smooth and shockless transportation to avoid further injury to the spinal cord.

Pain relieving medication in the form of codeine intramuscularly may be given for cervical fractures or dislocations. Demerol is slightly more apt to diminish respirations and morphine and atropine are to be avoided because of their artificial constriction or dilatation of the pupils, respectively, signs which

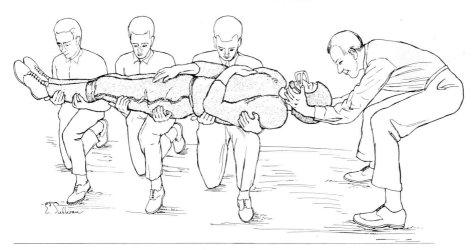

Fig. 58. In suspected cervical spinal cord injuries it may be more desirable to leave the football helmet in place rather than to struggle with its removal. In such instances the chin strap should remain in place; traction should be instituted in the plane of the body. At least three people should lift from the same side of the patient supporting the legs, buttocks, trunk, and shoulders.

are important in evaluation of the player who has an associated head injury. Most spinal fractures with complete transection of the cord require no pain medication.

Currently there has been a major advance in the treatment of spinal cord injuries. It has been demonstrated definitely in the experimental animal, and is reasonably well supported in man, as of this writing, that *the early use of steroids (14) in the treatment of some spinal cord injuries will cause a diminution of swelling and destruction of the cord with the prevention of neurologic deficit.* Experimental work has shown that the drug probably should be administered within 3 to 6 hours after the spinal cord is injured for the drug to be effective. Therefore the decision whether this form of medical therapy should be instituted should be made by the physician shortly after the player has been taken to the dressing room and the presence of spinal cord damage has been confirmed. It may be withheld if the patient definitely can be transported within 3 hours to the neurosurgeon so he can make the decision. If the time interval is longer than this, then Decadron, 10 mgm., should be administered intramuscularly and then 4 mgm. should be given every 6 hours. *This is a major and serious decision.* If the drug is administered it should be tapered over a prolonged period and not stopped abruptly, for fear of adrenal gland failure. In order to prevent gastric ulceration and hemorrhage from hyperacidity with its long time usage, antacids or milk should be given at regular specified intervals. *It is believed that once the drug has been administered in this manner, the patient must again receive it at the time of any later period of stress, such as an operation later in life, etc.*

The proper approach to spine injuries demands that the patient be moved as little as possible to prevent any distortion to the spine and further damage

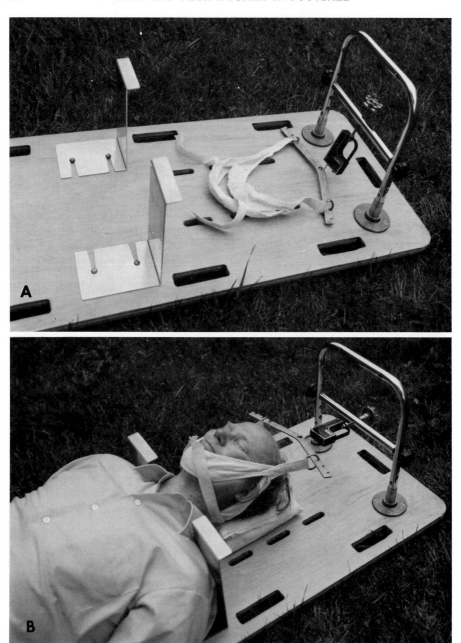

Fig. 59A. The emergency long board is shown with the removable shoulder supports *and the special calibrated spring traction apparatus in place*. [Taken from Gooding (14a).]

Fig. 59B. The patient is held in position by the shoulder supports. Traction is applied using a typical cervical traction sling and tension may be adjusted by turning the handle which is attached to the hook on the scale until the desired tension is noted (up to 25 pounds). *An additional chin sling may be slipped through one of the three slots in the board on either side of head and neck or sandbags may be applied to gently support the neck in the event that any slippage of the traction should occur.* [Taken from Gooding (14a).]

to the underlying spinal cord or nerve roots to a minimum. Consequently, the patient is maintained on the original stretcher in traction or with some other support until all x-ray examinations have been procured. If a cervical fracture is suspected the lower portion of the C7 vertebral body's relationship to T1 vertebral body must be demonstrated for completeness' sake. A "swimmer's view" may be necessary to demonstrate this region. If no fracture or dislocation of the spine is found the traction apparatus may be removed, and the patient may be permitted to go without support, or, if there is a painful muscle sprain or ligamentous injury, a collar or neck brace may be substituted for support.

On the contrary, if an unstable fracture or fracture-dislocation of the cervical spine is demonstrated, skeletal traction should be inserted under local anesthesia and the necessary amount of weight applied to maintain alignment or reduce the dislocation. The patient is most frequently placed upon a Stryker frame or Foster frame in order to ensure better nursing care with the least possible chance of displacement of the fracture. Operative intervention may be desirable or a conservative course of action may be elected.

The indications and contraindications for surgical intervention relative to spinal injuries. Over the past 20 years this author has constantly reviewed the cases of patients with spinal cord injuries attempting to establish a set of criteria for operation and another group of standards for which surgical intervention is contraindicated. These rules of thumb have been recorded at length elsewhere in detail (26), and are merely listed here for the sake of completeness.

I. Indications for operation
  1. A progression of neurologic signs.
  2. A blockage of subarachnoid space when the jugular vein compression (Queckenstedt) test is performed. This is mentioned only to comment that, if there is a block, operation is indicated. If there is no blockage, surgical intervention may still be desirable.
  3. The anterior cervical spinal cord injury syndrome, (Chapter 5). This is characterized by immediate complete paralysis with a sensory level of hypalgesia to the level of the lesion and with preservation of motion, position, and vibration sense. One may not be able to distinguish between anterior spinal cord compression, vascular insufficiency, or destruction. Thus operation is indicated.
  4. A compound fracture of the spine. (This author has no knowledge of such a lesion occurring in a football player; it is doubtful that it would occur).
  5. *Decompression of an important nerve root.* In some instances the decompression of a C6 or C7 nerve root may result in better functional recovery of the hand even though there is an immediate complete cord injury.

Any of the above criteria would dictate an urgent surgical approach. There are other factors to be considered, but in such instances time does not play as vital a part.
  6. Bone fragments in the spinal canal in selected cases. There is always 100% more bony damage than is visualized in the x-ray examination.
  7. The prevention of increasing deformity with subsequent chronic neurologic sequelae by proper stabilization of anterior lesions of the spine. The "tear-drop" fracture discussed in Chapter 5 is an example.
  8. Any lesion demonstrating neurologic involvement of the cauda equina or conus medullaris. Such injury is different from a spinal cord injury. Trauma to the cauda equina may result in a type of injury simulating peripheral nerve damage. If motor roots are merely contused but remain in continuity and are compressed by a bone fragment, which can be elevated, regeneration of the root may occur inasmuch as the cell body for the motor root lies within the anterior horn cell of the spinal cord.

II. Contraindications to surgical intervention
  1. A C3-C4 injury with complete areflexic tetraplegia. Such a patient already has difficulty

with respirations, for the intercostal muscles are paralyzed. Any surgical intervention at this level might cause irritation of the nerve roots, which supply the phrenic nerve, damage to which would result in the complete loss of diaphragmatic respirations, i.e., all voluntary respiration.

2. The acute central cervical cord injury syndrome (Chapter 5) is characterized by more profound motor loss in the upper extremities than the lower ones with varying degrees of sensory impairment. Recovery follows the set pattern of the lower extremities recovering first, the upper arms following, then motion returning to the forearms with recovery of the finger movement occurring last of all.
3. The patient who is in traumatic shock. Good surgical principles dictate the surgery should not be performed or the patient will succumb.
4. The situation where the proper facilities and instruments are unavailable.
5. A "hangman's fracture" (26) where healing with solid union may occur spontaneously with proper bracing. This lesion is an avulsion of the laminar arches of C2 from the body of that vertebra with possibly slight dislocation of C2 on C3 vertebral body. The advantages of the conservative treatment are the avoidance of anesthetic or respiratory problems with manipulation at this level and the dangers of an infection. The disadvantages are the discomfort of immobilization in a brace for a seven or eight week period while healing occurs. The patient may be ambulatory during this interval. (Incidentally, this author has never heard of a "hangman's fracture" occurring in football, The forces involved in this type of impact are probably insufficient to cause such a lesion.)
6. *The patient with the immediate complete tetraplegia or paraplegia without block on the Queckenstedt test. (The current use of Decadron may alter this criterion).*
7. The Dejerine "onion skin" pattern, which more recently has been associated by this author with cervical spine injuries, may indicate involvement of the trigeminal descending tract with traumatic lesions as low as the C5 level (27). If the pattern of hypesthesia involves the entire face and head except for the vermillion border of the lips, it suggests that the damage to the blood supply or the nervous system may extend as high as the medulla and thus warrant deferment of any surgical procedure.

This appears to be a complicated list of criteria but they have been found to be workable when followed carefully. They will never become popular with those surgeons who merely wish a single simple rule of thumb that can be used without an understanding of the neurologic and orthopedic factors involved in the diagnosis and treatment of such cases. Further discussion may be found in the chapter on treatment of the acute spinal injury (Chapter 12).

References

1. American Medical Association: Standard Nomenclature of Sports Injuries.
2. American Heart Association: Chart—Emergency Measures in Cardiopulmonary Resuscitation. 44 East 23rd Street, New York, New York 10010.
3. Beck, C. S., Pritchard, W. H. and Fiel, S. H.: Ventricular Fibrillation of Long Duration Abolished by Electrical Shock. *J.A.M.A., 135:* 985, 1947.
4. Calhoun, H. D., Crosby, E. C., Kooi, K. A. and Schneider, R. C.: Cortical and Subcortical Lesions Evoking Vestibular Symptoms. An Electroencephalographic, Anatomical and Surgical Study. *Clin. EEG, 3:* 6, 1972.
5. Carveth, S. W.: Resuscitation Program at the Nebraska Football Stadium. *Dis. Chest, 53:* 8, 1968.
6. Committee on Head Injury Nomenclature of the Congress of Neurological Surgeons: Glossary of Head Injury Including Some Definitions of Injury of the Cervical Spine. *Clin. Neurosurg., 12:* 388, 1966.
7. Cooper, T. Y.: Contact Sports and Cardiac Injury: What a Team Physician Might Be Called upon to Do. *J. Am. Coll. Health Assoc., 17:* 64, 1968.
8. Courville, C. B.: *Commotio Cerebri.* p. 63, San Lucas Press, Los Angeles, 1953.
9. Crosby, E. C. and Calhoun, H. D.: A Discussion of Some Interrelated Functions of the Vestibular and Ocular Motor Systems. In *Vestibular and Oculomotor Problems*, p. 15–20. Tokyo, 1965.

10. Day, W. H.: A Cardiac Resuscitation Program. *Lancet, 82:* 153, 1962.

10a. DeQuervain, F.: *Clinical and Surgical Diagnosis for Students and Practitioners.* p. 914, William Wood and Co., New York, 1921.

11. Elam, J. O., Brown, E. S. and Elder, J. D., Jr.: Artificial Respirations by Mouth-to-Mouth Method. *N. Engl. J. Med., 250:* 749, 1954.

12. Fisher, C. M.: Concussion Amnesia. *Neurology, 16:* 826, 1966.

13. Fors, W. J. Jr.: Personal communication.

14. Galicich, J. R. and French, L. A.: Use of Dexamethasone in Treatment of Cerebral Edema Resulting from Brain Tumors and Brain Surgery. *Ann. Pract. Digest. Treat., 12:* 169, 1961.

14a. Gooding, E. R.: A Specially Calibrated Spring Traction Apparatus for Immobilization of the Head and Neck on the Long Emergency Board. To be published.

15. Jamieson, K. G. and Yelland, J. D. N.: Extradural Hematoma. Report of 167 Cases. *J. Neurosurg., 29:* 13, 1968.

16. Kouwenhoven, K. B., Jude, J. R. and Knickerbocker, G. G.: Closed Chest Cardiac Massage. *J.A.M.A., 173:* 1064, 1960.

17. Marzia, V. D. B. and Randt, C.: Amnesia and Eye Movements in First Stage of Anesthesia. *Arch. Neurol., 14:* 522, 1966.

18. Penfield, W.: Vestibular Sensation and the Cerebral Cortex. *Ann. Othol. Rhinol. Laryngol., 66:* 691, 1957.

19. Quigley, T. B.: Personal communication.

20. Reid, S. F., Tarkington, J. A., Epstein, H. M. and O'Dea, T. J.: Brain Tolerance to Impact in Football. *Surg. Gynecol. Obstet., 133:* 929, 1971.

21. Rose, K. D. and Dunn, F. L.: The Heart of the Spectator Sportsman. *Med. Times,* October, 1964.

22. Russell, W. R. and Nathan, P. W.: Traumatic Amnesia. *Brain, 69:* 280, 1946.

23. Schneider, R. C., Calhoun, H. D. and Crosby, E. C.: Vertigo and Rotational Movements in Cortical and Subcortical Lesions. *J. Neurol. Sci., 6:* 493, 1968.

24. Schneider, R. C. and Kriss, F. C.: Decisions Concerning Cerebral Concussions in Football Players. *Med. Sci. Sports, 1:* 112, 1969.

25. Schneider, R. C.: Craniocerebral Trauma. In *Correlative Neurosurgery,* 2nd ed., edited by E. A. Kahn, E. C. Crosby, R. C. Schneider and J. A. Taren, Chap. 25. Charles C Thomas, Springfield, Ill., 1969.

26. Schneider, R. C.: Trauma to the Spine and Spinal Cord. In *Correlative Neurosurgery,* 2nd ed., edited by E. A. Kahn, E. C. Crosby, R. C. Schneider and J. A. Taren, Chap. 26. Charles C Thomas, Springfield, Ill., 1969.

27. Schneider, R. C.: Concomitant Craniocerebral and Spinal Trauma, with Special Reference to the Cervicomedullary Region. *Clin. Neurosurg., 17:* 266, 1970.

28. Schneider, R. C., Gosch, H. H., Norrell, H., Jerva, M., Combs, L. W. and Smith, R. A.: Vascular Insufficiency and Differential Distortion of Brain and Cord Caused by Cervicomedullary Football Injuries. *J. Neurosurg., 33:* 363, 1970.

29. Symmonds, C. P.: Concussion and Its Sequelae. *Lancet, 1:* 1, 1962.

30. Taylor, A. R.: Post-Concussional Sequelae. *Br. Med. J., 3:* 67, 1967.

31. Ünterharnscheidt, F.: About Boxing, Review of Historical and Medical Aspects. *Texas Rep. Biol. Med., 28:* 421, 1970.

32. Yarnell, P. R. and Lynch, S.: Retrograde Memory Immediately after Concussion. *Lancet, 1:* 863, 1970.

chapter twelve

Treatment of Acute Spinal Injuries

The cervical spinal area, which comprises the site for the major number of our neurosurgical injuries, is such a delicate one that there is no situation corresponding to that of acute expanding intracranial hemorrhage in which emergency operative treatment is justified other than by certain qualified neurosurgeons or orthopedic surgeons.

For some reason the prompt closed realignment of the dislocated spine provides a challenge that simply cannot be resisted by some impetuous or unscrupulous individuals. Ofttimes there is a failure to consider the consequences of manipulation of the cervical spine with the possible permanent sequelae of spinal cord transection or nerve root injury (Chapter 6). If relocation of the cervical spinal injury is to be effected it should be performed very cautiously with skeletal cervical traction without manipulation or at the time of operation, when the relationship between the distorted bone and the spinal cord and nerve roots may be visualized.

It is not within the province of this monograph to discuss the various kinds of operations or their application to specific types of spinal injuries. Nevertheless this author would be remiss in not even briefly mentioning for the student certain current exciting experimental and clinical work which may completely alter the acute treatment of spinal injuries in the future.

The methods of brain scans, radioactive iodinated serum albumin (RISA) studies, and special X-ray cerebral arteriographic and subtraction evaluations are gradually complementing or even replacing the use of the neuroanatomical examination in the diagnosis of head injuries. Similarly the newer techniques of x-ray polytomography, evoked potentials, and newer medical and surgical methods are tending to make reliance upon the neurologic evaluation of the spinal cord injured patient appear obsolescent, but the latter still has its place in diagnosis, the estimation of prognosis, and the evaluation of treatment (29, 33).

In this clinic during the past few years the use of the percutaneous instillation of contrast medium at the C2 vertebral level for cervical myelography using the translateral film in the prone position has eliminated anxiety concerning undue movement at the cervical fracture or dislocation site such as might occur with tilting of the patient if the radiopaque material was injected by the lumbar route. The increasing use of gas myelography (21, 24) with polytomography in some clinics (23, 28) has shown the presence of extruded disc or bone fragments anterior to the cervical spinal cord and has reinforced the clinical observation of the acute anterior cervical spinal cord injury syndrome (29, 30) with the necessity of urgent operation (33). On the other hand, if there is a smooth gas shadow anterior to the cervical spine cord and a fragment is excluded, there may have been destruction or merely vascular insufficiency without compression to the anterior portion of the cervical spinal cord and surgery may be contraindicated as suggested by Rossier (28) to this author.

Over a decade ago Turnbull et al. (34) reported their microangiographic study of the spinal cord of the cadaver describing the intrinsic relationships of the tiny vessels. In order to study the results of trauma to the spinal cord in the laboratory, the older techniques of Allen (1, 2) of dropping a given weight a specific distance directly on the cord has been used (3, 10, 25, 26, 36). However, a rather more realistic development of a lesion by Gosch et al. (14, 15) employing the impact track has been used in the Michigan Neurosurgical Research Laboratory (Chapter 14). Ducker and Assenmacher (11) studying trauma induced in monkey spinal cords emphasized the importance of the timing in the microvascular response. They believed that the subacute and delayed response due to alteration of the vessel wall resulted in a perivascular inflammatory response, vasomotor paralysis, intravascular stasis, and occasional intravascular coagulation which halted circulation and led to necrosis within the cord. These authors suggested that such a response was self-destructive and indicated that prevention of this phase was essential.

In other important experimental work Wagner et al. (35) believed that within 4 hours following contusion pathologic changes occurred in the microvasculature of the spinal cord which resulted in depleted circulation of the capillaries and postcapillary venules. In further work from that laboratory Dohrmann et al. (9) demonstrated by electron microscopy that, by 1 hour after the spinal cord was experimentally contused, the periaxonal spaces of the involved fibers were dilated and that, although the myelin sheaths of the fibers were attenuated, the axonal morphology remained intact. After 4 hours the myelinated nerve fibers had markedly dilated periaxonal spaces and the intact but attenuated sheaths had axons in various stages of degeneration. However, there still were only partially denuded axons. Since some of their animals only had a transitory paraplegia they postulated that the changes in these less injured fibers were reversible within the first two weeks after injury. Kelly et al. (19) found in studying traumatized dog spinal cords that low tissue pO_2 could be replaced with oxygen under high pressure and that following the use of hyperbaric oxygen recovery of neurologic function seemed equal to other treatment with hypothermia, steroids, etc. (20). From their observations on monkeys' spinal cords which were submitted to weight dropping technique, Osterholm and Mathews (25) discovered the rather rapid accumulation of norepinephrine after injury. The result was first a neural reaction of electrical depression or paralysis of fiber activity. The second response was a vascular one which was toxic tissue destruction. Their subsequent studies (26) demonstrated that alpha-methyltyrosine blocked the formation of norepinephrine and thus diminished the degree of spinal cord damage. However, alpha-methyltyrosine is extremely toxic and Osterholm and Mathews (26) have warned against its use in humans. Nevertheless, this chemical study provides the possibility of an improved outlook for the spinal cord injury patient of the future.

To Albin et al. (3) and to White and Albin (36) must go the credit for the current interest in experimental work due to their studies with local hypothermia. Their work suggested that local cooling of the traumatized spinal cord using Allen's (1, 2) old techniques effected remarkable neurologic recovery. Ducker and Hamit (10) and Black and Markowitz (4) found the administration of steroids in similarly produced experimental trauma to be at least equal to and usually superior to local cooling of the injured cord in attaining neurologic recovery. The report of Cole et al. (5), stemming from the long use of corticosteroids at Minnesota, suggested that if they are to be effective they should be administered early, for the effect is probably greatest in 3 to 6 hours.

Although Dawson studied cerebral responses following electrical peripheral nerve stimulation in 1947 (7) and improved his technique in 1954 (8), the use of evoked responses in studying the prognosis of traumatized peripheral nerves (22) and injured spinal cords in animals (6) and man (12, 13, 16, 27) has only recently been reinstituted. The future application of these techniques may be of aid in estimating the prognosis and the value of various medical and surgical techniques in the treatment of acute spinal cord injuries in man.

This author (33) and others (17, 18) have stated in the past that, if spinal cord injury is immediate and complete without block for 24 hours or longer, the prognosis for any functional recovery is hopeless. Currently as a result of the early treatment of such patients with corticosteroids this author believes this view is no longer tenable, for there has been effective recovery of neurologic function beyond the 24 hour interval in some instances (33a). In 1951 (29) the syndrome of "acute anterior spinal cord injury" was first described (Chapter 5) and was expanded upon in further reports (31, 33) as an indication for operation. Perhaps the early administration of steroids to diminish anterior cord edema is all that is necessary, provided the presence of a disc or bone fragment can be excluded by gas myelography or polytomography, as suggested by Larson (23) and Rossier (28).

From a discussion of the experimental data above it is apparent that the goal in the treatment of acute spinal cord injuries, whether it be on a biochemical or surgical basis, should be the diminution in hypoxia to the injured spinal cord by the improvement of the microcirculation. White et al. (37) reported applying their experimental cooling local techniques, which required operative intervention, to 10 patients, who had "complete or nearly complete" tetraplegia with some degree of satisfactory neurological recovery. This paper intimated that such recovery probably was related to the operation and the hypothermia technique which was employed. Inasmuch as this work was presented at a national meeting and numerous impressionable neurosurgeons may hasten to provide such therapy, a few critical comments are in order. A lesion is either "complete or incomplete." Since the recognition of the "acute central cervical spinal cord injury syndrome" (30, 32), this author discovered that patients with only a twitch of the quadriceps or minimal movement of a great toe may progress to complete recovery without operation. If surgery had been performed the return of function would have been attributed to the successful operative procedure. Attention to each detail in the neurologic examination is significant. This is the reason why large surveys of spinal cord injuries by a multitude of examiners, some thorough and others not so compulsive, may produce evaluations which are misleading.

Another consideration relative to surgery is that the jostling about necessary to introduce an intratracheal tube in a patient who already has an almost completely compromised respiratory function by a complete lesion at the C3–C4 level or higher may lead to tragedy (33). In the series of the 10 patients which were reported (37) there were four who were stated to have respiratory or/and cardiac arrest. It is difficult to understand what effect such occurrences can have on the microcirculation of the injured spinal cord other than a deleterious one.

Of what significance is all of this discussion to the treatment of the football player with a cervical spine injury? A glance at the pathologic specimens, Figure 57, A and B (Chapter 11), makes one realize that care in proper immobilization for transportation is more important, currently, than the speed at which one can take such patients to an operating room. If they arrive at the hospital with a further damaged spinal cord, surgery will be of little avail.

The most important factor to be gleaned from the experimental and clinical work is the fact that the early administration of steroids, at least at the present time, seems as effective as or perhaps even better than surgery. This is the rationale for the early administration of steroids on the field to the player with a broken neck. Prior to this era this author and many of his associates (18, 28) had never seen a patient recover motor function when *an immediate areflexic tetraplegia* had prevailed for 24 hours. During the past year he has had two 18 year old patients, a young girl and a young boy, who were *totally tetraplegic* for a period well beyond the 24 hour interval described above (33a). The girl received Decadron (a steroid) 9 hours after injury, but the boy was given his first dose of the drug 3 days after injury. The girl had an operative decompression and posterior spinal fusion 1 week after injury while the boy was operated upon 3 weeks following his accident. A 14 months' follow-up revealed the girl had loss of pinprick sensation only over her right leg which caused no handicap for she was teaching dancing 5 days a week and on a 6th day was taking ballet lessons. On the same date the boy had only residual deficit in the interossei muscles of his hand but had no difficulty performing his job as a heavy truck driver. Can one attribute these excellent results to Decadron any more than cooling of the spinal cord? The operations in both patients were deferred 1 week and 3 weeks after injury, respectively, thus avoiding the dangers of acute operation and possible vascular insufficiency in the microcirculation.

The administration of 10 mgm. of Decadron intramuscularly by the physician on the field to a player with a tetraplegia is certainly justified and probably indicated. Every 4 hours thereafter he should have another dose of 4 mgm. intramuscularly to maintain a high level of the drug in the body. After 4 days this dosage may be diminished to 2.5 mgm every 4 hours. However, there are certain features of the drug which must be considered. Decadron may cause hyperacidity and ulceration in the gastrointestinal tract so that it is necessary to administer antacids every 4 hours to prevent this complication. It is also important to realize that if the patient has been placed on the drug for a prolonged interval, additional dosages of Decadron may have to be administered if severe stress, such as an operative procedure, is anticipated. The steroids are not to be used lightly; there may be complications with them but the benefits of the drug far outweigh its contraindications when one considers the chance of preventing immediate complete areflexic tetraplegia or paraplegia.

References

1. Allen, A. R.: Surgery of Experimental Lesion of the Spinal Cord Equivalent to Crush Injury of Fracture Dislocation of Spinal Column. A Preliminary Report. *J.A.M.A., 57:* 878, 1911.
2. Allen, A. R.: Remarks on the Histopathological Changes in the Spinal Cord Due to Impact: An Experimental Study. *J. Nerv. Ment. Dis., 11:* 141, 1914.
3. Albin, M. S., White, R. J., Acosta-Rua, G. and Yashon, D.: Study of Functional Recovery Produced by Delayed Localized Cooling after Spinal Cord Injury in Primates. *J. Neurosurg., 29:* 113, 1968.
4. Black, P. and Markowitz, R. S.: Experimental Spinal Cord Injury in Monkeys: Comparison of Steroids and Local Hypothermia. *Surg. Forum, 22:* 409, 1971.
5. Cole, H., Long, D. and Chou, S.: Are Corticosteroids Effective in the Treatment of Spinal Cord Lesions? Presented at the 25th Annual Meeting of The Neurosurgical Society of America, Pebble Beach, Calif., March 22, 1972.
6. Croft, T. J., Brodkey, J. S. and Nulsen, F. E.: Reversible Spinal Cord Trauma: A Model for Electrical Monitoring of Spinal Cord Function. *J. Neurosurg., 36:* 402, 1972.
7. Dawson, G. D.: Cerebral Responses to Electrical Stimulation of Peripheral Nerve in man. *J. Neurol. Neurosurg. Psychiatry, 10:* 134, 1947.
8. Dawson, G. D.: A Summation Technique for the Detection of Small Evoked Potentials. *Electroencephalogr. Clin. Neurophysiol., 6:* 65, 1954.
9. Dohrmann, G. J., Wagner, F. C. Jr. and Bucy, P. C.: Transitory Traumatic Paraplegia: Electron Microscopy of Early Alterations in Myelinated Nerve Fibers. *J. Neurosurg., 36:* 407, 1972.
10. Ducker, T. B. and Hamit, H. F.: Experimental Treatment of Acute Spinal Cord Injury. *J. Neurosurg., 30:* 693, 1969.
11. Ducker, T. B. and Assenmacher, D. R.: Microvascular Response to Experimental Cord Trauma. *Surg. Forum, 20:* 428, 1969.
12. Ducker, T. B. and Perot, P. L. Jr.: Cerebral Somatosensory Evoked Potentials from Peripheral Nerve Stimulation in Spinal Cord Injuries. Presented at the 3rd Annual Edgar A. Kahn Neurosurgical Meeting, Ann Arbor, Mich., November 19, 1971.
13. Giblin, D. R.: Somatosensory Evoked Potentials in Healthy Subjects and in Patients with Lesions of the Nervous System. *Ann. N.Y. Acad. Sci., 112:* 93, 1964.
14. Gosch, H. H., Gooding, E. and Schneider, R. C.: Distortion and Displacement of the Brain in Ex-

perimental Head Injuries. *Surg. Forum, 20:* 425, 1969.

15. Gosch, H. H., Gooding, E. and Schneider, R. C.: Mechanism and Pathophysiology of Experimentally Induced Cervical Spinal Cord Injuries to Adult Rhesus Monkeys. *Surg. Forum, 21:* 455, 1970.

16. Halliday, A. M. and Wakefield, G. S.: Cerebral Evoked Responses in Patients with Dissociated Sensory Loss (Abstract). *Electroencephalogr. Clin. Neurophysiol., 14:* 768, 1962.

17. Kahn, E. A.: Spinal Cord Injuries (Editorial). *J. Bone Joint Surg., 41-A:* 6, 1959.

18. Kahn, E. A. and Rossier, A. B.: Acute Injuries of the Cervical Spine. *Postgrad. Med., 39:* 37, 1966.

19. Kelly, D. L. Jr., Lassiter, K. R. L., Calogero, J. A. and Alexander, E., Jr.: Effects of Local Hypothermia and Tissue Oxygen Studies in Experimental Paraplegia. *J. Neurosurg., 33:* 554, 1970.

20. Kelly, D. L. Jr., Lassiter, K. R. L., Vongsvivut, A. and Smith, J. M.: Effects of Hyperbaric Oxygenation and Tissue Oxygen Studies in Experimental Paraplegia. *J. Neurosurg., 36:* 425, 1972.

21. Klefenberg, G. and Saltzman, G. F.: Gas Myelographic Studies in Syringomyelia. *Acta Radiol., 52:* 129, 1959.

22. Kline, D. G. and DeJonge, B. R.: Evoked Potentials to Evaluate Peripheral Nerve Injury. *Surg. Gynecol. Obstet., 127:* 1239, 1968.

23. Larson, S. J.: Gas Myelography in the Management of Spinal Cord Injury. Presented at the 25th Annual Meeting of The Neurosurgical Society of America, Pebble Beach, Calif., March 22, 1972.

24. Odén, S.: Diagnosis of Spinal Tumours by Means of Gas Myelography. *Acta Radiol., 40:* 301, 1953.

25. Osterholm, J. L. and Mathews, G. J.: Altered Norepinephrine Metabolism following Experimental Cord Injury. Part I: Relationship to Hemorrhagic Necrosis and Post-Wounding Deficits. *J. Neurosurg., 36:* 386, 1972.

26. Osterholm, J. L. and Mathews, G. J.: Altered Norepinephrine Metabolism following Experimental Spinal Cord Injury. Part II: Protection against Traumatic Spinal Cord Hemorrhagic Necrosis by Norepinephrine Synthesis Blockade with Alpha Methyl Tyrosine. *J. Neurosurg., 36:* 395, 1972.

27. Perot, P. L. Jr.: The Use of Somato-Sensory Evoked Potentials in the Evaluation of Brain and Spinal Cord Injuries. A Preliminary Report. Presented at the 25th Annual Meeting of The Neurosurgical Society of America, Pebble Beach, Calif., March 22, 1972.

28. Rossier, A. B.: Personal communication.

29. Schneider, R. C.: A Syndrome in Acute Cervical Injuries for Which Early Operation is Indicated. *J. Neurosurg., 8:* 360, 1951.

30. Schneider, R. C., Cherry, G. L. and Pantek, H. E.: The Syndrome of Acute Central Cervical Spinal Cord Injury. *J. Neurosurg., 11:* 546, 1954.

31. Schneider, R. C.: The Syndrome of Acute Anterior Cervical Spinal Cord Injury. *J. Neurosurg., 12:* 95, 1955.

32. Schneider, R. C., Thompson, J. M. and Bebin, J.: The Syndrome of Acute Central Cervical Spinal Cord Injury. *J. Neurol. Neurosurg. Psychiat., 21:* 216, 1958.

33. Schneider, R. C. Trauma to the Spine and Spinal Cord. In *Correlative Neurosurgery*, 2nd ed., edited by E. A. Kahn, E. C. Crosby, R. C. Schneider, and J. A. Taren, Chap. 26. Charles C Thomas, Publisher, Springfield, Ill., 1969.

33a. Schneider, R. C., Russo, R. H., Gosch, H. H. and Crosby, E. C.: Traumatic Spinal Cord Syndromes and their Management. Presented at the 22nd Annual Meeting of Congress of Neurological Surgeons. Denver, Colo., October 20, 1972.

34. Turnbull, I. M., Brieg, A. and Hassler, O.: Blood Supply of Cervical Spinal Cord in Man. A Microangiographic Cadaver Study. *J. Neurosurg., 24:* 951, 1961.

35. Wagner, F. C. Jr., Dohrmann, G. J. and Bucy, P. C.: Histopathology of Transitory Traumatic Paraplegia in the Monkey. *J. Neurosurg., 35:* 272, 1971.

36. White, R. J. and Albin, M. S.: Spine and Spinal Cord Injury. In *Impact Injury and Crash Protection*, edited by E. S. Gurdjian, W. R. Lange, L. M. Patrick et al., pp. 63–85. Charles C Thomas, Publisher, Springfield, Ill., 1970.

37. White, R. J., Yashon, D., Albin, M. S. and Demian, Y. K.: The Acute Management of Cervical Cord Trauma with Quadriplegia. Presented at the Meeting of The American Association of Neurological Surgeons, Boston, Mass., April 16, 1972.

chapter thirteen

Treatment of Subacute and Chronic Spinal Injuries

**RICHARD C. SCHNEIDER, M.D. AND
GERALD A. O'CONNOR, M.D.**

Probably the best approach to a discussion of these spine and spinal cord injuries is to describe the neurologic patterns which initially are less serious but which may cause definite disability. Since many of these less spectacular injuries do not result in extreme neurologic deficit or death, they do not receive as much attention as they deserve. However, they are by far the commoner, every day, incapacitating lesions. It is essential to present some of this data under a heading which may prove familiar to those directly involved in training and treating football players.

The So-Called "Nerve Pinch Syndrome"

The term, "nerve pinch," as used by athletic team physicians, coaches, and trainers to refer to pain in the neck radiating to the shoulder, arm, and hand, frequently associated with numbness and degrees of weakness, has been the source of much confusion. To many it has been an entity the origin of which has been mystifying and the treatment has been uncertain since a clear understanding of the anatomical factors responsible for the symptoms has never been presented to them. This material may seem elementary to the neurologist, neurosurgeon, and orthopedic surgeon who specialize in the diagnosis of lesions of the spine and spinal cord, but too frequently the general practitioner of medicine does not have reference sources readily available on this topic.

Fundamentally, the differential diagnosis in the so-called "nerve pinch syndrome" should be made upon consideration of the following points.

I. Cervical nerve root lesions
    A. Flexion injuries with contusion or avulsion of the nerve root by:
        1. Protruded or extruded disc with transient or permanent compression or contusion of the nerve root
        2. Cervical spondylosis or osteoarthritis

3. Transient anterior overriding of facets
4. Permanent anterior overriding of one or both facets with dislocation (11)

B. Hyperextension injuries with foraminal encroachment and contusion of a nerve root by:

1. Transient posterior overriding of facets
2. Transient posterior inward wrinkling of the ligamentum flavum

II. Combined cervical nerve root and spinal cord injury due to concussion or contusion by a protruded or extruded disc
III. Brachial plexus injury due to contusion, compression, or stretch of the components of the brachial plexus
IV. Combined nerve root and brachial plexus injury

Football Survey. In this series of 225 serious and fatal injuries there were eight ruptured cervical discs and one brachial plexus injury reported, all of whom survived (16). These lesions are never considered to be quite as serious as head and spinal cord injuries; thus, very many more such injuries have remained unreported.

Evaluation

History. The history of how, when, and where the injury occurred is of great importance. Was there merely pain in the neck originally with the subsequent development of pain, numbness, and weakness in the arm, forearm, or fingers? What movements accentuated the pain? Were the symptoms increased by coughing, sneezing, or straining? What relieved the symptoms? Did cervical traction decrease the symptoms or make them worse? Were there previous injuries? Had x-rays of the neck or other studies antedated the current examination?

Examination. This evaluation should be concerned with neck pain either locally or in a radicular distribution on motion or percussion. With certain movements of the neck and downward thrust on the head with the chin rotated into either supraclavicular fossa or with the head and neck in hyperflexion or hyperextension, there may be a radiating pattern of discomfort, suggesting nerve root impairment. The strength and tonus in both the upper and lower extremities must be tested. All forms of sensation, and particularly pain or pinprick, must be checked. The deep reflexes of the upper and lower extremities must be compared. Any pathologic reflexes such as Babinski signs (pyramidal tract signs manifested by the upward movement of the great toes and flaring of the toes) suggest spinal cord involvement and must be carefully evaluated.

Laboratory Studies. Plain X-rays of the cervical spine may demonstrate fractures, dislocations, congenital lesions, tumors, or inflammatory diseases. Anterior-posterior, lateral, oblique and "open mouth" views are mandatory. The C7 vertebra must be plainly visible, and films should be made in hyperflexion and hyperextension. Special laminagrams often are of great value. Where cineradiography is available it should be used to identify undisclosed fracture-dis-

locations. Electromyography (EMG) is the graphic study of the muscles supplied by an involved nerve root by fine needle sampling, which may suggest evidence of transient compression or complete denervation of the root. Serial
sampling by EMG several weeks or months apart may indicate recovery or
further deterioration. Therefore it may present objective evidence of injury,
but the test is of no value until at least 18 to 20 days have elapsed after the injury. In abnormal states a spinal tap may show an elevated cerebrospinal fluid
protein. The instillation and flow of a radiopaque material into the subarachnoid
space with fluoroscopic and X-ray examination is termed a myelogram. An abnormality on this study may suggest encroachment on the nerve roots or the spinal
cord.

I. Cervical Nerve Root Lesions

As outlined above, any nerve root may be compressed in flexion by a protruded
or ruptured disc, by a bony spur, or by overriding of the facets with dislocation.
Such "pinching" of the nerve root may be transient or permanent, but all of these
pathologic conditions may present with the same symptoms. They are pain in the
neck, radicular discomfort, and numbness in a given dermatome and/or associated weakness depending upon the extent and site of the nerve roots involved.

In our experience the clinical findings in football players with lesions at the
three more common levels of cervical nerve root compression frequently may
vary slightly from those originally listed by Spurling (18) *due to the presence
of a prefixed or postfixed brachial plexus.*

Compression of the Fifth Cervical Nerve Root at C4-C5 Interspace

Compression of the C5 cervical nerve root causes pain in the tip of the shoulder
and lateral or radial surface of the arm to the elbow
    Hypalgesia over the C5 dermatome overlying the arm and forearm may
be present
        Weakness, fasciculations, or atrophy of the deltoid or biceps muscles, or both
        Impairment of biceps tendon reflex, or its absence

Compression of the Sixth Cervical Nerve Root at C5-C6 Interspace

Downward thrust on the neck with pain, numbness, and tingling in the thumb
and on the radial aspect of the hand
    Hypalgesia in the C6 dermatome of the thumb, part of the index finger, and
perhaps the radial part of the hand
        Possible weakness, fasciculations, and atrophy of the biceps muscle
    Impairment of the biceps tendon reflex or sometimes the triceps tendon re-
flex, or absence of either one

Compression of the Seventh Cervical Nerve Root at C6-C7 Interspace

Compression of the cervical spine causes pain, numbness, or tingling in the
middle finger

Hypalgesia in the C7 dermatome of the middle finger and center of the hand

Weakness, fasciculations, and atrophy of the triceps muscle

Impairment or absence of the triceps tendon reflex

Despite some reports an accurate diagnosis cannot be made on the basis of the neurologic examination alone. The history, signs, and studies must provide the information for proper localization.

A. Flexion or Torsional Injuries. *1. Protruded or Extruded Cervical Nucleus Pulposus (Ruptured Disc).* Between the vertebral bodies is a cushion of fibrous tissue, the annulus fibrosis, containing a centrally located nucleus pulposus. This material known as the intervertebral disc lies between the cartilaginous plates of the vertebral bodies (Fig. 60). Along the anterior margin of the spinal canal on the posterior portions of the vertebral bodies and the discs is the posterior longitudinal ligament. If the disc tissue, whether it is annulus

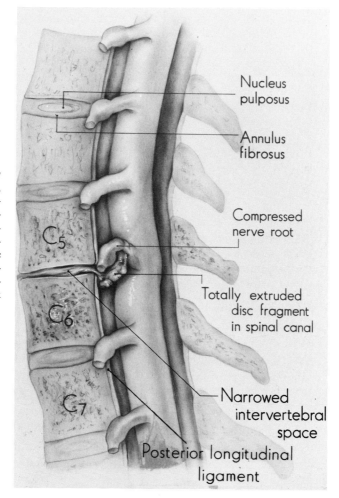

Fig. 60. A lateral view of the spine with the facets, lamina and lateral processes removed shows narrowing of the C5-C6 intervertebral space with extrusion of the cervical disc through the posterior longitudinal ligament with pressure on the C6 nerve root and/or the spinal cord.

Nucleus pulposus

Annulus fibrosus

Compressed nerve root

Totally extruded disc fragment in spinal canal

Narrowed intervertebral space

Posterior longitudinal ligament

fibrosis or nucleus pulposus, is wedged under the posterior longitudinal ligament, a diagnosis of a "protruded" disc is made. If the material has been completely displaced through this ligament and into the spinal canal, the lesion is referred to as an "extruded" disc. Since it is impossible to tell clinically whether the disc has burst through the posterior longitudinal ligament, most clinicians make a diagnosis of "ruptured" disc. This diagnosis is suggested by the history of neck injury, usually associated with a tilt of the head away from the affected side so that hyperextension of the neck causes pain to radiate into the arm, forearm, and hand, with or without numbness, extending into a single dermatome (sensory distribution of nerve root). Pain may be associated with weakness and reflex change and, if prolonged, there may be some muscular atrophy (shrinkage). The pain is usually accentuated by coughing, sneezing, or straining, or with flexion of the neck toward the involved side. The vast majority of football players who have radicular pain following an injury, without any evidence of deformity on X-ray examination, probably have a protruded or ruptured disc.

Case 49. A college football player reported to the team physician with neck pain and numbness in his right thumb and index finger of 3 weeks' duration. He had sustained six or seven such episodes. Two years before he had had a neck injury when he dove into 3 feet of water. He was not rendered unconscious but had pain in his neck with persistent numbness in his right arm for 2 months. When he reported for college football he did not record this event. He stood erect with a tendency to tilt his head toward the right side with a sagging of his right shoulder. When the neck was flexed there was no local tenderness on cervical percussion. When the head was upright with the chin rotated into the right supraclavicular fossa, downward thrust upon the head caused pain in the right arm and numbness in his right thumb and index finger. Similar findings were present when the neck was thrown into hyperextension with downward thrust on the head. With rotation of the chin into the left supraclavicular fossa, such downward pressure caused no symptoms. There was definite hypalgesia in the C6 dermatome and the right biceps reflex was diminished. The cervical spine x-rays showed evidence of an old compression fracture of the C4 vertebra with calcification of the superior portion of this body and a narrowed C5-C6 intervertebral disc space.

Comment. This is the classical history and the usual neurologic finding in a patient with a ruptured cervical disc at C5-C6 intervertebral space with compression or "pinch" of the C6 nerve root (19, 20). On the basis of 25 years of neurosurgical experience, this author is more inclined to follow, in part, the dermatome patterns for the upper extremities described by Foerster (5) than those of Keegan (8). Since it was at least 6 weeks after this patient's most recent football injury, further confirmation of the diagnosis could have been made by electromyography and a cervical myelogram could have been done if operation was contemplated. However, the majority of such patients will recover on conservative measures of cervical traction, muscle relaxants, physiotherapy, and analgesia, all followed by a judiciously planned exercise regime (17, 18).

The player adhered to this course of therapy and has made a good recovery; he has given up football on the neurosurgical consultant's advice.

2. Cervical Spondylosis or Osteoarthritis. Cervical spondylosis or osteo-arthritis is usually considered to be a disease of the middle-age or older-age groups. This type of bony spur is infrequently found in a patient of the age group of football players. The symptoms are similar to those described above for any nerve root compression or spinal cord compression.

> **Case 50.** A college football player sustained a hyperextension injury to his neck while blocking with his head. He had acute discomfort in his neck and numbness in his left arm and shoulder. There was no evidence of neuro-logic deficit, but he had marked limitation of motion of the cervical spine in all directions and had tenderness to palpation over the posterior cervical area and the left trapezius muscle. Cervical spine X-rays showed hyper-trophic changes posteriorly at the C3-C4 interspace (Fig. 61A). When laminagrams were made, the marked bony spurs at the C3-C4 and C4-C5 interspaces were readily visualized (Fig. 61B). Oblique views of the cervical spine revealed a marked cervical spondylosis or osteoarthritis at the C3-C4 interspace (Fig. 61C). Two years previously he had been doing neck ex-ercises when he heard a cracking sound but continued his exercises. Sub-sequently he developed triceps and trapezius muscle spasms with splint-ing of his neck toward the left side. X-rays of the cervicothoracic spine showed an avulsion fracture of the tip of the right T1 transverse process.

Comment. This football player developed a moderate degree of cervical osteoarthritis in spite of his relatively young age. Because of his position at cen-ter and the need for hyperextension of his neck, whenever he was struck on the head he had recurrence of his radicular symptoms in the C4 dermatome with pain in the neck and across the shoulders each time the lower posterior margin of the plastic helmet struck the neck. The hyperextension maneuver resulted in a squeezing of the C4 nerve root against the bony spur. His symptoms dis-appeared after a sponge rubber collar was applied so that the posterior rim of the helmet now struck it and prevented a direct blow to the neck.

This patient demonstrates a premature type of cervical spondylosis or osteo-arthritis. This condition may affect the spinal cord or nerve roots by impairment of blood supply or by direct compression of these structures. Frykholm (6) has indicated that actual fibrosis of the nerve root sleeve is responsible for the symptoms in such cases. Miller (12) has stated "the radiological signs of cervical spondylosis are so ubiquitous as to be valueless." The diagnosis as to which of the bony spurs is the offender must be made by history, physical examina-tion, electromyogram, and myelogram. Sometimes bony spurs at several in-terspaces may cause multiple nerve root compressions simultaneously.

3. Transient Anterior Overriding of Facets. The rounded articular facets, which are at the lateral portions of the vertebral arches, have smooth joint sur-faces lined with cartilage and synovial membrane so they may glide painlessly over one another and permit an even motion. The inferior facet of the upper ver-

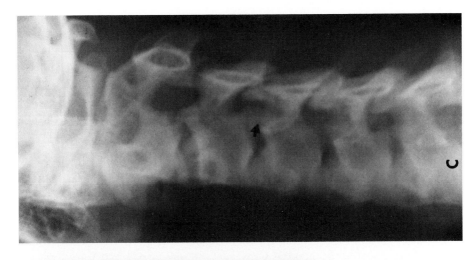

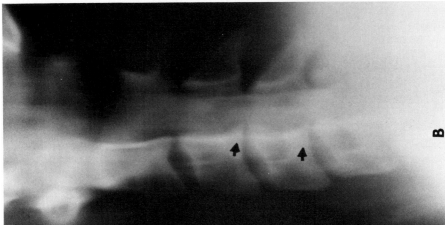

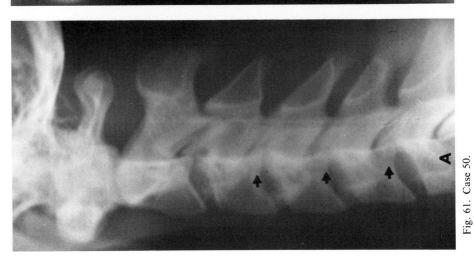

Fig. 61. Case 50.
Fig. 61A. The lateral cervical spine film shows cervical spondylosis or osteoarthritis with hypertrophic changes at C3-C4, C4-C5, and C5-C6 interspaces (arrows).
Fig. 61B. With laminagraphy the bony osteoarthritic spurs at the C3-C4 and C4-C5 intervertebral spaces were demonstrated to better advantage (arrows). The C5-C6 interspace is not well visualized on this view.

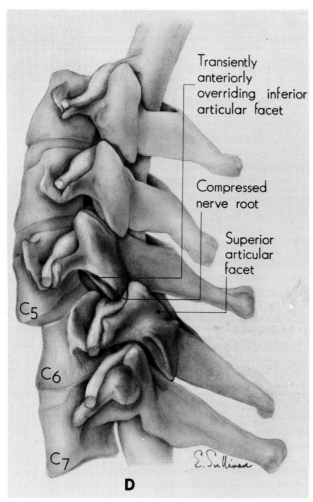

Transiently
anteriorly
overriding inferior
articular facet

Compressed
nerve root

Superior
articular
facet

C5

C6

C7

D

Fig. 61D. This diagram demonstrates the overriding of the superior articular facet of the C6 vertebra upon the inferior articular facet of C5. When this is transient, there is a temporary pinching of the nerve root in the cervical foramen. With a sudden realignment of the spine there is relief of nerve root pressure and a diminution of symptoms.

tebral normally overlies the superior facet of the vertebra below it (Fig. 61D). The joint itself is bound together by a firm capsule and tendons so that normal flexion, extension, or limited rotation of the neck may be achieved. In forced combined cervical flexion and rotation injuries of the cervical spine, the superior articular facet of the lower vertebra may become displaced backward over the inferior facet of the upper vertebra causing a transient unilateral dislocation of the joint. A compression of the cervical nerve root, which leaves the spinal canal through the neural foramen formed by these structures, may result. Thus the joint capsule or ligaments may become transiently overstretched or torn in order for this degree of displacement to occur. This episode may be noiseless or may be associated with a transient cracking or clicking sound as the facets override each other, and it may be accompanied by radicular symptoms limited to one nerve root as described above. Reduction *may* occur spontaneously or with gentle manual traction and rotation, with the relief of the symptoms. The X-ray examination with anterior-posterior, lateral, and oblique views may show no abnormality in such instances because of spontaneous reduction of these over-riding structures, and the symptoms subside until the player is injured on another occasion.

> **Case 51.** A 19 year old college football player received a head and neck injury in September 1955. Although he was dazed, he recovered on the field and noted pain in the neck radiating downward along the outer aspect of the arm into the right forearm with a tingling sensation extending into the thumb and index finger and with equivocal weakness in the grip of the right hand. Cervical spine X-rays were normal. He recovered and subsequently received another flexion injury on the cervical spine with similar symptoms and findings. Intermittently there was a recurrence of his injury and symptoms until he finally completed his collegiate football career.

Comment. There was a clicking sound of the neck on movement in flexion and extension with a reproduction of the player's symptoms. On checking his spinal X-rays on each occasion they were negative and his symptoms would sub-side. Local pain in the neck remained on each occasion for a short time. It was believed this pattern was due to a nerve root compression following a transient anterior overriding of the facets of the cervical spine because of the clicking noise, although this sound may be due to tendons sliding over joint surfaces. Symptoms usually subside rapidly on rest. Currently cineradiography would be used to evaluate the status of such a player's facets.

4. Permanent Anterior Facet Dislocation. The symptoms are identical with those described above and the diagnosis may be made only by the X-ray examina-tion and relocation of the facets may only be accomplished safely by open re-duction and spinal fusion (Fig. 87B).

B. Hyperextension Injuries. *1. Transient Posterior Overriding of Facets*

2. Transient Inward Buckling of the Ligamentum Flavum. Both are mech-anisms of injury which are overlooked but which have been noted by one of us (G.A.O.). The player's neck is forcibly hyperextended *toward* the side of the injury resulting in foraminal encroachment with nerve root contusion, causing temporary radicular pain and muscular weakness. Such as injury may be contrasted to the brachial plexus stretch injury incurred by forcible *contralateral* hyperextension of the cervical spine.

II. Combined Cervical Nerve Root and Cervical Spinal Cord Injury

Occasionally the ruptured intervertebral disc is sufficiently extruded so that it may cause a concussion or contusion to the nerve roots and/or the spinal cord causing instantaneous paralysis of all four extremities and impairment of bladder and bowel functions.

> **Case 52.** In September 1964, a right-handed high school player was crouched for a tackle when another player soared through the air striking the patient on the head so that the cervical spine was forced downward in severe flexion. The player did not lose consciousness but fell to the ground with immediate complete tetraplegia. After 3 minutes he regained the use of

his arms. A neurosurgeon who saw him at the hospital noted *a Horner's syndrome* and made a diagnosis of "spinal cord concussion." Within 12 hours of injury the player was neurologically negative although he still retained some numbness and tingling in his left arm. Thirty-six hours after his injury he was completely normal.

Two weeks later the player fell striking the top of his helmet on the ground and noted weakness, numbness, and tingling in the *left* arm, particularly in the little and the ring fingers. The symptoms lasted 10 minutes and disappeared. He continued to play football but wore a neck support for the remainder of the season.

In September 1965, during a scrimmage he was struck on the left side of his helmet by an opponent's shoulder. His head and neck were flexed sharply to the right and he immediately noted his right arm was weak and a hot tingling sensation was felt in the entire *right* arm, but this was most severe in the right little and ring fingers. He had no weakness but he had some difficulty in maintaining his balance for a few minutes. The arm remained functionless for an hour. The symptoms were on the side opposite the injury of the preceding season. X-rays of the cervical spine displayed a reversal of the normal lordotic curve at C4-C5 interspace. Because of the boy's intense desire to play football, he saw a neurologist and neurosurgeon who cautioned him against continuing to play the game. One consultant even had raised the possibility of cervical disc excision and spinal fusion by an anterior surgical approach so the boy might participate in the sport again! Fortunately, reason prevailed and when the seriousness of a possible permanent tetraplegia was explained to the player, he reluctantly abandoned football.

Comment. Initially this player had a severe concussion of the cervical cord with a possible ruptured disc at the C5-C6 interspace from which he completely recovered. The subsequent symptoms alternating between the left and right upper extremities suggested the presence of a degenerated extruded disc which might be migrating as a free fragment in the spinal canal. If symptoms persist in such a case, myelography and intervertebral cervical disc excision will become necessary.

The presence of the Horner's syndrome and unconsciousness described in the initial episode in September 1964 might suggest the possibility of a vascular insufficiency of the posterior inferior cerebellar branch of the vertebral artery. The symptoms following the third injury in September 1965 perhaps might have been due to a transient vertebral artery and posterior inferior cerebellar artery insufficiency for he had a few minutes when he had difficulty with his equilibrium. Nevertheless the tingling in the right little and ring fingers suggested a dermatomal distribution. Unfortunately the finer details of the neurologic examination, facts which would have enabled better localization, were omitted in the report.

III. Brachial Plexus Injury

The symptoms of a brachial plexus injury as described by the player following a blow to the shoulder or neck are an immediate "complete paralysis, numbness, and intense burning sensation throughout my entire arm, hand, and fingers followed by tingling in the hand and arm" (Fig. 63). When the neck is hyperextended forcibly, and the chin is rotated toward the side opposite the blow, and the arm extended and abducted particularly at the shoulder height, a blow to the cervicobrachial area will cause either a concussion, contusion, stretch, or, if very severe, actual tear of the nerve roots of the brachial plexus (Fig. 62B).

One of the authors (G.A.O.) has indicated that when the shoulder is abducted and extended the clavicle is lowered decreasing the space between the first rib and the clavicle. When a direct blow occurs over the clavicle there may be a compression of the brachial plexus as well as a stretch injury. Palpation in

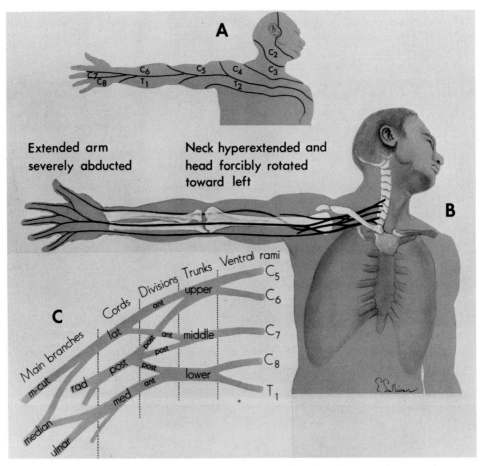

Fig. 62A. This diagram portrays the dermatomes of the head, neck, upper thorax, and upper extremity.

Fig. 62B. With the head hyperextended and the chin rotated to the left and with the right upper extremity extended to shoulder height and abducted, the brachial plexus is placed on stretch.

Fig. 62C. This diagram of the brachial plexus illustrates simply the nerve roots, trunks, divisions, cords, and main branches. From examination of this diagram a lesion of the brachial plexus may be diagnosed.

the supraclavicular fossa may elicit tnederness over the plexus.

Differentiation from a cervical nerve root lesion is usually made by the history of a burning pain with paresthesias not limited to one dermatome but spread throughout the entire intricate course of trunks, divisions, and cords of the brachial plexus with sensory changes in several dermatomes and multiple myotome involvement (Fig. 62C). This may be contrasted to the nerve root injury previously described with symptoms and signs confined to a single dermatome and myotome. Three weeks after such an injury the electromyogram may be of value in demonstrating the site and the extent of a brachial plexus injury. If myelography is performed a defect may be visualized in the dural sleeve of the cervical nerve root, suggesting the possibility of nerve root avulsion with irreparable damage. A player with an irreparable lower brachial plexus injury is portrayed (Fig. 62D).

IV. Combined Nerve Root and Brachial Plexus Injury

There may be some confusion whether the patient is suffering from isolated nerve root impairment versus brachial plexus injury. The injuries to this area occasionally cannot be sharply defined for there may be a combination of pathologic entities. This problem is best illustrated by the following case report.

> **Case 53.** During his junior year in high school a football player was injured in a game sustaining a blow to the right side of the neck and right shoulder which caused pain beneath the scapula, a numbness in the "entire" right upper extremity and a severe burning sensation in all the fingers of the hand and right arm, although he thought it might be worse in his index and little finger. There was also transient weakness in both the arm and shoulder. He stated "I could restore my circulation to the extremity by throwing it in a flailing motion in the air until strength and feeling came back into it." He continued to play football during his junior and senior high school years although these symptoms recurred an *estimated 50 or 75 times*. When asked why he did not give up the sport, he replied with obvious reluctance and embarrassment, "It was a small town high school and they didn't have enough players to make up a good team if I dropped out. They needed me." However, because of the pain in the neck and radicular pain in the arm, which was accentuated by coughing, sneezing, and straining, the boy gave up football. When he attended college and reported for wrestling, his symptoms recurred shortly after the beginning of the season, and for the first time he sought medical aid.
>
> On examination he stood upright with his head slightly flexed forward. Percussion over the cervical spine caused no pain. There was definite limitation of motion at 30 degrees rotation of the head toward the right side with the chin directed downward into the right supraclavicular fossa. Downward thrust on the head caused pain at the scapula and in the C4 dermatome. Rotation of the head toward the left caused pain in the same region of the scapula when downward thrust to the head was applied. Strength seemed good in all movements of the upper and lower extremities. There was absence of the right biceps reflex, but the left one was present. The triceps and radioperiosteal reflexes were equal and active. There was hypal-

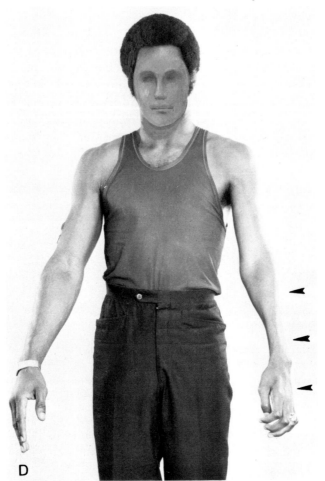

Fig. 62D. Two years previously upon tackling an opponent, this player sustained an immediate paralysis of his left hand due to a presumed lower brachial plexus injury. Electromyography at this time demonstrated paralysis of all of the left hand and wrist muscles with the exception of partial paralysis of the extensor carpi radialis and ulnaris and flexor carpi radialis. There was a complete loss of sensation in the index finger and thumb. Note the muscular atrophy of the musculature of the left upper extremity. The prognosis for further recovery after 2 years is hopeless.

It was recommended that an attempt should be made to stabilize the thumb and the wrist with a transfer of wrist flexors and extensor tendons to the fingers before considering an amputation of the hand.

D

gesia in the radial portion of the right neck, shoulder, arm, forearm, thumb, and index finger, as well as hypalgesia in the right little finger and the ulnar aspect of the right forearm (Fig. 63). The middle finger was spared. There were no pyramidal tract signs in the upper or lower extremities. The cervical spine x-rays appeared normal. An EMG suggested partial denervation of the muscles supplied by the right C6 nerve root. A lumbar puncture demonstrated a spinal fluid protein of 48 mgm.%. The cervical myelogram showed no abnormality.

A complete laminectomy was performed at C5 and C6 vertebrae on January 11, 1966. At the right C5-C6 interspace there was a small bony spur firmly adherent to the C6 nerve root so that fibrosis of the sheath rather than compression of this root had occurred. The small bony excrescence was chiseled away and a moderately degenerated disc was removed from the interspace. A partial foraminotomy was performed to completely free the nerve root. The right C6-C7 interspace was examined and the root was found to be perfectly normal. The wound was closed in layers.

Five months postoperatively, the player still had a dull ache behind his right scapula but had good freedom of movement of his neck toward the

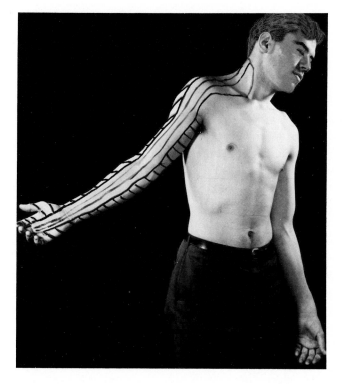

Fig. 63. Case 53. This position is the one in which injury may occur when further forceful separation of the head and shoulders occurs with a blow. The symptoms are further accentuated when the arm is extended at shoulder height with forceful abduction.

The pattern illustrated suggests cervical as well as brachial plexus impairment. The brachial plexus involvement includes injury to the lateral and medial cords of the brachial plexus as demonstrated by hypesthesia in the crosshatched areas along the radial and ulnar areas of the right forearm. The longitudinally demarcated area indicates a region of numbness without true objective hypersthesia. Functional overlay, although possible, seemed highly unlikely.

right side. Strength was good in the biceps and triceps muscles, but the right biceps reflex remained absent. He had residual hyperalgesia in the C5 and C6 dermatomes, but the previous ulnar hypalgesia had disappeared. His grip was strong. The boy felt so well that he wished to return to wrestling, but he reluctantly gave it up after being advised to do so and after seeing another wrestler who had sustained a tetraplegia.

Comment. In this instance the case history was particularly important. The fact that the patient had pain on turning the head toward the side of his involvement plus the fact that downward thrust on the head or coughing, sneezing, or straining accentuated his radicular pain suggested a lesion, possibly a ruptured disc, in the spinal canal compressing the C6 nerve root. A positive EMG indicating involvement of this root supported the diagnosis. However, burning pain in all his fingers with numbness in the whole arm on many occasions required a diagnosis of brachial plexus stretch injury to be made. Such a lesion usually is not influenced by head turning, coughing, sneezing, and straining. The combination of the history and the examination suggested a lesion of the lateral and medial cords of the brachial plexus plus an extension of the traction injury to the cervical plexus because of hyperalgesia involving the C4 dermatome distribution. Even though the myelogram was negative for a lesion at the C5-C6 interspace at operation a small foraminal bony spur and a degenerated cervical disc were found which were markedly adherent and fibrosed to the sheath of the C6 nerve root. In such combined lesions of cervical root damage and of brachial plexus stretch injury, exploration may be indicated. The disparity from the usual anatomical pattern was at first believed to be due in part to functional overlay. However, it must not be forgotten that in such injuries there may be not only encroachment on the cervical nerve root but also intraneural contusion, edema, and fibrosis of components of the brachial plexus (7). In such instances damage may not be complete and with a state of neurapraxia existing a major degree of recovery may occur after 5 months. The presence of significant objective findings on examination and definite abnormality on electromyography to a large degree aided in excluding a superimposed functional diagnosis.

In a fine review of 63 closed brachial plexus injuries in Great Britain after World War II, Barnes (1) agreed with the belief the essential mechanism in traction injuries was a forcible separation between the head and the shoulder. Most of these patients were motorcyclists. Barnes indicated the blow must be sufficiently severe to tear the deep cervical fascia, rupture the scalene muscles, and avulse the tubercles of the transverse process before stretching of the nerve roots might occur. The upper roots of the brachial plexus are most often injured with a forcible depression of the shoulder with the arm at the side, as occurs when a motorcyclist falls on his head and shoulder. Barnes (1) showed in cadavers that the tension on each nerve root of the brachial plexus varied with the position of the extremity; thus with elevation of the upper extremity and forcible abduction of the lower cervical roots, tension increased upon them with forcible thrust of the head toward the opposite side. However, in the hard driving live football player the neck may be so severely rotated and the extended upper extremity so forcefully abducted at shoulder height that lesions of the entire brachial plexus and even cervical plexus may be incurred. Such injuries may be sustained by a defensive player "clotheslining" a fast charging backfield opponent (Chapter 6, Fig. 36, A-C).

A moderate stretching of a nerve root causes temporary impairment of conduction which has a greater influence on motor rather than on sensory fibers. Distal degeneration of the nerve does not occur, and complete recovery takes place within 2 months of injury. It is suspected that this is what has occurred in this case. If traction of the plexus causes disruption of the axons there is damage to the blood vessels and fibers with intraneural scarring which may occur at multiple levels, causing irreparable damage and making excision of a scar and a successful operative result impossible (7). It is not the extraneural scarring of the other tissues impinging on the brachial plexus which is responsible for the damage as has been suggested by Davis et al. (3). Operation therefore should not be resorted to for this reason. It is generally believed the prognosis is best for recovery when the upper three nerve roots of the brachial plexus are involved and considerably less when the lower ones are injured (4).

Kerr (9) reported two cases of traction lesions of the cervical plexus in association with brachial plexus injury in which there was sensory loss and anhidrosis over the C2, C3, and C4 dermatomes and the muscular bundles to the deltoid, spinati, and diaphragm were involved. He noted three or four other cases in which the area of sensory loss extended to the supra-acromial area, but these were not regarded as cervical plexus lesions because of the variability of the distribution of the C4 and C5 nerve roots. There was no apparent accompanying nerve root damage. This author suggested that there might be direct contusion of the sensory nerve roots emerging from the deep cervical fascia along the posterior border of the sternocleidomastoid muscle in such instances. The patient presented in Case 53 fits into this pattern. It is not known whether the disability was due to combined cervical and brachial plexus traction or to direct contusion to the cervical sensory nerve roots.

Frykholm (7) showed by careful experimental studies at open operation in cases of brachial neuralgia that the dural sleeve was often thickened and rigid around the emerging nerve roots, even where no disc protrusion could be found. This pathologic change was believed due to traction, direct trauma, congenital maldevelopment of the nerve root pouch, or cervical osteoarthritis. Russell (14, 15) and Lishman and Russell (10) have found their studies of brachial neuropathy that there often are lesions separated at widely different points along the course of the nerve which have been blamed for one and the same syndrome. In a review of brachial plexus war injuries Nulsen and Slade (13) were of the opinion that surgery on intact neural elements in the brachial neuralgias was of little or no benefit. Drake (4) has indicated that the character and the site of traction injuries of the brachial plexus precludes surgical care. In lesions of the lower plexus the prognosis is bad. In upper plexus injuries, where rupture of the nerve roots has not occurred but where there has been neurapraxia, recovery of the muscular function of the shoulder girdle and arm may take place. No such case was found in this study. Bateman (2) stated these patients have "neurodynia" which requires attention. Such pain is not as severe as a causalgia, but prompt recognition suggests that early "handling" of the limb, reassurance, and encouragement are a most important part of the treatment. Frykholm (7) demonstrated that stimulation of the ventral roots can produce deep boring pain in the region of the scapula and shoulder girdle which is commonly felt in the muscles themselves, whereas stimulating posterior nerve root causes sharp shock-like radicular pain. This is probably the reason that the patient in Case 53 continued to have postoperative subscapular pain, although that pain which was localized to the ulnar nerve or the medial cord of the brachial plexus had disappeared. In two-thirds of his series of 63 blunt or traction injuries to the brachial plexus, confined to the C5, C6, and C7 roots, Barnes (1) found a fairly good return of motor power. This seemed to be the experience in this last case.

Summary

The various pathologic conditions which might cause the so-called "nerve pinch syndrome" in football players have been presented. Either single or multiple involvements of the various nerve roots or the more complex cords, trunks, or other components of the brachial plexus may be found. The essential thing is a good history and examination which aids one in the correct evaluation and the procural of the proper studies required to make a satisfactory diagnosis. These case reports may be of some solace to the general physician or specifically, team physician, in that he may know that not all of these lesions can be placed in a nice compartment even by specialists in the various fields. The multiplicity of lesions responsible for such confusion in the symptomatology is probably best illustrated in the final case presentation, Case 53. Perhaps the *Standard Nomenclature of Athletic Injuries* published by the American Medical Association may be of some aid in differentiating and recording the types of lesions responsible for the various nerve root or brachial plexus injuries. *In conclusion, it is obvious that there is no single nicely defined entity the "nerve pinch syndrome"; the term really describes a multitude of conditions.*

Lumbar Spine Lesions

Since the neurologic residual is not as devastating following lumbar lesions, such as a ruptured lumbar intervertebral disc or a lumbar fracture-dislocation, as the sequelae resulting from cervical ones, there is less tendency for the former lesions to be reported in athletic injuries.

Football Survey. There was only one ruptured disc injury in a football player reported by the neurosurgeons. He was operated upon and made a good recovery (Fig. 27). Many more of these lesions no doubt were not reported. For example, this author forgot to inculde two of his own ruptured lumbar disc cases, no doubt because they were less spectacular than the cervical injuries. Only one case of a patient with a lumbar fracture with partial neurologic deficit was recorded; he succumbed months after his injury due to a chronic ascending urinary infection. Although few in number in the survey, the frequency of the lumbar ruptured disc syndrome deserves further elaboration.

The Ruptured Lumbar Disc

History. The football player usually presents himself for examination with the story of lifting a heavy object or sustaining a sudden wrenching or twisting motion of his back. *This author and others have had several players (Case 54) date the onset of their symptoms to their attempts at conditioning by weight lifting or by the Royal Canadian Air Force exercises.* The player reports the sudden onset of backache followed shortly thereafter by the development of sciatica. The pain radiates from the back down the posterior portion of the thigh and may extend along the posterolateral aspect of the calf perhaps even to the heel or base of the great toe. It is a sharp pain classically accentuated by coughing, sneezing, or straining. These symptoms in athletes may be dubbed as the "nerve pinch" syndrome of the lower extremity. There may be numbness along the lateral border of the calf, heel, or some of the toes of the involved foot. Occasionally there will be a dragging of the great toe and/or foot with a tendency to trip over objects or a weakness in plantar flexion so that the patient cannot "take off," finding himself unable to forcibly plantar flex his foot and support his weight. The symptoms are usually confined to one lower extremity, but in rare instances with large lumbar disc extrusions both may be involved with incontinence of bladder or bowel. There may be remissions and exacerbations as the disc, the nucleus pulposus (the ball-bearing-like structure) shifts about in the annulus pulposus (the washer-like structure) which contains it. When the nucleus pulposus breaks through the annulus fibrosus and through the ligaments, it is said that the disc has "slipped," ruptured, or extruded. If the disc is merely protruded, i.e., has not been displaced through its associated supporting ligament, the posterior longitudinal ligament, chiropractic manipulation, or osteopathic adjustment may be capable of jostling it from beneath the nerve root within the confines of the annulus pulposus. The patient may then obtain some relief of his symptoms. However, the neurosurgeon or orthopedic surgeon frequently will see the patient, after a series of such manipulations or adjustments, with increasingly severe pain and/or foot drop. This author has had such patients referred to him as an emergency when the disc has extruded completely, resulting in severe compression of the cauda equina bilaterally. They had complete paralysis of both lower extremities and a loss of bladder and bowel function.

Examination. The player may stand upright but with a list of the trunk toward the side opposite to the lesion so that the intervertebral disc space is opened, thus relieving pressure on the nerve root. Often when the patient bends forward at the waist he will find it simpler to flex his lumbosacral spine than to return to the upright stance which is often achieved by a sort of cogwheel pattern in extension of the spine. Tilting the trunk to the side of the lesion or backward in hyperextension may cause radicular pain in the involved sciatic distribution. Apparent weakness in eversion or dorsiflexion of the foot or great toe is best elicited by having the patient first rock forward on the tips of the toes and then rock backward on the heels. The faltering great toe or foot clearly demonstrates the degree of weakness. Too frequently the strength of plantar flexion or dorsiflexion of the feet is not examined individually. This response is best tested by having the patient stand independently first on the toes of one foot and then the other, then rock backward on first one heel and then the other, separately. A positive straight leg raising test, consisting of elevating the leg without bending the knee to its limit of tolerance and then dorsiflexing the foot thus putting the sciatic nerve on stretch and causing sciatica, is the single best sign of nerve root compression. Such positive findings may be due to a ruptured disc, a cauda equina tumor, or a bony osteoarthritic spur.

There may be some atrophy or wasting of the calf with chronic recurrent difficulty. Hypalgesia, a loss of pain sensation over the L5 dermatome which may follow the posterior aspect of the thigh, posterolateral calf, the dorsum of the foot, and base of the great toe, suggests L5 nerve root compression at the L4-L5 interspace. If this sensory impairment is in the S1 dermatome, i.e., over the posterior aspect of the thigh and calf and perhaps radiating over the lateral aspect of the foot and the outer two toes, it suggests an S1 nerve root compression at the L5-S1 intervertebral space. The Achilles reflex is usually impaired with an L5-S1 lesion, more rarely with an L4-L5 involvement. The patellar reflex is most often diminished with an L2-L3 lesion, although it may be seen occasionally with L3-L4 ruptured discs and more rarely with nerve root compression as low as the L4-L5 intervertebral space.

Laboratory Studies. Anterior-posterior, lateral, and oblique x-rays are taken of the lumbosacral spine to exclude a congenital bony anomaly, a spinal tumor, a fracture or dislocation, or osteoarthritic changes. The findings of a narrowed intervertebral disc space does not warrant the diagnosis of a ruptured intervertebral disc being made. It may be extruded above or below this interspace. On lumbar puncture the cerebrospinal fluid protein may be slightly elevated. If it is much above 100 mgm. % a tumor may be suspected. If the lumbar root compression has been of a longer duration than three weeks the EMG may be helpful in showing evidence of changes in the muscles supplied by the involved root. This author uses the myelogram primarily as a localizing procedure when he is reasonably sure that the patient requires operation. Only under very exceptional circumstances does this author use it as a diagnostic study.

Case 54. A 20 year old, right-handed collegiate football player had the onset of backache while lifting heavy weights, approximately 180 pounds, during summer training. He subsequently developed pain in the right buttock which radiated down the posterior aspect of the right thigh to the calf and into the heel. The pain was increased by coughing, straining, and sneezing but was relieved by lying down. There was neither numbness, tingling, or weakness in the foot nor difficulty with bladder or bowel control.

On examination he had a lordotic lumbar curvature with a tilt toward the left side. Straight leg raising was possible to 30 degrees on the right side and dorsiflexion of the foot caused sciatic pain. Similar testing with the left leg was possible to 90 degrees without pain. There was minimal weakness in dorsiflexion of the great toe but no paresis on plantar flexion of the foot. There was impairment of pinprick sensation over the dorsum and lateral border of the right foot. He had an asymmetry of the Achilles reflexes with the right one markedly diminished compared to the left. A diagnosis of a ruptured disc at the right L4-L5 intervertebral space was made and the patient was treated conservatively with pelvic traction, analgesics, muscle relaxants, and physiotherapy for 8 days. At the time of discharge he was improved with his straight leg raising now possible to 60 degrees on the right side. He was given a back support and gradually started on Williams exercises, having been told he should not play football for the season.

Three months later he had a recurrence of his symptoms. An EMG was normal but his myelogram (Fig. 64, A and B) demonstrated an impingement on the L5 root. An L4-L5 hemilaminectomy was performed, and his ruptured disc was removed and the involved interspace was thoroughly curetted out. No spinal fusion was performed and he made an uneventful recovery while intermittently despondent and then jubilant watching his teammates on television win the Rose Bowl game in which he had hoped he would be playing.

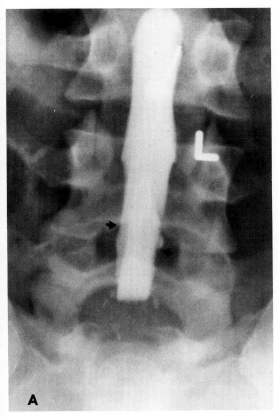

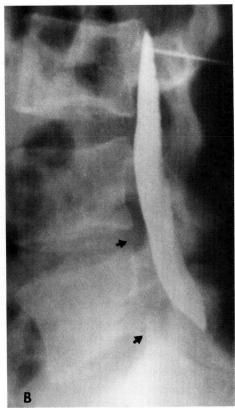

Fig. 64. Case 54.

Fig. 64A. The posterior-anterior view of the lumbar myelogram demonstrates the unequal filling of the nerve root sheaths (arrow) at the L4-L5 interspaces. There is some wasting of the right one as noted by the double shadow, suggesting nerve root compression. In most instances the deformity is more apparent.

Fig. 64B. The translateral view of the myelogram shows no defect in the pantopaque column but there is a large soft tissue shadow between the column and the posterior margins of the vertebral bodies. There is settling at the L5-S1 intervertebral space.

Comment. This player's case is presented for several reasons. His symptoms occurred while lifting weights in training for football and he developed classical ruptured lumbar disc symptoms in the first days of fall practice. Most of these patients will recover under ordinary circumstances if a similar conservative regime of 2 or 3 weeks is followed and if as was done in this case, analgesics, muscle relaxants, and immobilization with pelvic traction on a firm mattress during the acute phase are used. Later after muscle spasm has diminished, the transient use of a firm back support while strengthening the flabby or atonic muscles of the back with exercise is sufficient to carry the average patient through the usual stresses of life. The player elected to follow this course of action giving up that year of football and thereby preserving his year of eligibility. With careful complete removal of the lumbar disc, spinal fusion is rarely necessary and thus avoids months of disabling immobilization. The unfused lower back with proper training and rebuilding of the musculature provides adequate support in the vast number of these cases.

In this author's opinion the man who sustains a *ruptured cervical disc* should not be permitted to return to the game even if operated upon. The danger of a partial ruptured disc extrusion at the same or another interspace is ever present. If it were to occur, the extrusion of a cervical disc fragment into the quite narrow cervical canal with contusion of the cord might result in total permanent paralysis of all four extremities and in the loss of control of bladder and bowel function. Cervical spine stabilization by either anterior or posterior fusion in such players does not afford sufficiently adequate support to permit them to return to the game without the risk of such serious injury.

On the other hand, a player with a ruptured lumbar disc which has been completely excised and who has kept in excellent physical condition, should be allowed to continue to play football if he desires to do so. If a further problem arises and a fragment extrudes at another interspace, usually it causes a unilateral nerve root compression rather than involving all of the nerve roots, for the lumbar spinal canal is proportionately of much greater size than the cervical one. Most important is the fact that in the cervical region, if the spinal cord is damaged, it has no chance of repairing itself, resulting in permanent deficit in all four extremities. However, in the lumbar region, if the cauda equina (nerve roots), is damaged unilaterally or even bilaterally, weakness or paralysis of only one or both lower extremities with bladder and bowel impairment might result. If the player elects to return to the game after a lumbar disc operation he and his parents should be carefully advised of the risks of such sequelae.

Such players may still be successful as described in Case 54 above; the player accepted this responsibility of playing again under these conditions. He returned to football for 3 years of collegiate play and as a superb end caught many passes sustaining severe bone rattling tackles without any difficulty with his lumbar spine. This fine young man and excellent athlete achieved All-American status at his position, eventually receiving bilateral disabling knee injuries after playing a few years of professional football.

References

1. Barnes, R.: Traction Injuries of the Brachial Plexus in Adults. *J. Bone Joint Surg. 31-B:* 10, 1949.
2. Bateman, J. E.: *Trauma to Nerves in Limbs.* W. B. Saunders Company, *Philadelphia,* 1962.
3. Davis, L., Martin, J. and Perret, G.: The Treatment of Injuries of the Brachial Plexus. *Ann. Surg., 125:* 647, 1947.
4. Drake, C. G.: Diagnosis and Treatment of Lesions of the Brachial Plexus and Adjacent Structures. *Clin. Neurosurg., 11:* 110, 1963.
5. Foerster, O.: Symptomatologie der Erkrankungen des Rückenmarks und seiner Worzeln. In *Handbuch der Neurologie,* edited by O. Bumke, and O. Foerster, Vol. 5. Julius Springer, Berlin, 1936.
6. Frykholm, R.: Deformities of Dural Pouches and Strictures of Dural Sheaths in the Cervical Region Producing Nerve-Root Compression. A Contribution to the Etiology and Operative Treatment of Brachial Neuralgia. *J. Neurosurg., 4:* 403, 1947.
7. Frykholm, R.: Cervical Nerve Root Compression Resulting from Disc Degeneration and Root-Sleeve Fibrosis: A Clinical Investigation. *Acta Chir. Scand. Suppl. 160:* 145, 1, 1951.

8. Keegan, J. J.: Dermatome Hypalgesia with Posterolateral Herniation of the Lower Cervical Intervertebral Disc. *J. Neurosurg., 4:* 115, 1947.
9. Kerr, A. S.: Cervical Plexus Injuries as an Extension of Brachial Plexus Injuries. *J. Bone Joint Surg., 31-B:* 37, 1949.
10. Lishman, W. A. and Russell, W. R.: The Brachial Neuropathies. *Lancet, 2:* 941, 1961.
11. Melvin, W. J. S., Dunlap, H. W., Heterington, R. F. and Kerr, J. W.: The Role of the Faceguard in the Production of Flexion Injuries to the Cervical Spine in Football. *Canad. Med. Assoc. J., 93:* 1110, 1965.
12. Miller, H.: Discussion on Cervical Spondylosis. *Proc. R. Soc. Med., 49:* 200, 1956.
13. Nulsen, F. E. and Slade, H. W.: *Recovery following Injury to the Brachial Plexus, in Peripheral Nerve Regeneration: A Followup Study of 3,656 World War II Injuries,* edited by B. Woodhall and G. W. Beebe, pp. 389-408. Government Printing Office, Washington D.C., 1956.
14. Russell, W. R.: Discussion on Cervical Spondylosis. *Proc. R. Soc. Med., 49:* 198, 1956.
15. Russell, W. R.: Brachial Neuropathies of the Housewife. *Med. Press, 240:* 1151, 1958.
16. Schneider, R. C.: Serious and Fatal Neurosurgical Football Injuries. *Clin. Neurosurg., 12:* 226, 1964.
17. Semmes, R. E. and Murphy, F.: The Syndrome of Unilateral Rupture of the Sixth Cervical Intervertebral Disc, with Compression of the Seventh Cervical Nerve Root: A Report of Four Cases with Symptoms Simulating Coronary Disease. *J.A.M.A., 121:* 1209, 1943.
18. Spurling, R. G.: *Lesions of the Cervical Intervertebral Disc.* Charles C Thomas, Publisher, Springfield, Ill., 1956.
19. Stookey, B.: Compression of the Spinal Cord Due to Ventral Extradural Cervical Chondromas. *Arch. Neurol. Physchiatry, 20:* 275, 1928.
20. Stookey, B.: Compression of Spinal Cord and Nerve Roots by Herniation of the Nucleus Pulposus in the cervical Region. *Arch. Surg., 40:* 417, 1940.

chapter fourteen

An Experimental Approach to Head and Spine Injuries*

HANK H. GOSCH, M.D., ELWYN R. GOODING AND RICHARD C. SCHNEIDER, M.D.

An urgent need for comprehensive methods of study which may enhance our knowledge of serious athletic injuries has been recognized in the preceding chapters. If an experimental study helps to formulate a hypothesis of the mechanisms and causes, then certain facts may emerge which can improve the recognition and prevention of such injuries.

The experimental approach to studying the central nervous system trauma is not uncommon (1, 8, 12); however, one of the difficulties has been the development of a satisfactory method with the proper instrumentation for recording the event. Mechanical models, simulating the head (2, 8, 12), and cadaver skulls (11) have been used. However, the ideal method is to visualize and record events in their natural state with the brain in relationship to the cranium. Such conditions can only be approximated in an experimental animal which is sufficiently biologically advanced in the phylogenetic scale. In this laboratory, the live, but anesthetized, monkey has been used as the experimental model (3–7) and much of our investigative work has been directed toward simulating conditions illustrated in the collection of tragic fatal football cases (16, 17) which have been presented in the foregoing chapters.

Method of Production of Head and Spine Injuries
Instrumentation

All experimental studies were performed with monkeys, closely observing the principles of laboratory animal care as promulgated by the National Society for Medical Research. Rapid and reliable anesthesia was obtained by an intramuscular injection of 20 mgm. of phencyclidine hydrochloride (Sernylan) or 50 mgm. of sodium pentobarbital and maintained during the entire procedure when the head or spine was traumatized.

A considerable amount of ingenuity and engineering skill was used in the construction of an impact tract (see Fig. 71). The method by which trauma could be produced to the central nervous system with such equipment was more realistic in simulating injuries encountered in human subjects than by other techniques. The anesthetized animals were secured on a carriage and acceler-

---

* A part of this material was reprinted from Gosch et al. (4) by permission of the *Journal of Trauma* © 1970 The Williams & Wilkins Company, Baltimore and from Gosch et al. (6) by permission of the *Journal of Neurosurgery*.

ated by compressed air along a double track against a vertically fixed, rigid metal barrier, or impact anvil. The degree of acceleration of the animal along the track was preselected for the line pressure driving the piston and cable assembly of the carriage. The energy delivered to the head at impact was recorded by a transducer load cell mounted on the impact block. The electrical signal was monitored simultaneously on a dual channel oscilloscope and Honeywell 7600 tape recorder. The generated voltage amplitude, indicating the magnitude of impact at the head, was recorded on a Dynograph recorder and converted to foot-pounds of energy.

Directly over the impact site, a Hycam high speed camera was mounted and cinematographic recordings at 3000 frames per second were made of the head and neck region at the time of injury.

Head Injury Studies

In studies of the brain dynamics during head injury, direct visualization and photographic observations were made through clear Lexan polycarbonate calvarium (Fig. 65). A modification of the Lucite technique first devised and described by Pudenz and Sheldon (13) was employed using this newer type of plastic material. The animal's scalp was shaved and the head was secured in an adjustable holder on the operating table. The surgical site was then scrubbed with Phiso-Hex® and Betadine®, and meticulous aseptic techniques were followed. A Y-shaped incision was made, extending from the supraorbital ridges caudally past the inion, and the scalp flap was retracted laterally. The temporalis muscle was then stripped bilaterally from its bony attachment. Burr holes were placed on each side over the cerebral hemispheres and an extensive craniectomy was performed to expose the frontal, occipital, and a portion of the temporal lobes. An 8 mm. strip of bone directly over the sagittal sinus was left intact in order not to disturb the tight dural attachment in this region.

An impression of the craniectomy site was made with a steam-sterilized medical grade silicone compound. Polymerization to a semi-solid mass occurs in several minutes by the addition of stannous octoate catalyst. The silicone impression was then lifted from the craniectomy site after curing for 30 minutes. An industrial molding plaster was poured into the silicone impression, allowed to dry until rigid, and placed in an electric oven at 150 degrees F. for 30 minutes. Several 1/32 in. diameter holes were drilled through the cured plaster, for the escape of air during the thermoforming process of the Lexan calvarium. The surface was waxed and the mold was placed in a "vacuum box." An 0.008 in. thick polycarbonate sheet, heated to a temperature of 350 degrees F., was placed over the plastic mold and vacuum applied, thus forming the Lexan to the mold. The edges were trimmed and the calvarium was sterilized in 90% alcohol. The dura of the animal was excised to the bone edge and bleeding sites were carefully coagulated. The calvarium was then attached with nylon or stainless steel screws.

Cervicomedullary Junction and Upper Cervical Spine Injuries

Studies of the effects of injuries to the cervicomedullary junction were made on three groups of animals prepared for the experiment under three different protocols. 1) Anesthetized monkeys serving as controls had an extensive cervical laminectomy in which the dura was merely opened and re-approximated. 2) A second group had a similar operative procedure, but in addition to the control group had sectioning of the dentate ligaments bilaterally, from the foramen magnum to the C5 cervical segment. The dura was then closed and the paraspinous musculature was re-approximated. 3) A third group served for cinematographic observations of the cervicomedullary junction during impact. After cervical laminectomy and dural excision, complete exposure of this area of the central nervous system permitted observation of the dynamics at impact by the high speed camera.

Cervical Spine Injuries

Cervical spine and cord injuries were developed in animals with the impact directed to the vertex of the head and with the neck in flexion and extension and with the cervical spine aligned to permit only compression of this structure.

The injury mechanism and the effects of the trauma were studied by observing several criteria. Foremost was notation of the clinical state of the animal with the effect of trauma on the respiratory pattern and neurologic status. The cinematographic records were studied in detail for brain and spinal distortion. Radiographic studies of the cervical spine were made to show the degree and type of distortion, fractures, and subluxation. Gross pathologic observation of the brain and spinal

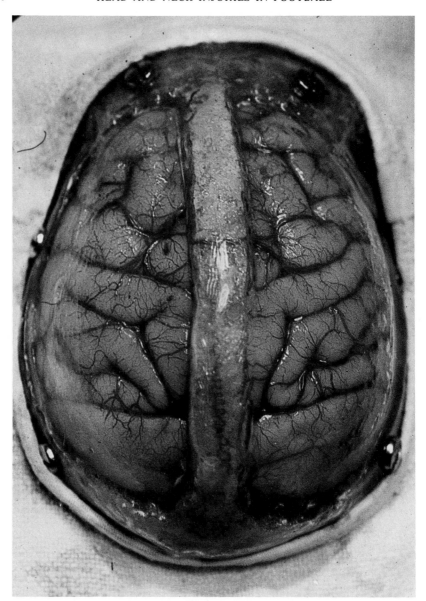

Fig. 65. The Lexan polycarbonate calvarium is shown attached to the monkey skull. Cranial bone over the midline saggital sinus is intact. The underlying cerebral cortex and pial vessels are visualized. [Reprinted from Gosch et al. (4) by permission of the *Journal of Trauma* © 1970 The Williams & Wilkins Company, Baltimore.]

cord were performed for determinations of contusion, hemorrhage, and lacerations. The brain and spinal cord were carefully removed in all animals, fixed in 10% formalin for 5 to 7 days, sectioned, and stained with hematoxylin-eosin. The pathologic condition of the traumatized brain and spinal cord was then examined microscopically. In the cervical spine trauma studies, some specimens were also frozen with gaseous nitrogen leaving the vertebral column, ligaments, and spinal cord intact. Midsagittal sections of these structures in toto were made which demonstrated the degree of compression or the extent of severance of the spinal cord by displaced bone fragments at the fracture-dislocation site.

Results

Head Injuries and Studies of Brain Dynamics during Trauma

The replacement of cranial bone by a clear, transparent Lexan calvarium was performed without any apparent neurologic deficits in most cases. One monkey was successfully observed for a period of 19 months with this type of cranial replacement. The integrity of the cortex was maintained, and no apparent interaction with the polycarbonate was observed. This observation was confirmed by electroencephalographic recordings which showed no gross pathologic deterioration of the cerebral cortex. The transparency of the calvarium for easy visualization of the underlying cerebral cortex and pial vessels is unique in this experimental method. Cerebrospinal fluid filled the "subcalvarial" space, and only gradual clouding with the formation of a yellowish exudate occurs over several weeks. However, with special techniques this may be cleared.

The value of this technique in studying impact injuries is suggested by the preparation shown in Figure 66. Brain movements are recorded with high speed cinematography at 3000 frames per second. The anesthetized animal received a linear impact force of 12 to 15 foot-pounds to the frontal skull region by sudden deceleration against a metal barrier. The cerebral mass maintains the momentum of acceleration in relation to the skull which results in compression of the intracranial contents, as is shown by the decreased distance at 1/200 second interval between two cortical vascular structures.

Cervicomedullary and Cervical Spinal Cord Trauma

A single direct vertex impact of only 25 foot-pounds caused hemorrhages in the upper cervical segments without fracture of the cervical spine. The average impact to the vertex of all animals in this group of experiments was 29 foot-pounds. It should be emphasized that the impact site and the vertebral canal,

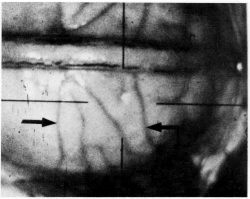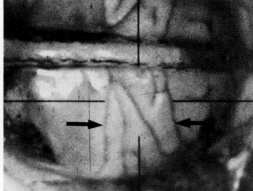

Fig. 66. The cerebral tissue between cortical vascular structures is seen just prior and after impact has occurred, and is noted to be compressed. These observations were made by high speed cinematography at 1/200 of a second interval at the same magnification. [Reprinted from Gosch et al. (4) by permission of the *Journal of Trauma* © 1970 The Williams & Wilkins Company, Baltimore.]

in this experiment, were placed in a straight trajectory. In this way it appears that a direct transmission of the impact occurs to the brain stem and cervical spinal cord.

The immediate postinjury period of the animals was usually marked by a transient extensor spasm and irregular respiratory excursions while the animal was under light Sernylan anesthesia. Some animals showed gradual respiratory recovery. The signs commonly cited as indicative of experimental cerebral concussion, namely paralysis of the corneal and pinna reflexes, were observed in our experiment. When the animals wore helmets under similar circumstances they showed no neurologic deficit.

Hemorrhages in the upper central cervical cord, varying from small discrete punctate lesions to gross destruction, were found in all animals subjected to an *impact of more than 25 foot-pounds* to the vertex of the head under our experimental conditions. The extent and amount of cord destruction varied with the magnitude of impact and also with the degree of muscular and bony absorption of the impact energy in each individual animal.

High speed photography at the time of injury showed marked dissipation of energy in the neck region. As the vertex of the skull struck the impact plate, the upper trunk, particularly the shoulder region, continued to move in the direction of acceleration with compression and telescoping of the head into the neck. Flexion or extension of the cervical spine was not visualized before the animal recoiled from the impact plate.

A cross section of the spinal cord at the C2-C3 level from an adult monkey (Fig. 67) is shown after the animal had received a vertex impact of 29 foot-pounds. The central gray matter suffered marked hemorrhagic destruction extending into the posterior funiculi. The external surface of the cervical cord showed no contusion and the surface vessels appeared intact. The only gross abnormality was a generalized mild hemorrhage in the cerebral and spinal subarachnoid space. No gross intracerebral lesions were found, and even microscopic sections of the hemispheres and pons revealed no structural changes. The zone of greatest cord destruction was in the third segment with extension rostral to the C2 and caudal to the C4 levels. This relationship is demonstrated in a sagittal section of a specimen taken from another animal (Fig. 68).

A total cervical laminectomy of the C1-C6 laminae and extensive posterior decompression did not alter the spinal damage. With sectioning of the dentate ligaments bilaterally throughout the extent of the laminectomy, hemorrhage was not produced with a vertex impact of 25 to 30 foot-pounds. In one animal only were there smaller central lesions at the cervicothoracic junction below the level of the cut dentate ligaments.

High speed cinematography at the time of injury aided in the study of the mechanical factors involved at the cervicomedullary junction. The cervical spinal cord showed minimal motion in the cephalocaudal direction, in contrast to the marked movement of the cerebral hemispheres as observed through the Lexan calvarium. At the time of impact the vertebral spaces were compressed, and the

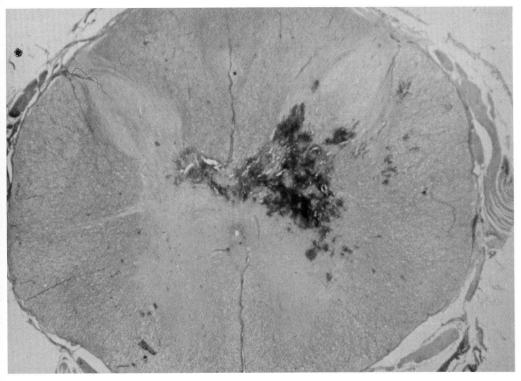

Fig. 67. Hematoxylin-eosin stain of the spinal cord cross section at the area of maximal trauma. Hemolytic necrosis is confined to the central structures of the cord. [Reprinted from Gosch et al. (7) by permission of the *Journal of Trauma* © 1972 The Williams & Wilkins Company, Baltimore.]

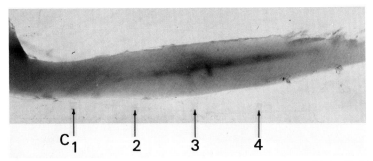

Fig. 68. Midsagittal section of the lower brain stem and upper cervical cord imbedded in paraffin. Central destruction is shown extending from the C2-C4 level. [Reprinted from Gosch et al. (6) by permission of the *Journal of Neurosurgery.*]

foramen magnum was telescoped over the upper cervical cord segments, while the cord itself remained relatively stationary. There seemed to be a direct transmission of energy from the vertex of the skull and cerebrum caudally to the cervicomedullary junction. However, when the dentate ligaments had been sectioned, the cord would not rigidly resist the cervical distortion and movement in the cephalocaudal direction so that there was a further distribution of the damage.

Cervical Spine and Cord Injuries

Cervical injuries with dislocation and fractures of the vertebral column can be produced by a vertex impact in the experimental animal. However marked dissipation of energy in the neck and shoulder musculature was noted by high speed photography at the time of impact. The anesthetized animal is in a totally relaxed muscular state. As the head strikes the impact site with the neck in either flexion or extension, the upper trunk and shoulder region continue to move in the direction of acceleration. This telescoping effect of the head and neck appears to afford some protection to underlying bone and neurogenic structures.

An impact of 25 to 35 foot-pounds to the vertex was delivered in one group of animals in which a rigidly aligned head and neck prevented flexion or extension. Detectable vertebral fractures with these impact energies and positioning of the cervical spine were rarely produced. Gross inspection of the cervical and upper thoracic spine by x-ray and necropsy showed intact ligaments and bony architecture.

An impact force of 40 foot-pounds delivered to the head with flexion of the cervical spine similarly had no effect on the vertebral body alignment as demonstrated by lateral cervical spine x-rays. However, a sagittal section of the cervical spine and ligaments of an animal with such an injury produced evidence of bone destruction as demonstrated in Figure 69. Compression of the C5 and C6 cervical vertebral body with disc space disruption was the usual result of an injury produced in flexion. A slight degree of posterior displacement of disc space content and bone fragments produced definite spinal cord encroachment. An impact of the same magnitude, however, with the cervical spine in flexion and rotation produced a different type of lesion. The simultaneous occurrence of these movements and forces during impact were confirmed by high speed cinematography. Cervical spine subluxation and vertebral compression was usually demonstrated on the lateral spine radiograph (Fig. 70, A and B). In order to produce such a lesion, disruption of the posterior spinous ligaments would be expected and gross inspection of such cervical spines always confirmed the presence of some degree of ligamentous destruction. Severance of the ligamentum flavum between adjacent laminae and facet dislocation was a frequent finding. In our experimental model, a greater force was required in order to produce vertebral disruption in a hyperextension injury. Again rotational force had to be present in addition to the cervical hyperextension in order to produce subluxation.

The pathologic studies of the injured spinal cords revealed exclusive hemorrhagic necrosis in the central portion of the cord substance. Compression, flexion, and hyperextension injuries showed localized nervous tissue disruption and hemorrhage directly under the site of vertebral fracture. The cephalo-caudal extent of the injury was noted to be localized to one or two spinal cord segments. Microscopic examination of these lesions demonstrated hemorrhagic destruction of the central gray substance. The external surface of the cord re-

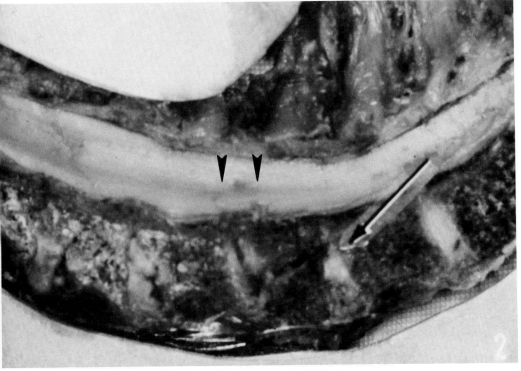

Fig. 69. Localized central hemorrhage is maximal at the C6 level, the area directly under the compressed and dislocated vertebral segment. Injury was produced at 40 foot-pounds with the head in flexion. [Reprinted from Gosch et al. (7) by permission of the *Journal of Trauma* © 1972 The Williams & Wilkins Company Baltimore.]

vealed no evidence of contusion and the pial circulation appeared intact.

The animals with these microscopic lesions exhibited marked neurologic dysfunction as was evident immediately by the labored respiratory pattern in some cases. The possibility of gradual recovery from our induced trauma to the cervical spine was not investigated at this time. The animals were sacrificed immediately after the postinjury examinations had been performed.

Discussion

A number of hypotheses for the mechanism of head injuries and concussion have been proposed in the past (1, 8, 12). Analysis of the various factors responsible for injury has differed among authors, but the significance of shear stresses as a cause of central nervous system damage has in general been accepted. Holbourn (12) stressed the significance of the relative incompressibility of brain tissue in contrast to its ability to change shape. The high ratios of these two properties, namely, compression and elasticity, are the cause for shear strains at predictable locations. The technique used in our laboratory has confirmed these findings by direct observation of the cerebral hemispheres through a plastic calvarium, at the time of injury. With sudden deceleration of the moving sub-

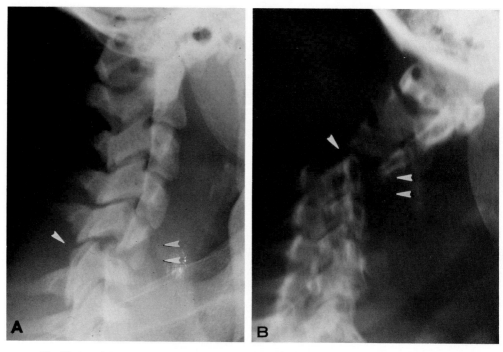

Fig. 70, A and B. Reprinted from Gosch et al. (7) by permission of the *Journal of Trauma* © 1972 The Williams & Wilkins Company, Baltimore.

Fig. 70A. Lateral cervical spine x-ray demonstrating a fracture-dislocation at the C5-C6 level with C6 body compression. An impact of 40 foot-pounds was delivered to the head with the neck in flexion and rotation.

Fig. 70B. Lateral cervical spine x-ray demonstrates the result of a hyperextension injury at 50 foot pounds to the head. Rotation of the head and neck was a necessary component to produce the C3-C4 fracture-dislocation.

ject (in this case an anesthetized monkey) the relatively low density cerebral tissue, in contrast to scalp and cranium, continues to move along the axis of acceleration. Maximum movement and deformation occur in the occipital region with a frontal impact, concomitant with displacement of cerebrospinal fluid, blood, and cerebral tissue through the foramen magnum. Evidence for such brain distortion at impact has also been demonstrated by flash x-ray techniques with implanted lead particles in the cerebral tissue (10, 11). It is therefore reasonable to believe that the greatest damage should be produced at areas where elastic flow or deformation is hindered. The frequent contusion of the temporal and frontal lobes found in severe human head injuries provides clinical evidence in support of this hypothesis (9). The undersurface of the brain moves across the sharp bone ridges at the base of the skull causing contusions. The formation of subdural hematomas is believed to be the result of hemorrhages from bridging cerebral veins in the parietal region when the torsional movement of the hemispheres from the midline stretches these vessels to the point of rupture.

The cervicomedullary junction and cervical spinal cord were similarly affected by stresses generated upon the nervous tissue by the impact. The cervical cord is firmly anchored to its dural covering by the dentate ligaments, which restrain this structure from cephalocaudal displacement. The direct transmission of energy along the brain stem and spinal cord was the cause of the cervical cord hemorrhages. These lesions are concentrated in the upper cervical segments where the initial absorption of shear strains occurs before dissipation of the impact energy. Relatively minimal cord movement occurred during impact because this region of the central nervous system is fixed. When plastic deformation was exceeded, tissues were subject to damage. This view is strengthened by the fact the sectioning of the dentate ligaments prevents hemorrhages under similar impact conditions when movement and deformation is permitted.

These data confirm the fact that shear strains in the central nervous system have a damaging effect. These strains may cause only a temporary neuronal dysfunction, as may occur with simple concussion, a condition not infrequently encountered on the football field. However, strains in a critical location and of sufficient severity may have a permanent or fatal effect as we have seen in some of the cases presented in the preceding chapters.

Summary

In this study we have also described an experimental approach to the study of cervical spinal cord injuries, simulating the mechanism of human spine trauma. Trauma was produced with the neck in flexion, extension and with direct cervical alignment to cause compression only. This model regards the cervical spine as an intact, functioning unit in which trauma is inflicted in a sequence of naturally occurring events by an impact. It encompasses any effect the gross and microscopic vasculature may have on the final neurologic and pathologic lesion. Both the intrinsic circulation of the spinal cord and the extrinsic vascular supply have profound effects on the end stage of the traumatic lesion. The importance of such vascular insufficiency resulting from trauma was stressed by Schneider and Crosby (16).

The state of muscular tone at the time of injury, which certainly is altered from the normal in the experimental animal by the use of pre-trauma anesthesia, had a notable influence on the ability to produce a cervical lesion. This observation has its clinical analog. In the human spine injury, which frequently results in cervical dislocation, muscle tone is set and the result of a relatively low impact force has profound neurologic sequelae.

It was discovered that rotation was a necessary component in addition to flexion or hyperextension to produce cervical dislocation.

The pathologic studies in the specimens showed the main lesion was hemorrhage in the central portion of the spinal cord. A mechanism for the occurrence of such a lesion with a characteristic symptom complex was described by Schneider et al. (15) as the syndrome of "acute central spinal cord injury." Anterior and posterior compressive forces, such as occur particularly in hyperextension, were demonstrated to distribute their greatest damaging effect upon the central portion of the cord substance. This points out the similarity of the pathologic findings of clinically encountered cervical spinal cord injuries and our observed experimental results. The question, "What significance can these findings have in regard to traumatic brain and spinal lesions among athletic injuries?" may be raised at this point.

The subdural hematoma, as stressed in the early part of this study, constitutes the most significant lesion among serious head injuries. The morbidity and mortality can be extremely high unless recognized and treated early. Brain movement and deformation as a result of a head impact have been observed in the experimental animals and a similar mechanism is very likely the cause for this lesion in participants of contact sports. Reid and associates (14) recently reported telemetric recordings of the mechanical and physiologic data obtained from instrumented football players. The maximum tolerable forces were recorded between 150 to 230 G's at a time duration of 310 to 400 msec. This indicates the tremendous forces transmitted to the central nervous system as a result of football trauma. Deformation of the brain can result in stretching and rupture of cortical veins and formation of the subdural hematoma. The authors believe that with an understanding of the mechanisms involved, efforts can be directed towards dissipating the forces which cause such brain deformation. The better design of protective equipment could be a step in this direction (Fig. 76E). Most important is the condemnation of the tactics of "spearing" and "stick-blocking."

The cause of sudden death among two football players, reported by Schneider et al. (17) as a result of a direct vertex impact, can be explained from this experimental data (see Fig. 32, Case 23; Fig. 43E, Case 34). The only pathologic findings, in both cases, were confined to the second cervical spinal cord segment. Petechial hemorrhages in the area of the ventrolateral reticulospinal tracts, the vital pathways for respiration, were reproduced in the laboratory animal. In the direct vertex impact, with the head and spine aligned, so as to allow transmission of the impact force to this region of the spinal axis, shear stresses are produced at the junction of the brain stem and spinal cord. The dentate ligaments attached laterally to the spinal cord prevent any cephalocaudal motion with resultant damage. Again, preventing the build-up of such forces in the brain and spinal cord may eliminate such tragedies. Improved protective headgear and perhaps some adjustments in coaching techniques could prevent this lesion.

Experimental cervical spine fractures were produced in the laboratory animal in flexion and hyperextension. It was observed that an injury in flexion required less impact force than an injury in hyperextension. This has long been an impression purely from clinical experience of some neurosurgeons (17). By physicians emphasizing to coaches and football players that a tackle with the head and neck in hyperextension will have a lesser chance of producing serious spinal injuries, some of these injuries might be prevented.

References

1. Denny-Brown, D. and Russell, W. R.: Experimental Cerebral Concussion. *Brain 64:* 93, 1941.
2. Eldberg, S., Ricker, G. and Angrist, A.: Study of Impact Pressure and Acceleration in Plastic

Skull Models. *Lab. Invest.*, *12:* 1305, 1963.

3. Gosch, H. H., Gooding, E. and Schneider, R. C.: Distortion and Displacement of the Brain in Experimental Head Injuries. *Surg. Forum*, *20:* 425, 1969.

4. Gosch, H. H., Gooding, E. and Schneider, R. C.: The Lexan Calvarium for the Study of Cerebral Responses to Acute Trauma. *J. Trauma*, *10:* 370, 1970.

5. Gosch, H. H., Gooding, E. and Schneider, R. C.: Mechanism and Pathophysiology of Experimentally Induced Cervical Spinal Cord Injuries in Adult Rhesus Monkeys. *Surg. Forum*, *21:* 455, 1970.

6. Gosch, H. H., Gooding, E. and Schneider, R. C.: Cervical Spinal Cord Hemorrhages in Experimental Head Injuries. *J. Neurosurg.*, *33:* 640, 1970.

7. Gosch, H. H., Gooding, E. and Schneider, R. C.: An Experimental Study of Cervical Spine and Cord Injuries. *J. Trauma*, *12:* 570, 1972.

8. Gross, A. G.: A New Theory on the Dynamics of Brain Concussion and Brain Injury. *J. Neurosurg.*, *15:* 548, 1958.

9. Gurdjian, E. S., Webster, J. E. and Arnkoff, H.: Acute Craniocerebral Trauma. Surgical and Pathologic Considerations Based upon 151 Consecutive Autopsies. *Surgery*, *13:* 333, 1943.

10. Gurdjian, E. S., Hodgson, V. R., Thomas, L. M. and Patrick, L. M.: Significance of Relative Movements of Scalp, Skull and Intracranial Contents during Impact Injury of the Head. *J. Neurosurg.*, *29:* 70, 1968.

11. Hodgson, V. R., Gurdjian, E. S. and Thomas, L. M.: Experimental Skull Deformation and Brain Displacement Demonstrated by Flash X-Ray Technique. *J. Neurosurg.*, *25:* 549, 1966.

12. Holbourn, A. H. S.: Mechanics of Head Injuries. *Lancet*, *2:* 438, 1943.

13. Pudenz, R. H. and Sheldon, C. H.: The Lucite Calvarium—A Method for Direct Observation of the Brain. II. Cranial Trauma and Brain Movement. *J. Neurosurg.*, *3:* 487, 1946.

14. Reid, S. F., Tarkington, J. T., Epstein, H. M. and O'Dea, T. J.: Brain Tolerance to Impact in Football. *Surg. Gynecol. Obstet.*, *133:* 929, 1971.

15. Schneider, R. C., Cherry, G. and Pantek, H.: The Syndrome of Acute Central Cervical Spinal Cord Injury. With Special Reference to the Mechanisms Involved in Hyperextension Injuries to the Cervical Spine. *J. Neurosurg.*, *11:* 546, 1954.

16. Schneider, R. C. and Crosby, E. C.: Vascular Insufficiency of Brain Stem and Spinal Cord in Spinal Trauma. *Neurology*, *9:* 643, 1959.

17. Schneider, R. C., Gosch, H. H., Norrell, H., Jerva, M., Combs, L. W. and Smith, R. A.: Vascular Insufficiency and Differential Distortion of Brain and Cord Caused by Cervicomedullary Football Injuries. *J. Neurosurg.*, *33:* 363, 1970.

chapter fifteen

A Method of Comparing the Impact Absorption Characteristics of Football Helmets*

GLENN W. KINDT, M.D., ELWYN R. GOODING AND RICHARD C. SCHNEIDER, M.D.

Although various types of protective headgear have been in existence for many years, the evaluation of the effectiveness of this equipment remains a problem. In the past 15 years a considerable amount of information has been derived from studies (1, 9, 10, 13). It is evident from this work that different types of helmets must be used to provide protection from the various degrees of trauma which are to be sustained. For instance, the helmet used in football should protect against the multiple types of blows received in that sport as contrasted to the protection afforded the snowmobiler who sustains a single impact.

The most common fatal injury in football is the acute subdural hematoma (11) which usually occurs following a horizontal blow to the cranial vault. Cerebral veins which bridge the subarachnoid and subdural spaces to the longitudinal sinus are torn during this injury, resulting in an expanding mass between the dural and arachnoidal membranes. If this condition is not relieved by surgical intervention, progressive impairment of the arterial blood supply to the brain will lead to cerebral swelling and brain stem distortion with eventual death. Usually there is no associated skull fracture with this lesion (11).

Another serious and tragic injury occurring in football is the cervical spine fracture with tetraplegia (11). The usual mechanism for such an injury is a blow to the vertex of the head with the neck in flexion. Excessive force is borne by the vertebral bodies which disrupt. Bony fragments and disc material may be projected into the spinal canal damaging the spinal cord, which if crushed or transected will not regenerate.

This study was performed to simulate the forces present during the production of these serious injuries and compare the effectiveness of various types of protective football headgear in attenuating these forces.

* Reprinted from Kindt et al. (7) by permission of *Medicine and Science in Sports*.

Materials and Methods

The simulated impact was achieved with the aid of an engineering complex involving sub-systems (Fig. 71, 1): Items 1 and 2 are the mechanical impact machine and control console; Items 3, 5, and 4 are the instrumented headform and impact anvil; Items 6 and 10 are the photographic documentation equipment; Items 7 and 11 are the pen recorder and x-y printing devices; Items 8, 9, and 12 are the electronic signal monitoring and recording equipment.

The specially designed and constructed impact machine consisted of a central power section and a horizontal carriage rail with air cylinders and supports. The central power section was composed of an air compressor, storage tank, air pressure regulator, and solenoid air control valves. The air pressure was delivered to two cable-type air cylinders with 14 ft., 5 in. strokes mounted on a 16 ft. horizontal track. At one end of the track there was a 600 pound concrete and aluminum anvil. An aluminum and steel carriage on drive blocks applied to cylinder cables was propelled horizontally down the rails on nylon rollers. A console was used to pre-program a series of events for an impact run. The air line pressure which regulated the carriage speed could be changed remotely from this console by push button switches operating solenoid valves. Photo cells and solid state interval timers were used to determine the distance through which the carriage accelerated to attain the required velocity.

An epoxy plastic headform size 7⅛ with a weight of 10 pounds was mounted on a sled with an aluminum holder containing an accelerometer at the center of gravity of the headform (Fig. 72, 2). For occipital impacts the muscular tone of the neck was simulated by supporting the headform with 5⁄16 in. diameter metal rods. A quartz load cell was bolted directly behind the front plate of the anvil at the site of the projected impact.

The electronic activating, monitoring, and recording equipment is exhibited in Figure 71, 1.

The load cells were connected through 100:1 attenuators to charge amplifiers, thence to two oscilloscopes, and finally to a magnetic tape recorder. The accelerometer was connected to an oscilloscope and the magnetic tape recorder. The calibration of each load cell was accomplished by applying a known load to the transducer and noting the signal intensity. A timing signal of

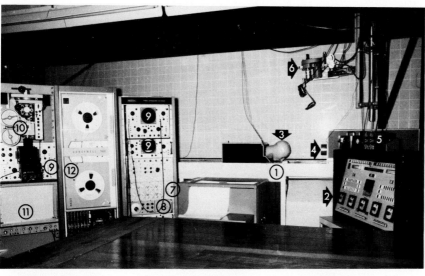

1. Impact Machine	2. Control Console	3. Headform
4. Metal Anvil	5. Charge Amplifiers	6. High Speed Camera
7. Pen Recorder	8. Function Generator	9. Dual Beam Oscilloscopes
10. Oscilloscope Camera	11. X-Y Printer	12. Magnetic Tape Recorder

Fig. 71. Equipment general arrangement. [Reprinted from Kindt et al. (7) by permission of *Medicine and Science in Sports*.]

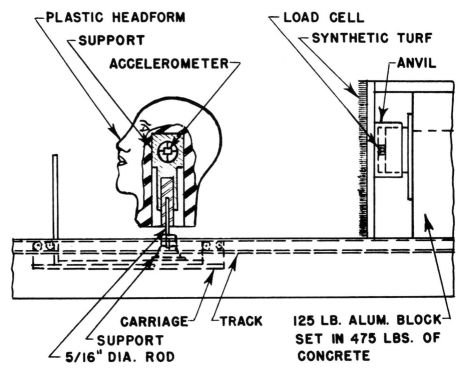

Fig. 72. Occipital impact arrangement. [Reprinted from Kindt et al. (7) by permission of *Medicine and Science in Sports*.]

1000 cycles per second, was recorded on the magnetic tape during each impact run. Two electrical impulses were recorded from the unit mounted on the carriage so as to be actuated over a measured interval to determine the final velocity of the carriage.

A multiple channel ink recorder printed out a permanent record from signals on the magnetic tape, and these signals were expanded from the tape to the recorder for better evaluation. An x-y plotter was also used to print expanded traces of the impact.

The high speed camera capable of obtaining 10 to 10,000 pictures per second was mounted on a movable carriage for positioning anywhere above or to the side of the impact machine. An oscilloscope camera was utilized to record impact traces and calibrations when desired. A 16 mm. camera, a 35 mm. camera, and an industrial camera were also used in the documentation of results.

This series of impacts was made at a typical playing condition ambient temperature of 72 degrees F.

Two types of impacts were studied for this report: 1) an impact to the occiput to simulate a blow producing a subdural hematoma and 2) an impact to the vertex of the head to simulate a cervical fracture with tetraplegia or a severe brain stem contusion or hemorrhage.

For one series of impacts to the occiput (Fig. 72, 2), the final velocity was equivalent to a man falling and striking his head on a hard surface. Such a fall has been known to produce an acute subdural hematoma. After the signal for this type of impact was recorded, using the bare headform against the rigid anvil, the study was repeated with several helmets of varying construction. All types of helmets attenuated the blow considerably when compared to that sustained by the bare headform against the plain anvil as demonstrated in Figure 73*. In order to approach a dangerous level, even with the helmet in place, a second series of impacts to the bare, rigid

* See appended list for description of numbered helmets (Appendix A).

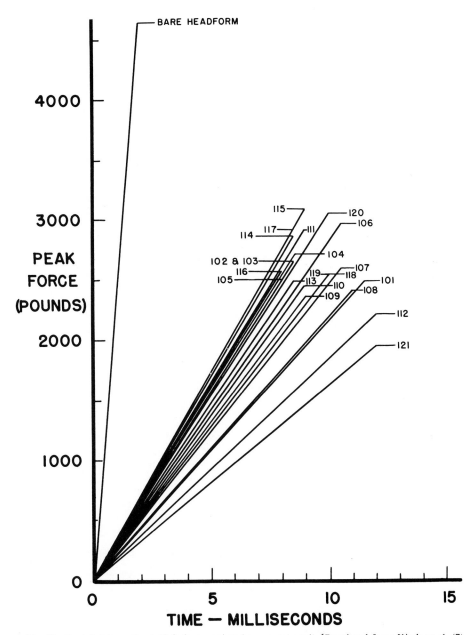

Fig. 73. Occipital impacts at 10 ft./sec. against bare metal anvil. [Reprinted from Kindt et al. (7) by permission of *Medicine and Science in Sports*.]

anvil was made at a higher velocity. Finally, a third series of impacts was performed using a synthetic turf over the anvil endeavoring to simulate to some degree the condition of the football field. (The authors grant that the comparison is certainly not identical because of the lack of other layers serving as a base for the synthetic turf.)

The impact machine and headform assembly then were rearranged to deliver a blow to the vertex in a direct plane with the body (Fig. 74). A sled in this series of tests was loaded with 75 pounds of sand to simulate the driving force of the upper part of the body such as might occur

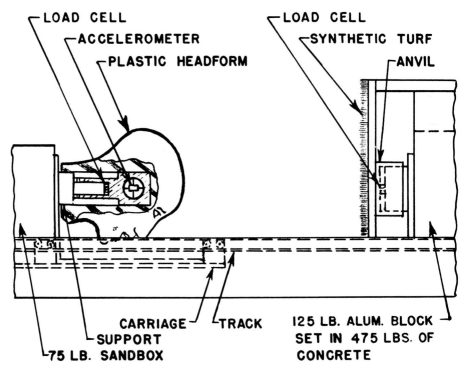

Fig. 74. Vertex impact arrangement. [Reprinted from Kindt et al. (7) by permission of *Medicine and Science in Sports*.]

in a football game. An impact which has often been demonstrated to produce a cervical fracture with tetraplegia is that sustained by a diver striking the bottom of a pool. Actually such a direct vertex blow to a football player without cervical fracture has resulted in spinal cord hemorrhages and death (12). An impact of such intensity was produced and studied using the bare headform and various types of headgear against a rigid anvil. The series of tests then were repeated using impacts of a higher velocity, as well as using the artificial turf over the anvil.

Results

An effort has been made to establish a test method and a specific procedure for the reproducible evaluation of all types of protective headgear for football players. The reproducibility of the results using this procedure were gratifying. The bare headform produced identical tracings on repeated impacts and the tracings from various types of headgear were similarly reproducible. All types of helmets markedly attenuated the impact compared to the bare headform with both the occipital and vertex blows.

One method of comparing the degree of protection afforded by various types of helmets is demonstrated in Figures 73 and 75, which contain both the peak force reached, as well as the length of time necessary to reach this peak force. Considerable differences are noted in the performance of various types of helmet construction. The inflatable multiple chamber, pneumatic-type helmet with more resilient areas in the outer shell seemed to be more effective in attenuating the impact forces in this series of tests. Although the figures illustrating the time-force curves for the various helmets show only one line for each helmet, it should be emphasized that all helmets were tested several times and the line shown is typical for that particular helmet. To show the time-force curves for all tests of each type of helmet would be too confusing if presented in the same illustration.

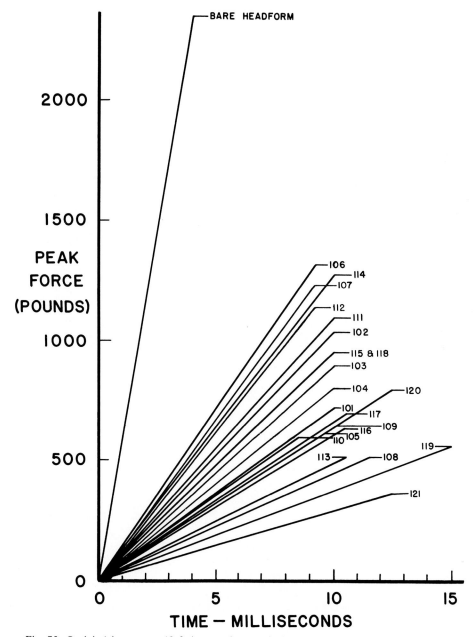

Fig. 75. Occipital impacts at 10 ft./sec. against synthetic turf. [Reprinted from Kindt et al. (7) by permission of *Medicine and Science in Sports.*]

In the "Description of Helmets" (see Appendix A), as numbered in Figures 73, 75, and 79, only one helmet was custom fabricated. All other helmets were donated by manufacturers and are typical of the quality available to coaches from a local supplier (Fig. 76, A–F).

The signals produced on impacts of the bare headform alone and with various types of headgear are shown in Figure 77. A sharp pointed signal such as that caused by the bare headform (Fig. 77, 1) would presumably indicate less protection than a lower rounded signal (Fig. 77, 2–5) as noted by Gurdjian et al. (4). An interpretation of a typical force-time curve is presented in Figure 78. Considerable differences were again shown to exist between the various types of headgear according to their construction (Figs. 73 and 75). The numbers used to identify the types of suspension systems are identified in each of these figures (see Appendix A). The interpretation of the force-time curve is shown

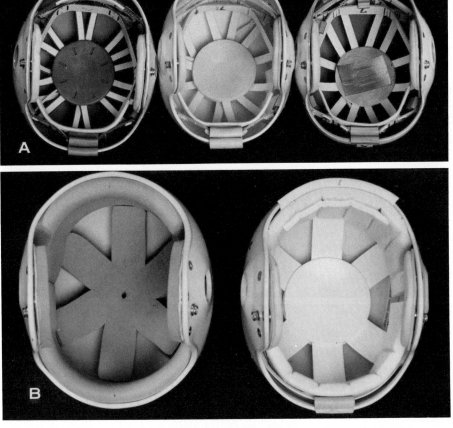

Fig. 76. Different makes of football helmets with various types of suspension systems.
Fig. 76A. Web type suspension systems.
Fig. 76B. Foam type suspension systems.

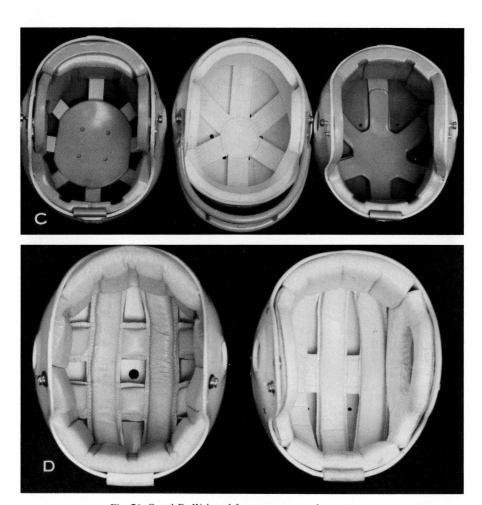

Fig. 76. C and D. Web and foam type suspension systems.

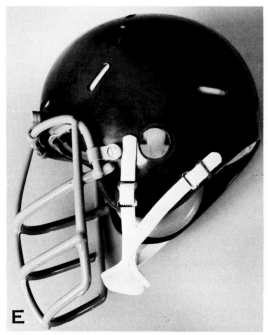
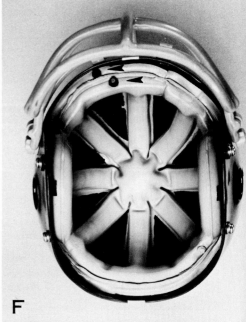

Fig. 76. E and F. The double pneumatic inner support crown helmet with the rigid shell containing more pliable inserts of lighter plastic is shown (Schneider, R. C. and Gooding, E. *Patent No. 3,462,763*. Any royalties are assigned to the University of Michigan Neurosurgical Research Laboratory). The component parts are demonstrated in Figure 85. This helmet seemed most effective in protecting against severe blows compared to other helmets when tested on the impact track as shown in Figure 77. The prototype is currently being field tested and has been found to be a superior headgear for protection and comfort. (See also Fig. 85 A–C, p. 251.)

Fig. 76E. The rigid outer shell is pictured with the more pliable inserts not visualized. There are strategically placed slits in the helmet to enable proper distortion, restitution, ventilation and comfort. A four point chin strap is used.

Fig. 76F. The outer and inner pneumatic crown supports are shown fused into a single unit. The outer crown lying against the shell is pneumatized to the same degree for all players. The inner support crown is pressurized to fit the individual for his safety and comfort. Note the only two valves molded into the crowns just to the left of the midline of the helmet (arrows).

in Figure 78. It was interesting to discover that, during the vertex impacts, the suspension system of three of the helmets studied failed and "bottomed out" (Fig. 79). A review of Figure 80 reveals the type of force-time curve in a helmet which failed.

Discussion

All current methods of testing the effectiveness of headgear are somewhat unsatisfactory. One reason for this is the difficulty in determining the limits of human tolerance (5, 8, 9). Because of the complex anatomy present and the human variability factor, a given impact can produce markedly different results. Even an identical impact to the same individual at the same site might produce a variation of the pathology if repeated at another time.

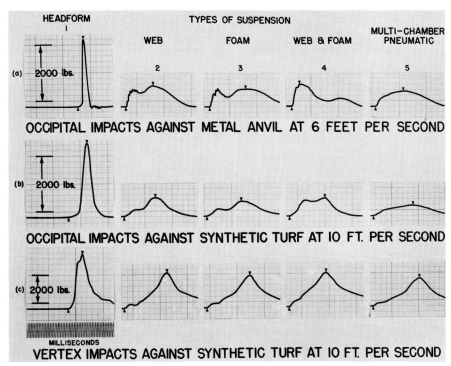

Fig. 77. Typical signal traces of impacts of the bare head form (1) and the various types of helmets (2–5) tested in Figures 76, A–E. The best head gear protection to the skull and brain is one in which there is the most gradual rise of the curve and the lowest peak. Such a curve is noted with the multichambered pneumatic helmet (5). [Reprinted from Kindt et al. (7) by permission of *Medicine and Science in Sports.*]

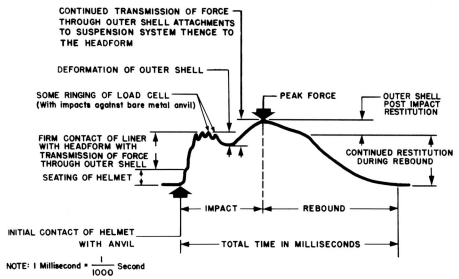

Fig. 78. Interpretation of force-time curve (analysis of segment 2a of Fig. 77). [Reprinted from Kindt et al. (7) by permission of *Medicine and Science in Sports.*]

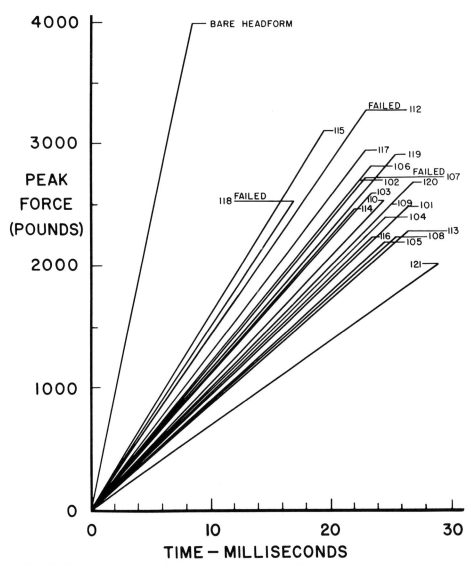

Fig. 79. Vertex impacts at 10 ft./sec. against synthetic turf. Note that in three helmets the inner suspension failed. [Reprinted from Kindt et al. (7) by permission of *Medicine and Science in Sports.*]

An attempt has been made in this study to begin with two types of severe injury and simulate the forces involved when these injuries occur. A plastic, semi-resilient headform was used to minimize the ringing noted with metallic headforms. The neck was simulated by the use of the metal rod which would bend similar to a neck with normal muscle tone. The same impact track and instrumentation have been used previously to produce successfully intracranial hematomas and cervical fractures in primates (2, 3).

When testing the effectiveness of football helmets, some limitations in helmet design must be considered. The smooth and firm outer shell is necessary to pre-

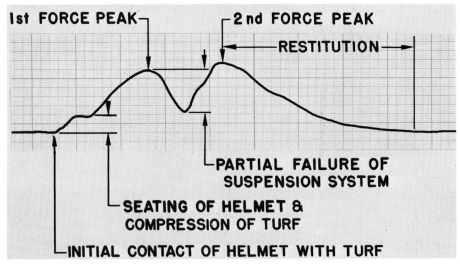

Fig. 80. Typical force-time curve of a helmet which failed. [Reprinted from Kindt et al. (7) by permission of *Medicine and Science in Sports*.]

vent "gripping" (the catching of one irregular surface of one helmet on a similar surface on the other helmet), which could produce serious rotational injuries (6). A certain degree of resiliency of the outer shell will enable dissipation of forces applied to the helmet at impact. The transverse distance between the head and the outer shell and the vertical distance from the vertex have been standardized at approximately one inch and two inches, respectively. To be of practical value the helmet must also resume its original shape following multiple impacts. One of the most important remaining variables is the type of padding and suspension within the helmet. In this study the multiple chamber pneumatic type suspension, in combination with the more resilient areas in the outer shell, gave the best protection for both the vertex and transverse impacts in the range tested.

Synthetic turf was incorporated in this test to better approximate the playing conditions. The "synthetic turf" attenuated the signals from the bare headform as well as from all types of helmets. Further factors being considered for subsequent investigation include the effect of temperature, hair, scalp, helmet mass, force time and duration, and the shape of the anvil against which the helmet is impacted.

However, the single most important fact to remember is not what happens to the helmet but what the effect is upon the underlying brain.

References

1. Ewing, C. L. and Irving, A. M.: Evaluation of Head Protection in Aircraft. *Aerosp. Med.*, *40:* 596, 1969.
2. Gosch, H. H., Gooding, E. R. and Schneider, R. C.: Cervical Spinal Cord Hemorrhages in Experimental Head Injuries. *J. Neurosurg.*, *33:* 640, 1970.

3. Gosch, H. H., Gooding, E. R. and Schneider, R. C.: Mechanism and Pathophysiology of Experimentally Induced Cervical Cord Injuries in Adult Rhesus Monkeys. *Surg. Forum*, *21:* 455, 1970.
4. Gurdjian, E. S., Lissner, H. R. and Patrick, L. M.: Protection of the Head and Neck in Sports. *J.A.M.A.*, *182:* 509, 1962.
5. Hirsch, A. E.: *Current Problems in Head Protection*. Head Injury Conference Proceedings, edited by W. Caveness, and A. E. Walker, J. P. Lippincott Co., Philadelphia, Pennsylvania. 37–40, 1966.
6. Holbourn, A. H. S.: Mechanics of Head Injuries. *Lancet*, *2:* 438, 1943.
7. Kindt, G. W., Schneider, R. C. and Robinson, J. L.: A Method of Comparing the Impact Absorption Characteristics of Football Helmets. *Med. Sci. Sports*, *3:* 203, 1971.
8. Lombard, C. F., Ames, S. W., Roth, H. P. and Rosenfield, S.: Voluntary Tolerance of Humans to Impact Acceleration of the Head. *J. Aviation Med.*, *22:* 109, 1951.
9. Rayne, J. M. and Maslen, K. R.: Factors in the Design of Protective Helmets. *Aerosp. Med.*, *40:* 631, 1969.
10. Roberts, J. B. and Hygh, E. H.: A Comparison of Methods for the Evaluation of Protective Headgear. *Aerosp. Med.*, *35:* 1044, 1964.
11. Schneider, R. C.: Serious and Fatal Neurosurgical Football Injuries. *Clin. Neurosurg.*, *12:* 226, 1965.
12. Schneider, R. C., Gosch, H. H., Norrell, H., Jerva, M., Combs, L. W. and Smith, R. A.: Vascular Insufficiency and Differential Distortion of Brain and Cord Caused by Cervicomedullary Football Injuries. *J. Neurosurg.*, *33:* 363, 1970.
13. Snively, G. C. and Chichester, C. O.: Impact Survival Levels of Head Acceleration in Man. *Aero. Med.*, *32:* 316, 1961.

Appendix A

Description of Helmets as Numbered in Figures 72, 75, and 77

101, 102, 103, and 104:
Web suspension system with web bands over crown and peripheral web band
105:
Same as above except has foam over band at front
106, 107, 108, 109, and 110:
Web suspension system with web bands over crown and peripheral foam band
111, 112, 114, 115, 116, and 117:
Web-foam suspension system with foam over web crown bands and peripheral foam band
113:
Foam suspension system with foam crown pads and peripheral foam band
118:
Web type suspension system with web bands over crown, with peripheral foam band and padded outside over midsection from front to back
119:
Web-foam type suspension system with web backed foam crown pads, with peripheral foam band and padded outside over midsection from front to back
120:
Pneumatic-hydraulic suspension system with multilayer foam and inflatable pneumatic cushions over crown and around perimeter
121:
Multiple chamber inflatable suspension system with resilient areas in the outer shell (custom fabricated)

Chapter sixteen

Recommendations for Improvement of the Game of Football

Head and Neck Protection

For centuries the use of headgear has been employed for the prevention of intracranial injuries. However, in the early days of football, 1890, the best protection afforded a football player was not a helmet but a bushy head of hair which not only cushioned the blow to the cranium but also afforded a fine handle for tackling. In the mid 1920's the non-padded leather headgear made its appearance and by the early 1940's a leather helmet with an inner suspension was developed. Finally in the early 1950's the rigid outer helmet with some type of inner suspension came into use.

Another contribution in the area of head, and particularly face, protection was the plastic face guard. About 30 years ago Coach Paul Brown (2) abandoned the old "nose guard" and provided the first "protruding face bar" face guard for the protection of one of his star players. This consisted of a single, simple plastic loop extending a short distance in front of the face for protection. At a discussion on football injuries during a meeting of the owners and coaches of the National Football League in New York in 1962 (2), he expressed amazement and some concern at the evolution which had occurred, perhaps haphazardly, in the intervening years. There had been the progressive development from the "single bar" to the "double bar" and the "middle line vertical" bar in association with either the single or double bar, resulting in the "bird cage."

Face Guards*

Clear and unobstructed vision is essential for any athlete participating in a contact sport so he may function at his best and with the greatest degree of safety

---

* Reprinted, almost in toto, from Schneider and Antine (15) by permission of the *Journal of the American Medical Association.*

(2, 14). This is particularly important where speed and heavy impact blocking are such vital factors in the proper execution of the plays (15). The plastic face guard has done much to protect the player from serious facial injuries and has permitted a more fearless type of tackling and blocking.

The authors have evaluated this equipment from the standpoint of good vision for the player. It is hoped that the data presented here may lead team physicians and surgical specialists to pay more attention to equipment with reference to the visual problem of individual players. Through their teaching they may encourage coaches, trainers, and helmet manufacturers to review these problems and perhaps correct equipment so as to prevent injuries.

For the purpose of this study, the subject, a reliable observer, had visual fields made with various types of headgear and face guards. All binocular visual fields were determined on an ordinary perimeter utilizing a 3 mm. white faced test object. A minor problem of head positioning was encountered in some cases necessitating the removal of the vertical maxillary rest bar. The subject was photographed in the helmet from an anterior and lateral aspect, and the visual fields were combined to show exactly what his binocular visual field deficit was with these types of equipment (Fig. 81, A–F). This varied to some degree with different combinations of helmets and face masks. In some instances the headgear was applied "slightly to the right or left of center" and the visual field charted. No attempt was made to correct this slightly untoward position for on the football field the player does not adjust the helmet perfectly during the heat of the fray.

When the plastic helmet, No. 20 (Fig. 81A), with the "single bar" plastic face guard was used, it may be noted there was a very slight visual deficit in the inferior quadrants of the fields. This visual defect cannot be attributed to the single bar but rather to the head position being too close to the arc center of the apparatus. This helmet was the type of equipment most frequently worn by the backfield player and probably the one which provided the best vision for the participant. It is said that one of the greatest disadvantages to such a face guard is the possibility of the overriding of one player's face guard on that of an opposing player's (Fig. 86). Melvin (9) has indicated that perhaps the player with the single bar type of face guard, when tackled and endeavoring to hyperextend his neck to prevent flexion injury to the cervical spine, occasionally catches the single bar in the mud, thus holding the head down (Fig. 40F). The result is that with further impact there is additional acute flexion causing a forced cervical flexion fracture.

The combination of double, or "double tube" face bar and rigid helmet, No. 67, gave a pattern showing two spike or pointed visual defects in the inferior temporal field bilaterally (Fig. 81B). Scotomata resulting from all bars could be plotted centrally in the visual field; they became less dense the distance of the bar from the eye increased. These scotomata, however, are not included in the field charts shown because the defects were small and the margins indefinite. Any slight bobbing movement of the head (as is the case during actual playing conditions) caused the scotomata to disappear or become so indefinite as to be impossible to

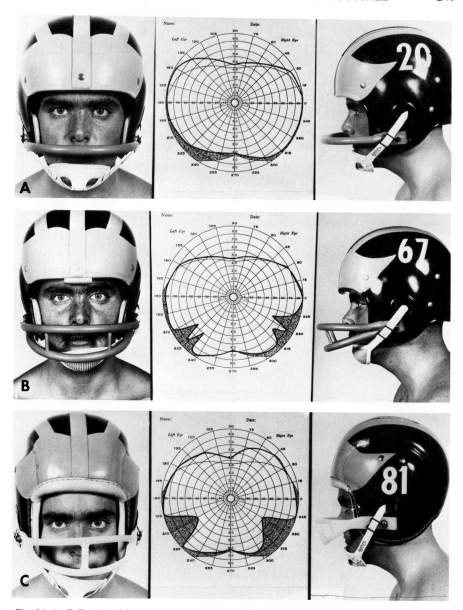

Fig. 81, A–C. Reprinted from Schneider and Antine (15) by permission of the *Journal of the American Medical Association*.

Fig. 81A. Single face bar probably provides the best vision but does not afford ultimate in protection. Loss of inferior visual field cannot be attributed to helmet bar but to head position being too close to arc center of apparatus.

Fig. 81B. Double bar, "double tube," face guard causes two definite defects in either inferior temporal quadrant of visual field inferiorly.

Fig. 81C. Double bar face guard with solid band attachment to helmets results in greater bilateral inferior temporal defect than previous piece of equipment. (Note careless but spontaneous slight offset of helmet and chin strap.)

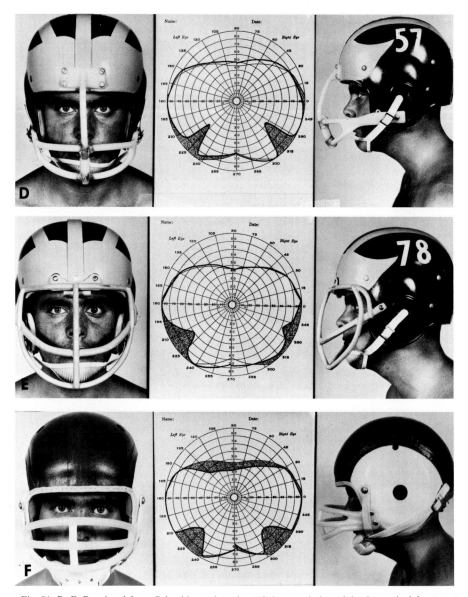

Fig. 81, D–F. Reprinted from Schneider and Antine (15) by permission of the *Journal of the American Medical Association.*

Fig. 81D. Vertical plastic midline bar is projected somewhat further outward in front of the nose than in Figure 81E, below, but no visible defect is noted. Usual bitemporal inferior quadrantic defects due to wide basal attachment are demonstrated.

Fig. 81E. Tubed vertical midline plastic bar attached to helmet causes no impairment of vision to individual with normal vision. Some bitemporal inferior quadrantic visual field cut is due to points of attachment of face guard.

Fig. 81F. Combined presence of external shock absorbing padding over vertex of helmet and firm plastic band attachment at zygomaticomandibular portion of helmet may cause bitemporal inferior quadrantic and superior visual field defects.

outline. The face guard portrayed in Figure 81B is more efficient in preventing facial injuries because of the greater area of protective coverage.

In another type of helmet, No. 81 (Fig. 81C) with a "double bar" face guard anchored by a broad band at the base of the helmet, there was a more significant cut in the player's inferior visual field bitemporally because of the solid bar. It may be noted the helmet may ride slightly higher on the head due to the peculiarities of its internal suspension mechanism or the helmet's fit. The entire headgear was displaced slightly toward the left side, while the chin strap was partially drawn toward the right side. Again, no attempt was made to artificially correct this situation for this is the way the player automatically puts on his helmet.

The evaluation of the headgear with the middle vertical plastic bar directly in front of the player's nose, as seen in helmets 57 and 78 (Fig. 81, D and E), showed it did not alter the visual fields centrally. There was good binocular vision with sufficient visual overlap from each eye as long as the player had no visual impairment on either side. Again, the bitemporal inferior quadrantic field cut is noticeable, more with the flat plastic band attachment in the mandibular region (Fig. 81D) and less with the "tube" type of face guard inserted high in the temporoparietal area (Fig. 81E). The latter type of equipment, however, does not appear to be quite so sturdy and it might conceivably break more readily. A few years ago one of the prominent college quarterbacks of the country was reported to have had severely limited vision in one eye. In such an instance the player wearing a helmet with the "bird cage" effect created by the vertical midline plastic "tube" would not have binocular vision and would sustain a sizeable central visual defect. If this were then coupled with the bitemporal inferior quadrantic defect, the total loss of visual field would indeed tend to be great. The player's effectiveness might be markedly hampered.

During more recent years there has been an added impetus given by physicians, coaches, trainers, and manufacturers to develop a safer type of headgear for football players. One of the most recent models to appear is shown in Figure 81F. The presence of an inner liner suspension, external ensolite (i.e., shock absorbable padding over the vertex of the helmet), the thickened plastic face guard with the firm zygomaticomandibular attachment, and a four point fixation nylon chin strap are some of the new features. Although many of these innovations are excellent, unfortunately, in this instance the added safety factors may cause further diminution in the field of vision. There may be not only the bitemporal inferior quadrantic field cut due to the wider band attachment of the guard to the helmet but also a bilaterally superior impairment of the visual field due to the forward projection of the helmet and its superimposed safety padding.

It is probable that transient obstruction of vision by the face guard may well interfere not only with the forward pass reception (Fig. 81G) but also with the ball carrier or tackler more frequently than is realized. Certainly the presence of a potential blocker or tackler approaching low and in a lateral plane may well fall

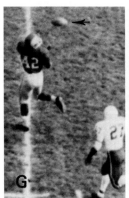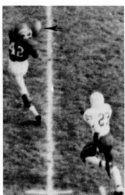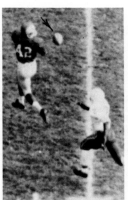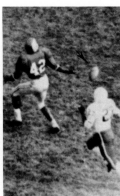

Fig. 81G. In this play the football struck the face guard and bounded away as though it was not seen by the player due to poor vision. The dark shirted player was in the clear, and if he had caught the pass would very likely have made a touchdown, placing his team in contention for the league championship. (Courtesy of Bill Shepherd, Staff Photographer, Dayton Daily News, Dayton, Ohio.)

within the inferior temporal quadrantic visual field cut, preventing the opposing player from seeing him. This could result in a greater chance for injury, particularly to the player's knees. Probably this is why the "roll-out" quarterback is so often smothered from his "blind side." A well known professional football player recognizes the importance of even the transient obscuration of vision for he will wear a helmet with a face guard during most of the game, but when called upon to punt the ball, he exchanges this helmet for one *without* the face guard so his vision remains unimpaired. Perhaps a reduction of defects in the inferior temporal quadrantic fields can be made by changes in equipment design.

Helmet

The rigid plastic football helmet with its various types of suspensions used for head protection leaves much to be desired in the prevention of head and neck injuries. In 1961 (13) after reviewing and analyzing the data on the mechanisms involved in the first 14 serious or fatal neurosurgical football injuries, the following suggestions were made by this author for a change in helmet construction (Fig. 84).*

"1. It might be wise to consider the use of a more resilient material for helmets to permit more deformation and more gradual deceleration of the head.

2. The face guard, if it continues to be used and is made of solid plastic material, should be shortened and placed closer to the face. This would provide the following advantages: a) a less accessible bar for the opponent to grab; b) cut down on the leverage available if backward thrust is employed; c) permit better vision due to less visual field cut; and d) provide less overriding surface of the bar which might injure the opponent's face.

3. There may be a place for the development of the chin strap which would release at certain safely determined pressures similar to the safety bindings on skis.

---

* Reprinted from Schneider et al. (13) by permission of the *Journal of the American Medical Association.*

4. Even with less rigid helmets than the present plastic ones, a skirt or flap of moderately firm sponge rubber or some other material should be incorporated into the back of the helmet so that its posterior margin will not administer a serious knife-like blow to the cervical spine when severe hyperextension of the cervical spine occurs suddenly."

In the intervening 11 years since the compilation of the initial survey of serious and fatal head and spine football injuries (13), the only major progress in the revision of the shell has been the cutting of the posterior rim of the helmet higher by a few manufacturers to eliminate serious cervical hyperextension injuries. Subsequent evaluation has shown that a pliable posterior flange of the helmet is unnecessary since it appears adequate protection is provided by proper fitting shoulder pads.

Within the past 2 years there have been some attempts to provide new inner supports for various types of helmets. Some of the older web suspensions served as a halo which upon impact actually absorbed the blow primarily at the points of its fixation. Other suspensions have consisted of isolated or individual pockets containing fluid, a shock-absorbing material, and a space to be inflated with air. Initially the wearers of such helmet suspensions complained of severe headache. Without the knowledge of the anatomy of the supraorbital and occipital nerves (the two main nerves supplying pain sensation to the scalp), the protective pads had been placed directly over them and inflated—causing the player to have a severe headache. In another instance communicating pockets partially full of fluid caused improved absorption of the blow but, like a boat which has shipped water, when there is a tilt of the head all the fluid rushes toward one side so that the inertia tends to carry the head to one side with an overswing to the heavy helmet. Ideally there must be a rapid distribution of the force of impact over the skull by a light material which will reconstitute itself rapidly ready for the next blow. There may be problems other than those related to headgear construction.

On one occasion this author learned that the sales department of a large manufacturing company overruled their group, which was doing what little research that had been transpiring, because the helmet "doesn't look like" that of another manufacturer. Therefore it presumably would not sell!

Probably one of the most alarming situations that has occurred has been the great upsurge in popularity of football among the little league age group resulting in a tremendous number of youngsters playing football at a grammar school age. The result has been the flooding of the market with flimsy headgear which are cheap and extremely dangerous. The parents buy the products and the youngsters wear these helmets because they state "authentic pro" on the liner and, what is most important, "they look like pros" (Fig. 82). In some instances the headgear are given away as a bonus for so many of father's cigar wrappers or at a gasoline station with the purchase of so many gallons of gas. The helmets not only are not constructed for safety but also do not carry any manufacturer's name to identify a source of liability.

Good football helmets must successfully withstand impact and function well in extreme ranges of temperature. A very cold day may have a devastating effect on any headgear (Fig. 83). Constant attention to these details is essential if better protective headgear is going to be available.

It was this author's opinion that newer football helmets should be constructed specifically on the basis of an anatomical knowledge of the skull and brain with an understanding of the mechanical principles involved in head injuries. The neuro-anatomical and neurosurgical facts had to be coupled with an extensive experience in mechanical engineering and the special adaptation of plastic materials to such uses. Six years ago Mr. Elwyn Gooding, who had this necessary expertise, joined

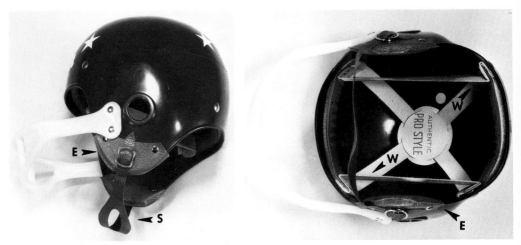

Fig. 82. A cheap type of helmet for "little league" players showing the sharp knife-like edges (E) of the helmet which would easily lacerate the little fellow or his opponent. The thin, loose strips of webbing (W) for the suspension would immediately bottom out on contact. The chin strap(s) is very flimsy. This is a death trap for the little league player and manufacturers of such headgear should be prevented from marketing them.

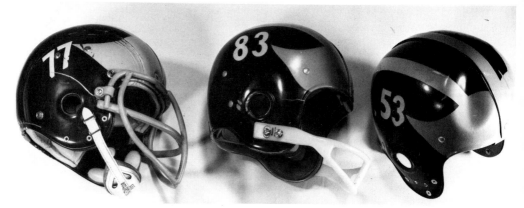

Fig. 83. Three helmets damaged in a collegiate football game on an unusually cold day. Nos. 77 and 83 show cracks in the plastic causing razor sharp margins. No. 53 demonstrates the failure of a knee imprint to expand. Two fiberglas faceguards were also fractured that same day.

this author in developing a headgear based on these principles.

To some degree an analogy may be drawn between the results of a blow to the head and its effect on the skull and brain comparing it to the sequelae of the impact to the rigid helmet shell and skull. The worst damage to the brain may occur in those closed head injuries in which skull fracture does not occur (Fig. 5A). For example, there is no dissipation of the impact of the blow but there is a direct transmission of the force to the underlying area of the brain with movement and impingement of it on the opposite side of the skull, resulting in a contrecoup injury (that is, damage to the skull or brain on the side opposite the side of the blow). This has been shown from experiments in previous pages by Dr. Gosch (Chapter 14). The pontine hemorrhages already described may be due to such a mechanism (Chapter 3). In occipital blows to the head the brain may rebound and on impact on a sharp bony sphenoid ridge may suffer frontotemporal injury with secondary clot formation within the brain. In closed head injuries where fracture occurs, there is some dissipation of the force of the blow as the bone breaks resulting in less damage to the underlying brain than if the skull had not been fractured (Fig. 5B). Currently, due to a lack of resiliency of the outer shell of the helmet and the inability of the present suspension systems to absorb the force of a severe impact, there is a transmission of such force to skull and the intracranial contents that tearing of blood vessels with fatal hemorrhage or destruction of the brain may result (13).

Ideally in designing a new helmet the rigid portions of the outer shell of the helmet should be constructed to overlie either the fragile areas of the skull, which might fracture, or to cover specific portions of the intracranial contents, which most frequently are vulnerable in head injuries (Fig. 84). For example, the branches of the middle meningeal artery are captives in a bony groove of the thin temporal bone. If this vessel is transected with or without a fracture of the skull, the result is a hemorrhage on the surface of one membrane surrounding the brain (i.e., an extradural hemorrhage; see Fig. 8, A and B). The lateral sinuses and the site at which they join the longitudinal sinus to form a reservoir (i.e., the confluens of the sinuses or torcula Herophili) must also be protected, for they too are a source of extradural hemorrhage, although they are less frequently a cause than the middle meningeal artery. The bridging veins which drain the blood from the upper surface (vertex) of the brain into the longitudinal sinus are thin walled and are the most frequent source of bleeding underneath the membranes which encircle the brain (i.e., subdural hemorrhage; see Fig. 11). The posterior walls of the bony frontal sinus or the base of the skull directly behind it (the cribriform plate) may be very thin and, if fractured, bone fragments may tear the membranes of the brain permitting a leakage of watery fluid (the cerebrospinal fluid which bathes the brain), providing a pathway for infection to enter the intracranial cavity with the possibility of meningitis or a brain abscess. All of the aforementioned structures should be covered by a rigid protective strip of the outer shell of the helmet.

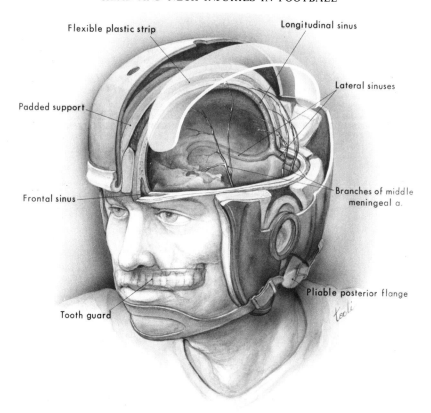

Fig. 84. In 1961 this cut-away view of the helmet and skull demonstrated the underlying cranial and intracranial anatomical structures, in addition to the brain, which must be protected. To provide more resiliency to the rigid plastic helmet, more flexible strips of plastic would be inserted over the relatively less dangerous regions on either side of the skull to permit dissipation or deceleration of the force.

The regions of the bony frontal sinuses, the thin temporal bone with its middle meningeal artery, and the areas of the superior longitudinal and lateral sinuses would be protected by the firm plastic, avoiding damage by a direct blow to these structures.

The high cut posterior rim may or may not have a pliable posterior flange to avoid the guillotining of the cervical spine by the rigid helmet margin.

In this diagram the face guard has been removed and the tooth guard inserted. This would prevent "spearing" and "stick-blocking," for the player would be reluctant to use his unprotected face for the impact.

The authors suggested a more flexible plastic material than the current rigid shell as a plastic strip which was to be inserted over the remaining areas of the brain (Fig. 84). Initially this was designed only with the thought of creating resiliency to dissipate the force of a blow. However, subsequent consideration proved this was impractical for two reasons: first, the motor strip of the brain was unprotected, and secondly, the plastic was difficult to mold satisfactorily with the more rigid surrounding material. The final design of this helmet shell was then altered so another rigid portion of the outer shell would overlay the motor strip laterally on either side of the helmet (Fig. 85C). As a result further protection was given to the more vital areas of the brain and the softer or more pliable portions of the helmet overlay the more "silent" regions (i.e., those areas which might absorb a direct blow without the danger of as much residual neurologic deficit). As has been shown in previous pages, the firm posterior margin of the outer shell of the helmet should be cut high to avoid the guillotining effect of this part of the helmet driving it into the cervical spine in severe cervical hyperextension injuries which may result in cervical fractures or spinal cord damages (Fig. 30B).

The inner suspension system was devised to distribute more uniformly over the head the force generated by the impact. The system consists of two crowns, one within the other (Fig. 85, A and B). Each crown is a hemisphere of hollow plastic material with arches extending from the apex to the base or circumference of the crown. Air or gas injected through valves into these structures may diffuse throughout all parts of each individual crown. In the completed helmet the two crowns are injection molded and high frequency electrically sealed together as a single piece. The inner crown (Fig. 85A) is pneumatized to fit the individual player, but the outer crown (Fig. 85B) coapting to the helmet is inflated to the same pressure for all wearers. The presence of the two separately pneumatized systems avoids the problem of the headgear bouncing on the head. The helmet is maintained in position on the head with a four point attached chin strap (Fig. 76E). Subsequent testing on the impact track (Fig. 71, Chapter 13) revealed that the peak impact force was lower and it was arrived at over a longer period of time than in other combined shell and suspensions which were tested under similar conditions. The prototype helmet has been field tested successfully. Not only is this headgear

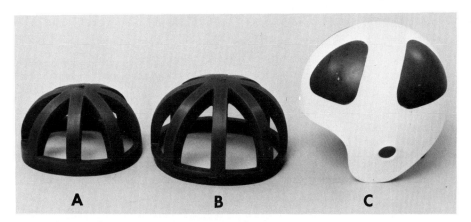

Fig. 85. Double inner crown pneumatic suspension system.
Fig. 85A. Inner crown support—inflated to individual head.
Fig. 85B. Inner crown support—inflated to same degree for all wearers.
Fig. 85C. Outer shell—firm plastic shown in white to protect vital cranial and intracranial structures (see Fig. 82). Black areas of more resilient material over relatively silent area permit some deformation of the shell with dissipation of impact forces. Schneider, R. C. and Gooding, E. *Patent No. 3,462,763*. (Any royalties are assigned to the University of Michigan Neurosurgical Research Laboratory.)

lighter than others, but also it is more comfortable because of the lack of reverberation of noise on impact, a significant problem in some helmets.

More recently Robey et al. (11) have suggested from their studies on football players that the hard or rigid helmet has been responsible for numerous injuries to their opponents. Therefore, they have recommended that consideration be given to applying outer absorptive padding over the crown of the non-resilient or rigid shell. Several colleges have used this type of helmet for many years and deem it satisfactory (4). However, there is always danger of the exterior padding on the helmet causing binding with another helmet or some other object resulting in injury to the wearer's neck. Further studies using the impact track to check these concepts are contemplated. However, continued research on helmets (7, 10, 12) can only be properly evaluated when carefully screened test values are obtained and are standardized on a national basis.

The Combination of the Face Guard and the Rigid Helmet

Since the innovation of the face guard there has been a tremendous diminution in the number of teeth lost, a decrease of the fractures of jaws, noses, and other facial bones, and presumably lessening of concussions. This has been well illustrated by several surveys, and one cannot fail to be impressed by these important statistics. Nevertheless the presence of this piece of equipment may give a player a false sense of security. The face protector has been reported as a "groove director" actually leading the elbow into the space between the helmet and face guard resulting in a severe facial injury with a fractured nose and multiple lacerations (Fig. 86). A similar situation was reported to have occurred in Case 6 (Chapter 3), resulting in a severely fractured nose, a skull fracture, and subsequent death from an intracerebral and intraventricular hemorrhage. This type of tragic result may be prevented by the addition of the midline vertical bar to the face guard between the anterior rim of the helmet and the face guard.

Mr. H. O. Crisler, the Athletic Director Emeritus and formerly the Head Football Coach at the University of Michigan, was for years the Chairman of the Rules Committee of the National Collegiate Athletic Association. He estimated that there was a four- to fivefold increase in neck injuries following the inception of the use of the face guard and the rigid non-yielding plastic helmet (5). The dangers of this combination in cervical hyperextension injuries resulting in paralysis from the neck downward and death have been elaborated upon in the chapter on "Mechanisms of Injury" (3).

The current practice of "stick-blocking," i.e., the tackler thrusting his head forward and upward with the neck in hyperextension and planting the face guard directly on the oncoming ball carrier's numerals, is regarded by coaches as "*the most scientific*" way to stop the ball carrier. If the latter were to feint to the right or left the head could follow easily, but if the shoulder were used to make the tackle a good ball carrier will see that his opponent has committed himself and will swing away in the other direction. Two other techniques, "spearing" and

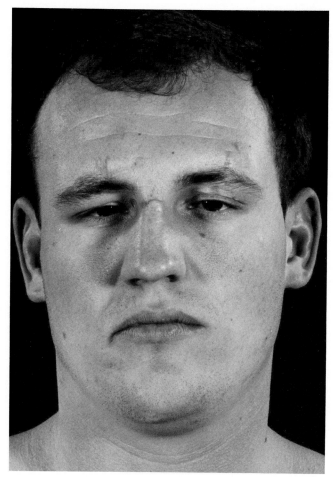

Fig. 86. Occasionally the face guard without the metal bar serves as a director. In this player's case there was an overriding of the face guards between the upper rim of the helmet and the face guard causing a compound fracture of his nose.

"head-butting" may also cause severe injuries. "Spearing" is usually defined as the driving of the head into the body of an opponent who has already been tackled and is on the ground. "Head-butting" is the deliberate blow of a player's head against an opposing player's head or body such as is used in trying to force the opponent out of bounds. The football player should be taught that his head is not invulnerable even with the best of headgears and that this technique is no substitution for a good tackle. Very serious brain damage in one player has been demonstrated (Case 28) and death from an acute subdural hemorrhage in another one (Case 29) with the use of "head-butting."

Recommendations

These suggestions are presented by a neurosurgeon, who is not attempting to try to tell a coach how to teach football, but who is endeavoring to decrease serious and fatal head and spine injuries.

This author realizes the storm of criticism and protest he is incurring but believes that the ideal method of treating the problem is the removal of the face guard, the use of a well-fitting mouth guard on the teeth of the upper jaw, and new instruction in blocking and tackling. The advantages would be: 1) remove the hazard of the upward thrusted torsion of cervical injuries due to tackling by, or a blow against, the face guard; 2) prevent the player from using a "stick-blocking" or "spearing" technique, for no man would dare try it without a face protector or he would deliberately injure his face and teeth; and 3) insure better vision for the pass receiver and kicker and permit them to see the blocker and tackler, thus cutting down on injuries of the knee and ankle. From the neurosurgical standpoint it is better to lose any number of teeth than to have the patient sustain a severe head or neck injury. The sequelae are much greater and it is a question of life or death rather than disfigurement due to losing some teeth or having a distortion of the nose. As far as the game is concerned it would be returned to the realm of an agile sport rather than the steamroller mayhem type of game which is currently practiced.

Eight years ago a young coach heard this work presented and after a careful review of the above recommendations he was sufficiently impressed and courageous enough to make alterations in his coaching methods. He removed the face guard from the players' helmets, returned to the old shoulder tackle with the head to one side, and reassured his men that they have a great advantage over their opponents because of much better vision.

He has kindly authorized me to publish the letter which was in answer to my query as to how this new system was faring. (Because of the policy of retaining anonymity his name unfortunately cannot be mentioned here.)

"In answer to your letter of October 2, I will give you a report that you probably would not believe if you were not vitally interested in this problem of spinal injuries to football players.

"Four years ago I was a member of the N.C.A.A. Rules Committee and heard Fritz Crisler give a report on your study at that time. It was then that I became actively aware of the cause of some facial injuries that my past players had been receiving. After thinking the thing through, I realized that these injuries had not occurred to any extent until we donned helmets with face masks in 1958. After returning from the Rules Committee Meeting mentioned above, I started my Spring practice using the old style, Notre Dame leather helmet with no face mask. The players were apprehensive at first and received a number of bloody noses and black eyes, etc., during the first week of practice; however, I had prepared them for this psychologically by impressing upon them that since they had always played with face masks they had learned to block with their heads down and that it would take time to correct this situation. At the end of ten days practice we got off a week for Spring Holidays. When we returned all the abrasions and bruises on their faces had healed and to this day this type of injury is very scant on our squad. *We have been through four Spring practices and are almost through our fourth season with this type headgear and have received no head and spinal injuries. Our dental bill over the past four years has been about one-tenth of what it was four years previous to this date.* We have had only two boys get their teeth knocked out, and this was probably my fault for I knew these two boys had not learned to block with their heads up, and they were slow learners, and I realized and often mentioned to my assistant coaches that they would probably receive facial injuries when we put them in a ball game. Actually, one injury occurred between plays when our boy was so unalert that he let a boy deliberately kick him in the mouth in a scuffle.

"As far as the psychological thing is concerned, we are at a great advantage because we have sold our kids on the idea that they can see 33 per cent more than the opposition and they firmly believe that we have a one-third advantage before the ball game starts. They are actually more aggressive than the opposition week in and week out. In talking to the boys and in viewing game movies we have found that our defensive linemen have a particular advantage over the opposition because when a boy with a face mask fires out on one of our kids he is at a great disadvantage since our boy can utilize 100 per cent of his vision. Also, our passers and pass receivers feel that they have a great advantage in completing passes. We have led (our league) in this department for the past three years.

"You may quote me if you wish. I firmly believe you are on the right track. I wish you every success in the world, and if there is anything I can do to help you please feel free to call upon me.

"P.S. This year I started an experiment which seems further to prove your theory of the face mask business. We gave the kids a choice of wearing or not wearing a face mask. Several of them have had to wear them because they have bridges of three or four teeth that they got knocked out in high school while wearing face masks. *All the boys who are wearing face masks this year, except one, have received either knee or ankle injuries.* Only one boy on the squad who does not wear a face mask has received a sprained ankle and not one has suffered an injured knee. I will keep a close record of this equipment and send you an accurate report when the season ends."

Unfortunately this author learned on follow-up that one of the boys had sustained a fractured mandible. The parents became adamant that the face guards be restored, and the coach had to comply.

This unusual experiment was an interesting one and one wonders whether it might not be tried again perhaps on a larger scale in spite of the anticipated protest to the suggestion.

Intraoral Mouth and Tooth Protector

For many years football players have worn mouth and tooth protectors, but in spite of the many studies and reports that have been issued showing their effectiveness, there has been some reluctance to accept their use. It has been almost eight years since Stenger et al. (16) presented a five year study suggesting that properly fitted mouth guards not only protected the teeth but protected against shock to the head and neck as well. Although this author is a bit skeptical as to their effectiveness for the extraoral structures, other studies have shown their value (8). Finally, an excellent resolution has been passed by the Joint Commission on Competitive Safeguards and Medical Aspects of Sports of the National Collegiate Athletic Association, effective 1973, "each player in competitive football shall wear an intra-oral mouth and tooth protector...." and these are then described in more detail (4, 6).

Perhaps a word of caution should be uttered. With severe jolts the mouth guard may slip into the pharynx causing respiratory or/and cardiac arrest as described in Case 45 (Chapter 11). The need for the "0" bolt cutter to remove rapidly the face guard as shown in Figure 49, A to D, should be a more readily available instrument to prevent tragedy.

A Central Injury Registry

Consideration should be given to the development of a nationwide football registry in which the injuries sustained in all player groups may be recorded. The fine work which is already being performed by the Committee on Serious and Fatal Injuries of the American Football Coaches Association on a somewhat limited scale would then be augmented (1). The current work of this group is outstanding, but it does not have the power to procure all reports referable to the problem; medical details may not be available or, if they are, the essential and proper interpretation may often be lacking. A combined Board consisting of coaches to review the moving pictures of the games and scrimmages and analyze the plays together with a group of physicians interested in athletics and specialists certified in certain medical specialties might do much to aid in the prevention of injuries. On one occasion this author was privileged to be present when a group of coaches representing a large national football conference considered the measure. Due to a fear that such a type of reporting of current injuries might give valuable information to an opponent, there was hesitation in adopting such a measure. Not until the provision was made that the registration of this type of material should be withheld until the end of the season so that unfair advantage might not be taken of the team in question was agreement reached and the plan supported. The question will immediately be raised as to how such an institution would be supported. It would seem that, for any national sport in which 2½ million individuals participate, the Federal Government might subsidize such a project with funds under its "Physical Fitness for Youth Program" and the National and American Professional Football Leagues might contribute.

Consideration of Enforcement or Alteration of Rules

A large number of the serious and fatal injuries take place on the kick-off and on the punt returns. The reason for this is that the two players are charging at each other at top speed and often suddenly collide head-on. If the high driving knee strikes the tackler's head or if there is a head to head collision it may result in instantaneous or rapid death. One wonders whether the extension of the Canadian regulation of tackling in such instances might limit the number of serious injuries. Under this rule when the ball carrier receives the ball on the punt or kick-off, a tackler may not be within 5 yards of the line at the time of catching the ball. Although it would cut down on the speed and possibly increase the skill of some broken field running, primarily it would eliminate the tremendous momentum generated and the force of the impact when the football players crash head-on.

The dangers of the techniques of "stick-blocking", "spearing," and "head-butting" have already been referred to in the discussion on helmets. Although some legislation has been passed against the use of teaching and employing such techniques, the enforcement of such rules has been given mere lip service.

Tackling by the face mask as shown on previous pages is a dangerous technique. The continued enforcement of the 15 yard penalty rule for grabbing the face mask has no doubt aided in eliminating serious neck injuries.

Consideration probably should be given to "high elbowing," a technique which has received less attention since the innovation of the face guard. The defensive use of the elbow above the shoulder level driving it under the face guard causes an increased leverage and may result in a severe hyperextension injury. The deliberate hard driving upward thrust of a defensive player's rigid helmet against an opponent's face mask may have a similar effect. A penalty for such a maneuver might be beneficial in preventing injury to the player.

The current use of the earlier whistle by the officials at the time of cessation of forward movement of play and the more liberal calling of the "piling on" penalty or "unnecessary roughness" penalty has been of increasing benefit in prevention of unnecessary injuries.

Improvement in Selection of Players

From the previous discussion it is obvious that one of the most important features in preventing injury is the selection of the players for football. The increasing tendency to select the grammar school student with a lack of physical development, clamp a cheap dangerous helmet on him in addition to other inadequate or improper equipment, and permit him to attempt to play the type of football which he sees on television is a catastrophe. Parents and other people who foster such folly often do so to satisfy their own egos at the expense of the child. Perhaps they seek to capture the athletic recognition which they themselves did not achieve or realize. Although there may be a place for little league athletics— it certainly is not in the sport of football.

The proper selection of players is a key point. The youngster with the long thin neck who is tall and gangly without adequate musculature is a poor candidate for the rigors of football, particularly as it is now played and taught with the head and neck used as a battering ram in "stick-blocking" and "spearing." One of the more fortunate players is pictured (Fig. 87A). He was a high school tennis player, was 6 ft. 3 in. tall, weight 135 pounds, and had the neck musculature de-

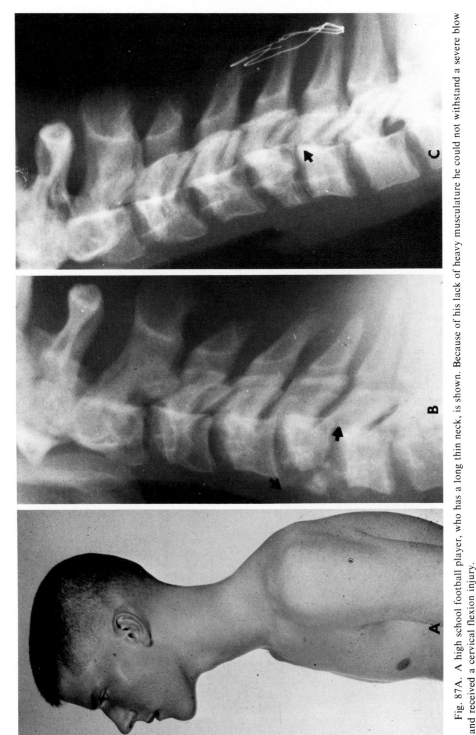

Fig. 87A. A high school football player, who has a long thin neck, is shown. Because of his lack of heavy musculature he could not withstand a severe blow and received a cervical flexion injury.

Fig. 87B. The "tear-drop" fracture of the 5th cervical vertebra which he sustained is an unstable one and is often associated with severe neurologic deficit when the posterior margin of the vertebra (lower arrow) impinges on the anterior portion of the cord.

Fig. 87C. This x-ray taken months later shows partial realignment and stabilization by wire.

velopment of a great blue heron. When he dove at a ball carrier he sustained a
"tear-drop" fracture-dislocation of the cervical spine, fortunately without neurologic deficit (Fig. 87B). He was operated upon with decompression of his cervical
spine and successfully fused without sequelae (Fig. 87C). Long ago, Coach "Red"
Blaik recognized the importance of building up the neck musculature by constant
conditioning exercises in football players to withstand severe blows. Picture the
high school player above playing the same type of football as one of the outstanding professionals with a neck requiring a size 19 collar (Fig. 88A). Please note his
relatively good looking spine after years of excellent rough professional football
play (Fig. 88B). The destroyed spinal cord does not regenerate but merely forms
a scar through which no functional fibers pass (Fig. 41D) with the result that

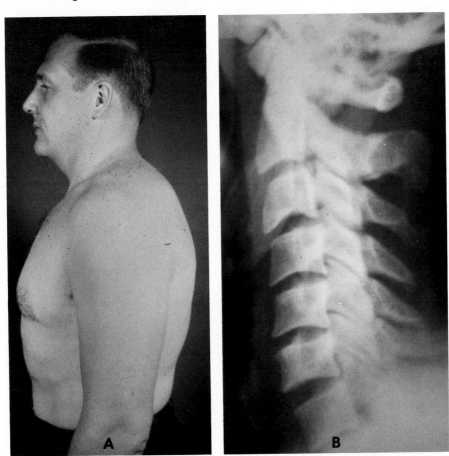

Fig. 88A. Note this professional football player's physique with the tremendous neck musculature.
This may be contrasted to the player in the previous photograph.

Fig. 88B. This man was an excellent linebacker for many years, sustaining many blows to the head
and neck. However, X-rays of his cervical spine show a relatively good bony configuration considering
the terrific impacts he has withstood. (The indentation at the lower part of the third cervical vertebral
body is due to a normal Schmorl's node.)

immediate complete total paralysis persists. The ability to survive in such a game depends not only on seasonal conditioning but also is best achieved by the athlete remaining in condition throughout the year.

To encourage the boy with convulsive seizures to play the game and expose him to chronic recurrent head injuries is folly as has already been indicated. However, to endeavor to fuse a cervical spine on a player who has already sustained neurological deficit in the hope of returning him to football seems to be an unbelievable choice by a coach or even to be considered by a physician.

Case 55. Early one fall the patient was in a football scrimmage when he was struck and fell to the ground, conscious and able to talk, but totally tetraplegic with generalized paresthesias in the extremities. He was carried from the field and recovered promptly except for some generalized tingling throughout his body and his lower extremities. However, he was "*able to re-enter the game and continued to play in subsequent games.*" Later he fractured a leg and recovered after 7 weeks to return to football. His trainer and the attending physician were informed about the transient paresthesias which he began to have in his upper and lower extremities, but they did not force him to abandon the game.

During the *next summer* while playing football he again developed tetraplegia similar to the initial episode in the preceding year. Following this he could not stand for a short period of time without help. The cervical spine x-rays appeared normal and he resumed playing professional football the rest of that fall. Finally after his third episode of tetraplegia he was released by the professional team. The player was seen by a neurosurgeon who had another set of cervical spine x-rays taken which were normal, and he was started on a program of cervical traction. He now had paresthesias in his left thumb, index, and third fingers, with these symptoms being most noticeable at the tip of the left index finger. The player was a well developed muscular man who had full movement of his cervical spine in all directions. There was hypalgesia in the left thumb, index, and third fingers. The brachioradialis reflex was slightly diminished on the left and normal on the right. The biceps and triceps reflexes and all other deep reflexes, sensory modalities, motor and coordination examinations were within normal limits throughout the body. He had no extensor plantar reflexes or Hoffmann's signs. An electromyogram revealed a left C6 nerve root involvement. The neurosurgeon diagnosed a cervical spine strain and a protrusion of the C5–C6 intervertebral disc with transient cervical cord compression. At this time the patient showed only residual nerve root injury. The player was treated conservatively with cervical traction and advised to give up football. His recovery has been good.

Comment. This player was extremely fortunate to have *survived three episodes of tetraplegia* and made a good recovery; any one of them might have resulted in a lifetime of complete paralysis. The patient made a good recovery on a regime of conservative management demonstrating that surgery is not always necessary in the treatment of such lesions. Such a patient should never be operated upon with the hope of returning to the game. Such a course of action would be too dangerous for fear of reinjury and tetraplegia.

The suggestions printed here are those of the physician looking at the problem of the safety of the football player, but this approach obviously will not be with the approval of some of the coaches and trainers. At times there is a tendency for a coach to fear consultation with a physician believing he will unnecessarily intrude into the sport and perhaps will withold a key player in a crucial game. If true, this is a sad commentary on the sport and its supporters. For the most part this author has enjoyed a very harmonious relationship with any coaches or trainers he has met. His suggestions have been kindly discussed and usually medical advice has been followed. On the other hand, the physician or consultant must always be cognizant of the many psychological factors with which the coaching personnel must cope (Chapter 8). He must realize that, just as in a time of war, he must assume some attitude of toughness in certain instances and not make too overly apprehensive and unwarranted concessions—for there might not be a football team just as there might not be an army if all the soldiers were sent home on the basis of minor or simulated complaints. An atmosphere of understanding with mutual respect between the coaches, trainers, and medical profession will do much to provide the best for our favorite national sport, football.

References

1. Blyth, C. S. and Arnold, D. C.: Thirty-Seventh Annual Survey of Football Fatalities: 1931–1970. American Football Coaches Association and National Collegiate Athletic Association, Chapel Hill, N.C., 1971.
2. Brown, P.: Head and Spinal Cord Injuries. In discussion before Meeting of Owners and Coaches National Football League, New York, May 21, 1962.
3. Clark, O. V.: Perceptual Moron. Read beofre the Michigan Chapter American College of Surgeons, Flint, Mich., March 8, 1960.
4. Cooper, D.: Personal communication.
5. Crisler, H. O.: Personal communication, May 29, 1972.
6. Fuenning, S. I.: Report of Chairman, Joint Commission on Competitive Safe-Guards and Medical Aspects of Sports, National Collegiate Athletic Association, 1972.
7. Kindt, G. W., Schneider, R. C. and Robinson, J. L.: A Method of Comparing the Impact Absorption Characteristics of Football Helmets. *Med. Sci. in Sports, 3:* 203, 1971.
8. Logan, T. E.: Prevention of Serious Injuries. Mouth Guards for Athletes. *J. Ken. Med. Assoc.,* p. 228, March, 1966.
9. Melvin, W. J. S.: Cervical Spine Injuries in Football Players. Read as part of the Donald Starr Athletic Symposium, Vancouver, British Columbia, Nov. 29, 1963.
10. Perini, H. M. and Abbott, B. W.: Investigation of Requirements for Protective Football Head Gear: Report of Armour Research Foundation of Illinois Institute of Technology, Chicago, June, 1962, p. 51.
11. Robey, J. M., Blyth, C. S. and Mueller, F. O.: Athletic Injuries. Application of Epidemiologic Methods. *J.A.M.A., 217:* 184, 1971.
12. Ryan, A. J.: Proceedings of the National Conference on Protective Equipment in Sports, Department of Postgraduate Medical Education, University of Wisconsin, Madison, June 1968.
13. Schneider, R. C., Reifel, E., Crisler, H. O. and Oosterbann, B. G.: Serious and Fatal Football Injuries Involving Head and Spinal Cord. *J.A.M.A., 177:* 362, 1961.
14. Schneider, R. C.: Report on Study of Football Helmets and Face Guards. In *Proceedings of the National Conference on Head Protection of Athletes*, pp. 44–48, May 19, 1962.
15. Schneider, R. C. and Antine, B. E.: Visual-Field Impairment Related to Football Headgear and Face Guards. *J.A.M.A., 192:* 616, 1965.
16. Stenger, J. M., Lawson, E. A., Wright, J. M. and Ricketts, J.: Mouth Guards: Protection Against Shock to Head, Neck and Teeth. *J. Am. Dent. Assoc. 69:* 19, 1964.

Author Index

Subject Index*

* Italic numbers denote references to figures.

267